Hildegard Peplau
Psychiatric Nurse of the Century

Barbara Callaway, PhD, is Professor of Political Science at Rutgers University in New Brunswick, New Jersey. She earned her BA at Trinity University in San Antonio, Texas and her MA and PhD at Boston University. For many years she served in academic administration at Rutgers, including a term as Acting Dean of the College of Nursing. She is the author of several books on Africa and Nigeria as well as many articles on Africa, Nigeria, women and Islam, women and development, and women and politics.

Hildegard Peplau
Psychiatric Nurse of the Century

Barbara J. Callaway, PhD

 Springer Publishing Company

Photos on pages 108, 109, 110, 418, and 419 were reprinted with the permission of Letitia Anne Peplau.
Photos on page 420 were reprinted with the permission of Neil Smoyak.

Copyright © 2002 by Springer Publishing Company, Inc.

Springer Publishing Company, Inc.
536 Broadway
New York, NY 10012-3955

The author and publisher have made every attempt to check the contents of this book for historical accuracy. Because history is often based on personal interpretation and memories as well as the "hard" data found in archives and publications, some of the information in this book may differ from the recollections of individual readers. Springer Publishing Company does not assume liability for these differences or any consequences that may arise from them.

Acquisitions Editor: Ruth Chasek
Production Editor: Jeanne W. Libby
Cover design by Joanne E. Honigman

02 03 04 05 06 / 5 4 3 2 1

Library of Congress Cataloging-in-Publication Data

Callaway, Barbara J.
    Hildegard Peplau : psychiatric nurse of the century / Barbara J. Callaway.
        p. ; cm.
    Includes bibliographical references and index.
    ISBN 0-8261-3882-9
        1. Peplau, Hildegard E. 2. Psychiatric nurses—United States—Biography.
    I. Title: Psychiatric nurse of the century. II. Title.
        [DNLM: 1. Peplau, Hildegard E. 2. Psychiatric Nursing—United States—
    Biography. WZ 100 P422C 2002]
    RC440.P423 C35 2002
    610.73'68'092—dc21
    [B]
                                                              2001057795

Printed in the United States of America by Maple-Vail Book Manufacturing Group.

Contents

Foreword

Hildegard Elizabeth Peplau is an icon of modern nursing. It has been 50 years since her book, *Interpersonal Relations in Nursing*, was published, and it seems fitting that at this time her biographer Barbara Callaway gives us this rich portrayal of the complexities of her life.

First and foremost, this is the story of a woman of uncommon intellect and great passion. By the power of her intellectual work, Peplau transformed nursing from an occupation where nurses did to and for patients, to a profession where nurses worked with patients. This underlying change in nursing practice has been 50 years in the making, the span of time that most social scientists agree is needed to accomplish a true paradigm shift.

The perspective in this book is informed by the depth and breadth of Peplau's archives, as well as from taped interviews with Peplau and other central figures in her life story. It is greatly enriched by Peplau's predilection for keeping records and notes of events and activities and reflections about her life and experience. Peplau, perhaps reflecting her thrifty "Pennsylvania Dutch" roots or the fact that she experienced the effects of the depression, kept nearly everything she ever committed to paper. She also kept a journal and wrote regular entries. Peplau lived the discipline of the examined life, and she expected it of her students too. When she began to develop the program of study for advanced students in psychiatric nursing at Teacher's College, she required verbatim records of the nurse-patient interaction. These notes then were analyzed for themes and patterns and thus began the development of theory for the field.

Readers will be held by the power of this narrative as it unfolds against the landscape of profound changes in America and indeed in the world. From the Great Depression to World War II, the civil rights movement and the Vietnam War era, the author follows Peplau's life and brings the experience to the reader in human terms. The life that unfolds in these pages will be of interest to students of women's history, to students of the history of nursing, and indeed to all women who have struggled in American society to meet the challenges posed by inherently sexist norms.

Most of Peplau's professional career was experienced in organizations that were largely all-women—hospitals, colleges of nursing, and nursing associations, particularly the American Nurses Association. Callaway faithfully narrates the vicissitudes of Peplau's experiences with these organizations. What results is a "warts and all" account of the dynamics of these particular organizations, as experienced by Peplau. I would expect that these dynamics are not unique but a pattern in the everyday lives of hundreds of thousands of women who work in such organizations. Perhaps careful study of Peplau's experiences will be useful to others who find themselves in similar situations. She would have liked that.

GRAYCE M. SILLS, PhD, RN, FAAN

Author's Note

Early in 1976, I was appointed Acting Dean of the Rutgers University College of Nursing in Newark, New Jersey. The College had been experiencing serious problems that were not helped by the fact that over the preceding decade there had been several changes in college deans. In reviewing the history of the College, I came across the name of a distinguished professor who had retired from her faculty position as recently as 1974, and I wondered why such an eminent person had never been offered the deanship. That professor was Hildegard Peplau. Upon inquiring, I was told that Dr. Peplau's ideas about nursing education were quite controversial and that as a colleague she had been most opinionated and difficult.

My first face to face meeting with Dr. Peplau occurred 10 years later, in 1986, when I was serving as an Associate Provost on the Rutgers New Brunswick campus. I was immediately taken by Dr. Peplau's quick wit, strong spirit, and trenchant comments concerning her profession. For the next several years, I met her for a meal whenever she was in New Jersey. In 1990, I somewhat jokingly suggested that I write her biography. Dr. Peplau took the suggestion seriously, and immediately began sending me packets of "vignettes" or descriptions of incidents in her life as she remembered them. These vignettes were accompanied by copies of relevant published materials she had in her possession, and by lists of names and telephone numbers of colleagues around the country who could verify Dr. Peplau's memories *or* who might present a different interpretation of events.

By 1992, I had decided that I would indeed undertake the challenge of writing a biography of Hildegard Peplau. I took leave of my administrative responsibilities at Rutgers and went to Los Angeles, where Hilda had lived since 1981. I met with her in her breakfast room for 3 hours a day, 3 days a week, for the first 4 months of that year. It was upon the base of these extensive personal exchanges that this biography was built. In addition to the material derived from these exchanges, I garnered further detailed information from a study of her diaries, and from the letters and papers that are deposited in the Schlesinger Library at the Radcliffe

Institute of Harvard University. In addition, I also spent considerable time with members of Hilda's family, seeking their corroboration of facts and events of Hilda's early family life as she had described them. The family was exceedingly helpful, and they, like Hilda, emphasized their desire for an honest, forthright, and objective account.

Hilda herself was most emphatic from the very beginning that I seek outside verification of her understanding of the facts and events of her life. To meet this goal, I made a great effort to check the accuracy of the details recorded in this account. I conducted more than a hundred interviews, read stacks of notes and memoranda, reviewed pertinent material in the ANA archives, checked current memories against materials written at the time of an event, and wherever possible, sought alternative interpretations of the more troubling aspects of Hilda's story. Unfortunately, I found that in many cases memories had faded or interviewees were simply reluctant to reexamine many events of the past that are at the core of this biography. As a result, I was given no choice but to present many of the potentially controversial parts of Hilda's life story solely from her perspective.

Hilda wanted her life story told and that could not be done in any way that would honestly portray her life without describing events in a manner that some may find unusually forthright and candid. Hilda undoubtably was a most controversial figure throughout her career in nursing. Her life involved a seemingly endless set of struggles and conflicts, both intellectual and interpersonal and, it is likely that those opposed to her position saw situations differently than the way they may be recorded here. Hildegard Peplau was in many ways a solo act.

Introduction:
A Life of Significance

This is the story of a controversial woman, whose life made a difference, not only to her profession, but to the lives of the mentally ill in this country.

Hildegard Elizabeth Peplau's descriptions of her childhood and interactions within her very patriarchal family suggest early on that hers would not be an ordinary life. As a young teenager, she made the decision to do what very few women did in her day: she decided to pursue an education and a career. She made this decision out of a passion to be her own mistress, to determine her own future, to live her life differently than anyone around her. Within her lifetime, she earned not only the celebrity of being recognized by the American Academy of Nursing as a "Living Legend" but also the unofficial designation, bestowed by the College of Nursing of the University of California at Los Angeles, as "Psychiatric Nurse of the Century."

Peplau was an imaginative innovator who left an indelible stamp on the theory and practice of psychiatric nursing. Known as "The Mother of Psychiatric Nursing," she devoted herself to the redefinition, clarification, and expansion of nursing services for psychiatric patients—and left an enduring mark on graduate education for clinical specialization in nursing. Although her contributions continue to stimulate debate and discussion, there is no doubt that Hildegard Peplau almost single-handedly led psychiatric nurses from the confinement of providing custodial care in public mental hospitals to theory-driven professional practice.

Her work always involved great risks, both personal and professional. It took a woman of uncommon courage and resilience to continually push forward the boundaries in nursing education, to test radically new approaches in nursing theory and practice, and in the process to challenge and ultimately revolutionize entrenched practices in psychiatric care. Such a career was not without controversy. Peplau was both vilified and exalted over the 50-year span of her active work. Always at the center of conflict, and often enduring great personal hardship, she earned

1

her nursing diploma and then baccalaureate, master's, and doctoral degrees, and ultimately rose to the very top of her profession. Disappointed by the lack of vision among her colleagues, continually betrayed by professional friends and sabotaged by nursing's leaders, she retired in 1974 from the faculty of Rutgers University, saddened that her years of effort had seemingly come to naught.

Such was not the case. In the 25 years between her retirement from Rutgers—though never from her work—and her death in 1999, she was awarded no less than nine honorary doctorates and was honored by the American Nurses Association with the establishment of the Hildegard Peplau Award, recognizing continuous contributions to the nursing profession. She received both nursing's highest honor, the Christiane Reimann Prize, and was designated one of "Fifty Great Americans" (the only nurse so recognized) by Marquis' Who's Who in 1997. Yet, surprisingly, the story of her life in professional nursing is not well known.

Hildegard E. Peplau was born in Reading, Pennsylvania, in 1909. The second child and middle daughter of immigrant parents who gave her little outward sign of affection, she was both typical and was to become very atypical of working class young women of her generation. She was the child of an authoritarian father, and a dedicated but emotionally remote mother who persevered in a difficult marriage with the comfort of music and religion and, more acceptably for her time and place, by immersing herself in baking and meticulous homemaking. From an early age Hilda was determined to escape her mother's fate. Most certainly her childhood and her perceptions of her parents' circumstances shaped her outlook and fueled her ambitions. She was open to experiences and had a deep passion for learning and growth, but in later life was often impatient with those who did not meet her own high standards of performance.

Her childhood and adolescence reveal a struggle for autonomy that focused initially on breaking away from the customary filial obligations that threatened to limit her opportunities. Hilda Peplau decided that, unlike her peers, she would not leave school, go to work, hand over her wages to her father, marry, and live forever after in Reading. She was determined, although she did not understand it in these terms, to develop an independent professional identity. In adulthood she would find a more fulfilling focus, balancing her professional life with motherhood and child care.

In her dream of rising above the circumstances into which she was born, Hilda was not unlike many first-generation children of immigrant parents who would achieve great success in later life. The difference in Hilda's case was her gender. She was young, of an independent mind, and blessed with both intelligence and ambition. Because she was a woman, however, she was entrapped both by the economic limitations of her working-class background and her sex. Viewing her limited opportunities, Hilda pursued one of the few options then open to women: a career in nursing.

Hildegard Peplau's entry into nursing had little to do with romantic notions of caring for the sick. In Reading she had worked as a store clerk, payroll clerk, and bookkeeper while completing courses at a business school and then graduating as class valedictorian from evening high school in 1928. Given that the alternatives, as she later described them, were "marriage, teaching, or becoming a nun," the promise of "free room and board and a monthly stipend" made nursing an attractive option. She maintained that the considerations behind her decision to enter nursing were largely irrelevant. What mattered was why she stayed: "My reasons for staying and making a career of it—intense interest in the work itself, the opportunity to develop my capabilities, helping to advance the profession in the public interest—were what was most important," she explained in retrospect.

The decision to leave the constrictive environment of her home and her community having been made, Peplau launched herself into a career—and in fact a life—that in every respect would prove to be quite *atypical* of anything that her background would predict. After completing her training as a nurse, Peplau did not continue along the usual path into hospital or private-duty nursing. Instead she found a position as a staff nurse at Vermont's new elite, but very progressive, Bennington College. There, her work was so impressive and her intellectual hunger so apparent that the college president decided to suspend admission requirements and admit her as a degree student, with a major in psychology. This was at a time when very few young women of her background, and virtually no nurses, were among the nation's college students.

When World War II intervened, Peplau accelerated her graduation to enlist in the U.S. Army Nurse Corps, with the intention of serving not on the home front but in Europe where the war was being waged. Posted to a military psychiatric hospital in England, Peplau pioneered innovative approaches to treating emotionally scarred and battle-fatigued soldiers sent back from the front lines. At war's end, she seized the opportunity presented by the G.I. Bill to pursue postgraduate degrees at Columbia University's Teachers College in New York City—and this at a time when the prevailing values for those women who had entered the workforce during the war were to resume traditional roles, returning to family life, preferably in a new home in a new postwar suburb. By then Hildegard Peplau was, by choice, a single parent raising a child in an era when such a role was entirely outside accepted social norms.

Three themes that emerge in a study of Hildegard Peplau's life and work serve to illuminate the changing position of women over the span of her lifetime. These include, first, the inherent conflict among women of Peplau's generation between marriage and a career; second, the unique place in an evolving social fabric played by women such as Hildegard Peplau who dared, in behalf of their own fulfillment, to confront the malicious stigma of unwed motherhood; and third, the role that the force of a woman's personality—a formidable one in Peplau's case—may play in effecting remarkable change in such conservative institutions as the nursing profession.

Peplau was determined to have both a career and a child when most women with children did not work. She was equally determined to make an important contribution to her professional field. She was raised in a time and a place where women were taught to believe they had to make a choice between marriage *or* a career. They could not do both. Hilda did make the decision that she would not marry, but she also made the even more unlikely decision to raise and cherish a child alone. In this, her work and her home were closely connected. Growing recognition in her profession notwithstanding, for many years Peplau managed both motherhood and a career—on a meager salary. For her there would be no full-time child care or part-time cleaning lady. During her daughter's childhood and teenage years, Peplau became prominent locally, nationally, and internationally, and whenever possible her child traveled with her. The style of parenting was both affectionate and cerebral. Hilda was intensely interested in theories of child rearing and stages of child development; and she implemented what she learned from these theories as she observed every aspect of her daughter's growth with genuine joy and delight. Fortunately, she was blessed with an uncommonly bright child.

In the course of pursuing these goals we see how over the years a shy young girl with a negative self-image became a professional mentor to decades of psychiatric nurses. Tall, willowy, blonde, and fun-loving as she was, Peplau nonetheless would come to be seen as a commanding, even domineering professor and intellectual mentor, and a demanding professional colleague. No shrinking violet, she was seemingly unable to avoid alienating her colleagues and friends alike when ideas were at issue. The adoring responses of those interviewed for this study compared to the anger found in Peplau's collection of the written record testify to the complexity of her personality. She was both a romantic and a rationalist who managed to keep both her idealism and unflinching realism intact. Her uncompromising integrity and the extraordinary demands she made of herself shaped both the professional career she forged for herself and the changes she brought about in the nursing profession.

Peplau assumed leadership roles from the time she entered the army, and she rose to the highest offices in her profession during the 1960s and early 1970s. This was the time when the women's movement was changing the lives of millions of American women, but hardly making a ripple within the closed circle of professional nursing. Peplau identified with the feminist movement, but was not a part of it. In nursing, the movement had little impact during her career. Hilda herself generally did not see the perennial struggle between nursing and physicians in gender terms, although she accepted an appointment at Rutgers in the 1950s primarily because it did *not* have a medical school. She did not want medical faculty interfering in her work. It is significant, however, that the most direct encouragement for her groundbreaking work almost always came from doctors, seldom from nurses.

Peplau's professional life was a four-ring circus. She held herself to high standards, whether in practice, teaching, publishing, mentoring, or mothering, and she demanded the same of others. Her professional life includes 6 years of general and private-duty nursing, 7 years as a student and the nurse in charge of the health service at Bennington College, 3 years in the Army Nurse Corps, 5 years at Teachers College of Columbia University, 1 year as a practicing therapist, 20 years as a professor at Rutgers University, and 1 year as Executive Director and 2 years as President of the American Nurses Association—the only person ever to serve in both positions.

During these years she also served as consultant to the World Health Organization, the National Institute of Mental Health, the Southern Regional Education Board, the Division on Nursing of the U.S. Public Health Service, and Nurse Adviser to the Surgeon General of the United States, as well as to the U.S. Air Force. She published hundreds of articles in professional journals; wrote three books; and over a 12-year period conducted annual summer workshops in 17 states that literally transformed the way nurses tended to patients in state mental hospitals. Throughout her career she traveled to foreign countries to consult on nursing education and in her later years worked tirelessly through the International Council of Nursing to raise the quality of nursing education and professional practice worldwide.

Publications of Peplau's clinical, scholarly, and empirical research are numerous, far-reaching, and were still widely used in schools of nursing even 20 years after her retirement. Her work has appeared in more than 30 professional journals, in organizational proceedings, university and conference proceedings, alumni quarterlies, and state nurses association journals. Reprints of her book chapters are found in texts edited by nurses, psychiatrists, and psychologists, and her books continue to be reissued, both in the United States and abroad. In the late 1960s, Smith, Kline Laboratories made an Oscar-nominated documentary film of her work.

Throughout her life Peplau was eager, if not driven, to seek to understand her own learning processes as well as to make a true contribution to her chosen profession. Until her death in March, 1999, she continued her habit of recording her thoughts about anything that affected her current experience. Her practice of writing, examining, and exploring intellectual and professional problems continued over the years after her retirement to enrich the correspondence of an ever widening circle of young admirers, as she was sought out for guidance on dissertations, for journal editorial boards, and for honor at professional plenary sessions.

The archival record of her career, deposited in the Schlesinger Library at the Radcliffe Institute of Harvard University, is both rich and extraordinary. From the time she was a high school student in Reading in 1924, Hilda preserved a written record of her life. The collection contains a complete genealogy of the Peplau and Loth families, early childhood photographs, school papers, report cards, and teenage diaries. It contains most correspondence with her family and letters received by her from 1933 to 1982, when her papers were given to the Schlesinger. Included are all her lecture notes over a 25 year career of teaching; clinical records of her own private practice, as well as those kept by students over the years; committee meeting minutes, many annotated in her own hand; professional papers; and voluminous professional correspondence.

The diaries and papers record daily appointments, details of family events, visits from friends and relatives, trips all over the world, course materials developed for seminars and workshops, and clinical observations made during the 1960s at every major mental hospital in the United States. The diaries document a private life as well as professional achievement. The papers reveal the day-by-day development of a professional career, and indeed of a profession. This remarkable archive makes it possible to trace both one woman's life work and major professional currents in nursing.

From the beginning of her career in the late 1930s, Peplau worked tirelessly to push the frontiers of nursing education and practice. Always, her fiercest opposition came from within her own profession. Nursing in the second half of the 20th century did not treat well women who tested the boundaries, who blazed new paths, who were true leaders. The roadblocks placed in her way by nursing's leadership as she tried to bring the American Nurses Association back from the brink of bankruptcy and self-destruction, while striving to move it in the direction of professional and scientific recognition and respectability, were monumental.

Hildegard Peplau was not a political feminist who actively supported the women's movement, but she was determined to mold her own destiny in the world—to achieve personal autonomy. Thus, although she did not use the word, her life is an example of feminism as a life process. By looking more closely at the struggles within nursing, as these are exemplified in the life and personal struggle of Hildegard Peplau, we are given a fresh lens through which to view conflict and growth within the nursing profession.

An American Childhood 1

Mother did adjust to this country. She spoke beautiful English. She made ends meet where there were no ends. They [father and mother] were both assimilated. But, educated women were beyond them!
—Bertha Peplau Reppert
October 19, 1994

Monday was wash day and all the neighbors looked forward to it. Ottylie Peplau, a tall, straight immigrant woman from Poland, but of German descent, would be out in the backyard of 1232 Church Street early, hanging up the family wash and singing powerful opera at the top of her lungs. Ottylie didn't mind the hard work, washing the coal and soot out of her husband's work clothes, or those of her children, or the towels and the sheets. She loved the physical exercise, the clean smell of the laundry, the outside air, and the space to let her voice soar. She loved her music; and she loved the town.

The town was Reading, set among the rolling hills of eastern Pennsylvania in the verdant Pennsylvania Dutch countryside. Reading was a city in a valley, with sturdy brick houses rising like stair steps up the hillsides. Reading at the beginning of the 20th century was a good place, solid and secure, with durable brick streets, handsome stores around Penn Square, and booming factories.[1] The thriftiness, frugality, order, and religiosity of the Pennsylvania Dutch were regional values with which Ottylie Peplau could identify, values in which she found comfort and reassurance. She was comfortable, too, with the dialect spoken here, "Pennsylvania Deutsch," a mixture of German and English that was unique to this area and is still spoken.

Reading was a railroad center, and the Peplau home was only half a block from the gigantic railroad yards that dominated the town. By the early 1900s Reading, with a population of 100,000, had become the third largest industrial city in Pennsylvania, with over 700 manufacturing plants. It was known not only for the railroads but also for its many garment factories and for the breweries that produced such brands as Old Reading Beer, Sunshine Beer, and Lauer's. Not surprisingly, seven pretzel factories were among Reading's hundreds of plants.[2] Most importantly to the immigrant families, the railroads and their shops meant work for every able-bodied man. Women were able to find work in the sewing factories.[3]

IMMIGRANT FAMILY

Ottylie Peplau was happy in Reading. She did not have an easy life, but she was grateful to be in America, to have a good husband, Gustav ("mein Mann" as she referred to him), and five healthy children.[4] Life could have been so much worse. Ottylie Elgert was born in 1883 in the small village of Kochanow near Warsaw, Poland. She was the firstborn of 13 children. Gustav Peplau, whom she did not meet until both were adults living in America, may have been a distant cousin. Gustav, who was a year older than Ottylie, was born in the nearby village of Boguchwala. He was the first son in a family of 8 children. The people of these beleaguered villages had seen a constant shift of national boundaries as the 18th century wars between Prussia, Austria, and Russia swept back and forth across Poland. Each invading army destroyed all before it, and the peasantry were forcibly moved from place to place, their possessions destroyed and looted. In the 19th century, people of German descent were granted land in the former state of Poland to resettle. Gustav Peplau's great-grandfathers, Christian Prill and Karl Peplau, were among these settlers.

Christian Prill ultimately worked himself to death. "His arms became stiff from overwork; he was even an invalid in the last years of his life. But he kept a joyful heart until the end."[5] The same grit, stoicism, and dedication to one's own responsibility and lot in life lived on in his great grandson, Gustav Peplau. The Prill and Peplau families remained on the land until the Germans—as many as 10 million human beings—were again chased from Poland during World War II and the village of Boguchwala disappeared altogether. Fear of displacement and severe hardship were deeply rooted in the minds of generations, even of those who escaped the villages. These were not happy memories.

Gustav's father, Karl Peplau, was able to emigrate to America in 1894. His wife, Julianna Prill, followed in 1896, leaving the couple's sons, Gustav, age 12, and Adolph, age 8, on the farm with their maternal grandparents in Boguchwala. Three years later the boys joined their parents in Reading, Pennsylvania, where they lived in a rented house at 933 Laurel Street. Karl, an ironworker, died of a heart attack in 1910, and Julianna bought a house at 1330 Buttonwood Street.[6] A hardworking farm boy, Gustav

Peplau did not have the luxury of attending school. Later in life he would teach himself to read, but in 1899 when he set out with his younger brother to find his family in America, he was essentially illiterate. He spoke German and Polish and would learn English, but remained fundamentally anti-intellectual all his life. His mother, Julianna, came from a family of teachers and preachers, yet she, too, was suspicious of education.[7] In Reading, the young Gustav lived with his parents and worked building cabinets and doing other odd carpentry jobs on commission.

Ottylie Elgert's background was more privileged than Gustav Peplau's. Her father was educated and had been a schoolteacher at one time. He sent his sons to school and taught the girls to read at home. Thus, although Ottylie was literate, she lacked formal schooling. One of her brothers, Gustav, went on to earn two doctorates and taught at the University of Warsaw until forced out of Poland during World War II.[8] Ottylie was 20 years old when she refused to marry the unattractive and domineering man of her father's choice. Instead she traveled alone from Tulowicz, Poland, to Hamburg and from there set sail for the United States abroad the S.S. Waldersee, arriving in the Port of New York on May 8, 1903. The ship's manifest recorded that she could read and write and that her nationality was "Russian."[9] Ottylie's destination was Bristol, Connecticut, where she would work as a housekeeper for a Lutheran minister who had come from the area near Ottylie's home village in Poland. Her sisters Olga and Amelia would follow her to America in 1906 and 1911.

Immigrants from the Boguchwala-Kochanow region tried to keep in touch, and immigrant Lutheran ministers of the day felt a responsibility to play matchmaker. Ottylie was 5 feet, 6 inches tall with blue eyes and a cloud of blond, curly hair. She was intelligent and energetic. In Bristol, she worked in the church manse, baking and cleaning. But the days were long and lonely, and she was getting older. The good minister took it upon himself to introduce the industrious, attractive worker in his home to the tall, quiet, and hardworking carpenter from Reading. Gustav then was entering early manhood and very much wanted to marry. Assured by his own minister that Ottylie Elgert would indeed make a "suitable wife and mother," Gustav was most anxious to travel to Bristol, Connecticut to meet her. In time he made the trip. Although she had several other suitors, Ottylie, a good judge of character, picked the quiet, steady, kindly Gustav to be her husband. On February 12, 1907, they were married in the Immanuel Lutheran Church in Bristol.[10] Immediately after the wedding the couple returned to Reading where they lived in a rented house at 537 Wunder Street.

Gustav Peplau was a handsome man. Six feet tall with black hair and grey-blue eyes, he was physically well built. Shortly after his marriage to Ottylie, he began working as a fireman at the Reading Railroad yards, stoking the great train engines with coal. He was proud of his employment, and worked 12-hour days, 6 days a week. Stoking steadily in the bitter cold of winter and unbearable heat of summer, he logged no sick days in his 31 years on the railroad. He came home at night, exhausted and covered with coal dust mixed with sweat, washed up, and settled into his favorite Morris chair to play rounds of solitaire and, in later years, listen to the radio. When his collected pennies permitted, he went to the local pool hall at Sixth and Robson to play poker with the boys. Sometimes, he and Ottylie would sit quietly and talk together, he in the Morris chair, she in her comfortable mission oak rocker. The conversation was always in German, quiet and companionable. Ottylie and Gustav were devout Christians and read the Bible every day. They never raised their voices at each other, and they didn't converse with their children.

Gustav and Ottylie had five children, all born at home, and they raised a sixth, a foster child, as their own. Their first daughter, Clara Julianna, was born November 11, 1907. Their second daughter, Hildegard Elizabeth, always known as Hilda, was born 2 years later, on September 1, 1909. Their two sons, Harold Gustav and Walter Carl, arrived on September 22, 1911, and September 14, 1913. Their last daughter, Bertha Ottylie, the baby, was born on November 26, 1919. Ottylie's foster child, John David Forster, born April 13, 1931, came into the household when Bertha was 12 years old.

In May 1908 the Peplaus bought their brick home at 1232 Church Street. Church was a narrow, short street, six blocks long, sandwiched between Sixth Street and the railroad yards and the larger homes lining Fifth Street across from the Charles Evans Cemetery. From the Peplau home to Penn Square and downtown was a pleasant walk through residential neighborhoods, across a gentle bridge spanning the railroad tracks, and into downtown Reading. It appears the Peplau home at 1232 Church Street was paid for many times over before the mortgage was finally paid off in 1953. On January 28, 1908, an "indenture" in the amount of $1,200 was recorded to William E. Fisher, a lawyer and the owner and publisher of the *Reading Eagle*. The interest on the principal was 6%, and payments were set at $10 per month.[11] At the beginning of every month one of the Peplau children would be sent around to Mr. Fisher's mansion at 216 South Fifth Street with whatever amount of money could be spared that month. Sometimes as little as $2 would be paid on the mortgage; other times it might be as much as $15. The money was accepted by Flora Miller, the live-in cook and maid for Mr. Fisher. Miss Miller always gave the child a receipt, and Gustav kept them all in his desk in the dining room at 1232 Church Street. Bertha, in particular, enjoyed this responsibility. Miss Miller welcomed the cheerful, youngest Peplau child, inviting her into the kitchen, giving her hot chocolate, and enjoying the wide-eyed wonder with which the child viewed the valuable glass and china in the kitchen and dining room.

When the Peplaus bought the house on Church Street, it was a narrow, two-story brick structure with a mansard roof. The first floor had two parlors, one for the family and one for guests. The rooms were small— about 8 x 10 feet—and the furniture was massive. Ottylie had a piano installed in the first parlor, filling the space in that room. The original oak dining room furniture, restored by John Forster, was still in place when he finally sold the house in February 1999. The second floor had three small bedrooms. Gustav and Ottylie were in the back, facing the alley. A middle room, where all the children were born,[12] belonged eventually to the boys. Clara and Hilda shared a small front bedroom that had bow windows looking out over the street. When Gustav and Ottylie bought the house there was room for a bathroom upstairs, but there were no fixtures or plumbing. The Peplaus, like all the families on Church Street, had an outhouse in the backyard. Once a week Ottylie heated water to fill one of her two large tin washtubs, and all the children bathed in the kitchen, in order of seniority but sharing the same water. At some point, a claw-foot bathtub was installed in the small upstairs washroom but there was still no running hot water. Ottylie would heat the water for Gustav's bath and he would carry it upstairs, but the children still bathed in the kitchen. Ottylie was thrilled when sewers were connected to the property by the City of Reading in 1932 and, wonder of wonders, an indoor toilet was installed.

Monday was wash day, and Ottylie washed in the two tin tubs that were kept in the backyard in summer and in the small kitchen during the winter. Tuesday was ironing day. The piles of laundry from Monday's wash were placed in two reed wash baskets and brought in, a bundle at a time, to the kitchen where the ironing board had been set up. Before electricity was installed in the 1920s, two flatirons sat on the coal stove at the ready. Ottylie ironed all day, separating out the pieces to be mended and distributing the clean, ironed clothes to the bedrooms upstairs. Ottylie was an expert seamstress, and Wednesday was the day for mending or, when need be, the day for sewing and making new clothes. The children wore her beautiful hand-made clothes until their confirmation at age 13, at which time "store" clothes were bought for the occasion. The trundle sewing machine was placed in front of the kitchen window for better light, and sewing projects and materials were piled on the kitchen table. Ottylie made virtually all the family clothing—dresses, skirts, tailored shirts, overalls, pants, and suits. Sheets and pillowcases were made from muslin sacks that had contained sugar, flour, or salt. Thursday was baking day. On baking day the dining room sideboard would be loaded with pies and cakes. Neighbors and teachers soon learned that Thursday was the day to visit, for they would always be offered some of Ottylie's incomparable baked goods. She was particularly noted for her fausnachts—pastries shaped as donuts, deep-fried in lard, and sprinkled with powdered sugar.

In summer, canning as well as baking filled the day. Gustav built long shelves at the back of the cellar, and by summer's end these shelves would be filled with jars of jelly, preserves, applesauce, and apple butter, canned peaches, pears, blueberries, peas, beans, pickles, corn, and red beets. There would be several large crocks of sauerkraut, pickles, and pickled eggs. Friday was cleaning day, when every room was swept, every windowsill wiped, and every corner thoroughly dusted. As they grew older, all the children had assigned chores. In spring and fall, rugs were taken up and hung outside for their semiannual beating; curtains were washed and hung to dry on curtain stretchers; bureau drawers emptied, cleaned, and lined with paper; kitchen cabinets were emptied and everything washed or polished. Ottylie was particularly sensitive to anything that didn't "smell right." Her house was always in perfect order, even with four, and later five, then six, children. On Saturday, with a bonnet on her head and a basket on her arm, Ottylie walked up to Penn Street and to the farmers' market for fresh produce. She was a naturally graceful woman, who held her head high and had a sprightly and graceful walk.[13] Sunday was a day of rest, for all but Ottylie. She was up early, long before church, preparing the Sunday dinner—and dinner it was. On the oak sideboard there would be pies, two of each: custard, lemon meringue, berry, apple. There would be a cake sometimes, too. A roast would be simmering in the oven, potatoes mashed, a jar of home-canned vegetables heating up, cucumbers pressed in brine and swimming in cream set out.

Christmas was a big holiday in America, and so it would be in the Peplau household. As the children came, Gustav honed his carpentry skills. Preparations began well in advance. He would carve toys and faces and limbs for dolls, and would construct cradles and cribs, wagons and buggies. Ottylie would bake large batches of cookies and store then in lard cans for the big day. On Christmas Day there would be a goose—the bigger and the fatter the better. Goose grease had many uses, and would be collected and stowed in glass jars for later use for cooking if lard were in short supply, to mix with camphor ice to rub on the head and chest of a sick child, or to put on second daughter Hilda's head in a vain attempt to straighten her curly hair. Ottylie's hair too had been curly, and she'd endured many a whipping herself as a child for not getting it combed out straight. Her father associated curly hair with frivolity, and Ottylie tried valiantly to spare Hilda this burden, but to no avail. When the children arrived, Ottylie tamed her own ring of blond curls, pulling her hair straight back into a neat bun on the nape of her neck. No curling irons or hairdressers for her.

Ottylie had no complaints. She had a hard life, but she knew how to count her blessings. Not for her the brooding or depression that came to so many women forced to suppress their intelligence as a part of the bargain of a secure marriage. She was an obedient wife and watchful mother whose abundant talents were expressed in her baking, sewing, and housekeeping. During depressed economic cycles, the Reading Railroad would rotate the men into and out of work, rather than lay them off. While this meant that jobs were preserved, it also meant some very hard times for the families involved. During these periodic stretches of unemployment, Ottylie did housecleaning for the more affluent families living on Fifth Street. Her thorough and conscientious housekeeping was well known, and she was much sought after. On the request of her neighbors, she also made extra money by selling home-baked bread, donuts, and cruellers. While she took pride in her talents and loved earning money on her own, she always ceased immediately when Gustav went back to work. She understood how important it was to him to feel able to support his family.

Ottylie enjoyed her garden, her rosebushes, and "working the soil." There was also her music. Her oldest daughter, Clara, and in later years her foster son, Johnny, would give her many hours of pleasure by playing the piano for her. She had few, if any, pleasures outside her home and didn't seek any.

A Child in Reading

Life on Church Street was active and safe for children. Toys were few but improvisation was great. What toys there were, were left out on the stoops and shared. The children would find a jump rope at one house, chalk to mark out hopscotch at another, skates at another, a set of jacks and ball at still another house. Someone one day had a baseball bat and ball. The neighbors had indoor games—cards and checkers—and encouraged children to gather at these homes on cold or rainy days. Two neighbor mothers, Mrs. Koch and Mrs. Delaney, frequently gave children's parties, and there were block parties on May Day, the Fourth of July, and special events at Halloween.

Much of the time, the days on Church Street were fun for children, but little of that fun actually took place at the Peplau home. Inside 1232 Church Street, children were quiet. They were taught to sit still with their hands folded and "look pious." All sorts of sins, such as dancing, card games, or anything that made noise, were forbidden. The Bible was read, obedience practiced, and serious attention paid to decorum. Health, cleanliness, good food, and fresh air were stressed. Ottylie was doing her best to understand America and to raise American children who would marry and become productive workers in the Reading factories—a life better than she or any of her family had known in Europe.[14]

Although she loved all her children, physical expression of affection felt alien to Ottylie. Hugging and kissing were not a part of this culture.

The Peplau family unit was a strong one, but childhood for Hilda Peplau was a stressful and often confusing time. Her home was a secure place, built on the solid foundation of Gustav and Ottylie's marriage, but this home was not a happy one for a child with great intellectual curiosity. From early childhood Hilda seemed to challenge every authority. She took herself and her life very seriously. Her constant refrain was Why? Why? Why? She was curious about everything, curious to know how things worked, curious about people and their motivations, curious about the world beyond Reading. Such curiosity was not appreciated by her parents. A child who constantly questioned was bound to run afoul of adults whose lives were too hard to leave time for inquisitive children. Hilda was frequently disciplined for her inability to just accept the world as it was. "Just do as you are told, obey the teacher, don't get in trouble, don't get noticed," were her mother's constant refrains.

Ottylie was confident that Clara and Harold, who were quiet and obedient, would be all right, but she worried about Hilda and Walter. She feared they would "get into trouble" and bring disgrace if not worse to the rest of the family. Thus Hilda, and later her equally inquisitive brother Walter, were the ones who most often felt the sting of the wide leather strap, kept behind the cellar door for just such use. Ottylie meted out punishment swiftly and forcefully, and sometimes let her anger get the best of her. Gustav worked from early morning until evening, so was less frequently available to wield the strap. Any form of disobedience, however slight, was punished. "Talking back," refusing a task, not coming home immediately when called, or getting into mischief were causes for a whipping. Physical punishment was not unusual in this time and place. When it came to disciplining children, whippings intended to "lick them into shape" were the norm in working-class families. Fear of the "wrath of God," preached in church and threatened by parents, relatives, and neighbors, together with the leather strap, helped ensure proper behavior and restraint. Children were spanked, whipped, or beaten at school as well as at home. Any neighbor could discipline any child, if discipline was called for.[15] A curious and verbally inquisitive child such as Hilda, who liked to wander and explore new things, was in constant trouble. Both parents were fearful of the development of intellectual interests, believing that no good could come from such curiosity. Learning what was prescribed was good; asking questions about it was not.

Their daughter Hilda—who would find unsurpassed success in an academic profession, who would travel throughout the world, and who would never marry—did not fit easily, or ever, into this mold. Ottylie clearly was a gifted, bright, creative, and talented woman. She learned English, and spoke German, Polish, and Russian fluently. She insisted that her children read to her from their school books, so that she could learn what they learned. From her housekeeping her children learned to be systematic and ordered in all they did. She was, though, a conventional and obedient wife. She loved music and sang opera when her husband was not at home. Once he came in the door, however, these talents were submerged; he had her full attention.[16] Their marriage no doubt was an intellectual mismatch, but respect for the husband was deeply ingrained. She lived within her husband's parameters and, thus, endorsed his antiintellectualism. Ottylie did not encourage her children to go beyond the clear boundaries set for those of her class and status in this country at that time. Her own experience suggested that life at best was difficult, and her upbringing taught her that no one should tempt fate, or call attention to themselves. Her children were bright, and she wanted them to finish high school, but Gustav wanted the older children to work as soon as it was legal. In this respect, Ottylie prevailed. Her children, she declared, would finish high school before going to work.[17] There was no discussion of education beyond that. As Bertha explained it,

> Mother did adjust to this country. She spoke beautiful English. She made ends meet where there were no ends. They were both assimilated. But, educated women were beyond them! My father told me I had to get a job as soon as I finished high school. Mother was clearly educated. But, love, honor, and obey was taken very seriously and personally. My picture of Mother is of her serving him, standing and attending, feeding and waiting on him. She would give him the meat, and then chew away on the fat herself. In the end, that's what killed her. Hilda fought with my father, so mother couldn't have taken her side, whether she agreed or not. It was just not possible for her.[18]

In later life, Hilda came to understand that her mother was afraid that a child who caused "trouble" would somehow lead to the family "being evicted from the country."[19] She realized that her parents were doing the best they could, that they were frightened on her behalf, that they sought to protect her the only way they knew—by compelling conformity.[20] For Ottylie and Gustav, the process of learning about freedom in a new country was indeed frightening and painful. They wanted to be accepted and to be seen as "good" people. Above all they wanted the security of knowing they belonged, that they would not be evicted. They feared that education would lead to "godlessness." They viewed American ideas of individual freedom with suspicion because they did not understand the concept and did not trust its promises. They were particularly frightened and bewildered during periods of labor crises when the family income was threatened.[21]

The young Hildegard did not understand any of this, however. Instead, she felt only rejection and derogation of her natural inclinations. Hilda remembered her mother as fair, but distant—unsmiling and serious—with clear blue eyes that did not invite intimacy. Hilda grew up feeling the isolation of her mother's perceived remoteness and expressed disapproval.[22] With five children, there were bound to be tensions. The tension between Hilda and her older sister, Clara, was the most pronounced and was felt most deeply by Hilda. Clara was quiet, unassuming, and desperately sought approval. Hilda always felt Clara, who was instinctively a "pleaser," was the favorite. Part of pleasing was to keep her parents informed about the activities of her siblings. When something went wrong, Clara would accuse Hilda, even if Hilda had nothing to do with the matter at issue. Clara had learned early that she could feel approval if Hilda and sometimes Walter were being punished. Hilda was also the victim of gender stereotypes. While her brothers were expected to conform to the authoritarian routines of the household, the young Hilda was given even less leeway. She was constantly punished, often whipped, but she remained ever inquisitive and competitive. She would not be squelched.[23] As she remarked,

> You learn fairly early that you cannot be first within the family, so you take the struggle where you're more likely to win it. You go out and play with other kids. You spend most of your time out with other groups, as soon as you've completed your chores, of course.[24]

Ever observant, she explained that when you are a second child you become a "watcher" and develop a repertoire of adaptive strategies to use to secure your place in the family, to survive the ordeal of childhood.[25] Because Clara was quick to tell of any activity that might cause concern on any level, Walter and Hilda were up and out of the house as soon as possible. They performed their assigned chores quickly and efficiently in order to spend as much time out of the home as they could. Hilda and Walter on at least one occasion did perpetrate a minor act of rebellion. The object was the dreaded leather strap. One winter day, while Ottylie was shopping, they seized the strap and threw it into the furnace. The smell of burning leather permeated the house, and the children ran from room to room trying to fan away the fumes. When Ottylie returned, they claimed ignorance of the source of the horrible smell. They were not punished on this occasion, but the act of defiance did not end the whippings. Outright rebellion, however, would never occur to them. They aspired only to leave.[26]

Hilda's feelings of isolation were reinforced by the fact that her grandmother, Gustav's mother, was a strong presence in the family, and not a kind one. No one could have been less grandmotherly than Hilda's "Grossmutter." Julianna Prill Peplau was a stern woman, very tall for that time—nearly 6 feet—thin, and gaunt. Grossmutter had narrow and strict ideas about children. They were to be seen and not heard, they were to honor and obey their parents until they could go to work and support those who had supported them. She had little if any use for education for children, thinking it was a waste of time, particularly after an age at which they could go to work. She was opinionated and a relentless disciplinarian. Grossmutter regularly arrived at Church Street to inspect the premises. She would sweep in, tall and austere, demanding, in German, "Come Ottylie, we go upstairs." Every closet and bureau drawer was duly opened, while Grossmutter inspected, criticized, or gave advice. After Bertha was born, Ottylie became gravely ill and was confined to her bed for nearly a year. That year, while Ottylie fought typhoid fever and phlebitis, Grossmutter moved into the home at 1232 Church Street to see to the running of the house. It was a grim time. Gone were the days of singing and baking, the good smells and bountiful meals. Quiet and fear seemed to pervade the house. Ottylie recovered and Grossmutter returned to her own home, but the pain caused by her presence remained in the hearts of the older children.

In spite of physical resemblances between the two, there was no rapport between grandmother and granddaughter Hilda. Julianna Prill Peplau was not a kindly grandmother who made up for the remote Ottylie's aloofness from her second daughter. If anything, she exacerbated the loneliness of the child. She had a loud, rasping voice, and complained often about the dirt and disorder in Ottylie's spotless house, and about the noise and disobedience of her cowed children. Although Gustav visited his mother often, both before and after Ottylie's recovery, his children were not welcome in her home. Visiting grandchildren were relegated to the backyard to play while adults visited in her kitchen. No matter how cold it was outside, Hilda was made to wait in the small, dreary backyard while her father visited with his mother. Hilda, much later would say, "My father thoroughly disliked me, perhaps because Grossmutter disliked me. Early on, he tagged me as a 'bad child.'"[27] Grossmutter approved of the obedient, docile Clara, but subjected Hilda to unfavorable comparisons, frequent shaming, and belittlement. Not until her grandmother was on her deathbed in 1938 did Hilda finally see the inside of her house. The house was impeccable and full of beautifully restored antiques. Presumably, Gustav spent his time with his mother refinishing her furniture. It was then that Grossmutter told Hilda, "If I had a chance to do it all over again, I wouldn't be so mean to you."[28]

There were the usual childhood diseases on Church Street for which there was no cure and for which quarantine cards (notices to post on front doors) were routinely issued and were routinely ineffective. Measles, mumps, chicken pox, scarlet fever, or diphtheria would start at one end of the block and move from house to house until almost all the children had been stricken, one after the other. When a child was out of school, it would be reported to the City Health Department, which would send a visiting nurse to check up on the family. Doctors were rarely consulted. When a "baby welfare station" opened at Spring and Church streets, Ottylie dutifully took the children to be weighed.

When Hilda was 9 or 10 years old, a particularly virulent flu epidemic broke out. Ottylie went out to the store, and Gustav to work, but the four children, Clara, Hilda, Walter, and Harold, were strictly confined to the house and the backyard. The Peplau family escaped the virus, but others on Church Street were not so fortunate. There were several deaths, and neighbors could be seen wandering in the street delirious. Walter and a friend rigged up a pulley so that they could send messages back and forth across the street. A few of their young friends died, and their bodies were on view at home for several days, sometimes displayed in the windows of the front parlors. Hilda and her friends would look through the windows where the bodies were laid out and Hilda would ask, "Why?"[29] The children on Church Street realized that this was a serious disease and intuitively understood the importance of preventive isolation from the victims. There were no arguments about staying indoors. The 1918–1919 influenza epidemic killed an estimated 550,000 Americans, a ghastly toll. New research places global mortality from the pandemic at 30 million people.[30] It ranks as the 20th century's most readily forgotten global disaster, and almost certainly the deadliest epidemic in recorded history.

Church, School, and Neighborhood

Church provided the primary social life for the family, and St. John's German Lutheran Evangelical Church was at its center. Gustav joined first, in 1902, and Ottylie joined when she came to Reading as his wife. Located on Walnut between Fifth and Sixth streets, St. John's was built directly over a colonial cemetery, and tombstones lay undisturbed in the church basement. All the Peplau baptisms, confirmations, marriages, and deaths are recorded at St. John's. The pastor during Hilda's childhood was the Rev. Phillip Kirchner, a rotund man with a ruddy face and a cheerful countenance. Ottylie was particularly fond of him, and prepared for his visits to her home with pleasure. He often dropped by on Sunday afternoons to listen to Ottylie play the piano and to enjoy her excellent baking. A jolly man of kind spirit, he was the only guest allowed to sit in the small front parlor.

While church and Sunday school was a large part of her early life, Hilda looked forward to entering "real school" where she had heard one "could learn things." Her parents, too, looked forward to sending her to school where, they believed, she would at last learn discipline. In 1914, Hilda, like Clara before her, started school at the St. John's church day school, where classes were taught in German. A year later, with the onset of World War I, the German school was closed, and Clara and Hilda were enrolled in the public school. Hilda hoped that public school would fill the lonely void she sometimes felt at home, but this was not to be. School in Reading only contributed to the confusion of her childhood.

Unwittingly, the public school teachers added to Hilda's pain and sense of isolation in an unexpected way. In those days, it was the custom for teachers to pay home visits, not only to report on their pupils' progress but also to give advice to immigrant families in regard to such matters as sanitation and proper food. For her part, Ottylie was proud of her beautiful English and welcomed the opportunity to use it. She encouraged Clara's teachers to visit. Once they discovered that at the Peplau home they would be served fresh bread or wonderful pastries, they came often and continued the practice when Hilda entered school. In her case, they most likely thought they were carrying favorable reports about the child who was so excited about learning, so full of questions. Little could they have known that these visits led to a seemingly unending cycle of punishment, that arose from Ottylie's fear that Hilda—in school as she had been at home—was too inquisitive, too inclined to attract notice. When Hilda brought home report cards with good grades, these too were rewarded with whippings. "It was believed that I had cheated or changed the grades en route home."[31] From that point on, Hilda faced an ongoing internal struggle. Family disapproval had to be weighed against her natural desire to do well and compete for grades with other students. This conflict laid the foundation for an emotional ambivalence that would never leave her. The teachers' home visits were not the only problem. School in Reading in the early decades of the 20th century was not a challenge to a bright child. According to Hilda, it was "mainly a matter of penmanship and addition so that you could be a good clerk." They expected their students would stay in Reading, and they aspired only to make them into good clerks or factory workers. It was an insulated world, not a world from which one expected, or usually even desired, to escape.

Although disappointed in school, Hilda was excited to discover the grand library at Fifth and Franklin streets, where you could actually take out books and take them home to enjoy. But this was not to be either. Alerted by Clara, Ottylie was so upset to discover a pile of books in Hilda's room, that she tore them up and then burned them for good measure. She feared it was illegal to bring the books home and burned the evidence, not understanding the concept of a lending library. Never again did Hilda bring books home, but she did sneak into the branch library after an acceptable waiting period, there to browse and read and dream. The librarian, however, had heard about the book destruction and so required Hilda to sit directly in front of the desk where she could conspicuously keep her eye on her. Hilda continued to read in the library even though she keenly felt the disapproval.[32]

The Church Street neighborhood offered comfort. It was friendly. Most of the homes were occupied by immigrants, and most bothered about the others' business. The Koehlers lived next door. Klothilde Koehler was 47 when the Peplaus moved into 1232 Church Street, and became a sort of mentor and mother substitute for Ottylie, who was then in her early 20s and a new mother. "Old Mrs. Koehler" over the years was a mellowing influence. The whippings that Hilda received were sometimes severe. Ottylie would become enraged and yell at Hilda about her presumed offenses, and Hilda would cry out in pain. Occasionally Mrs. Koehler would hear one of these whippings in progress and would come over, cautioning Ottylie, "That's enough!" The Koehlers had six children. Emma and Amelia, who were both more than 10 years older than Hilda, became registered nurses, a fact that did not escape young Hilda's attention. After nurses' training, the two sisters took jobs as private duty nurses in New York City. When they came home to Reading, they brought cast-off clothing from their wealthy New York City clients. Hilda had great fun dressing up and daydreaming of a life, such as theirs, beyond Reading. The Kinseys lived on the other side of the Peplaus, at 1234. The Kinsey sons, Paul and Raymond, were also older and would become good friends to Hilda. Mrs. Harriet Koch lived down the street and enjoyed visits from the tall, studious Peplau girl. Even then Hilda was a good listener, and Mrs. Koch liked to talk, particularly about sex. And there was Mrs. Delaney, a wonderful friend to all children on the block, provided her husband was not at home. He was an alcoholic, given to alcoholic rages. There were no battered women's shelters at that time to which a woman could turn for protection, and everyone knew when Mr. Delaney had been drinking because his wife would appear on the street bruised black and blue.[33]

Holidays were good times. Halloween in particular was a special day. Often three families—Koch, Kinsey, and Delaney—rented a barn on the next block over from Church Street and invited all the neighborhood children for a great Halloween party. Neighbors would pitch in to decorate the barn with pumpkins, corn shucks, and witches and goblins. The children would dress in their most creative attire and come to bob for apples, play games, eat cookies, drink cider, and have a grand time. There were other diversions for the neighborhood children, including the parades around Penn Square and the weekend open markets. Everyone loved the medicine man, who came once a year. His horse-drawn wagon would come bumping down the street to the vacant lot between Marion and Robson streets, where he would set up shop for a few days. He would have liniments, salves, cough medicines, and "pain killers" (juice laced with a healthy slug of alcohol and probably also opium which was freely available at the time). He stood on the back of his wagon to pitch his goods, telling risque stories and performing simple acts of magic to entertain the children. He was a fast talker, quick to spot the vulnerable, and he charmed the children with his stories, jovial appearance, and free balloons. He added variety to daily life, and his visits were anticipated with pleasure.

Ottylie and Gustav were German Protestants in an Irish Catholic neighborhood, and wanted desperately to blend in and be accepted. The advent of World War I exacerbated Ottylie's innate fear that the family might not be secure in America and her desire that her children should, above all else, be trained to "fit in." Indeed, there was a shadow of reality to these fears. Anti-German sentiment mounted when the United States entered the war in Europe. In spite of their long residency and general good standing in the neighborhood, the Peplau home was stoned. Ottylie was terrified that they would have to leave America, as her forbearers had been forced from their homeland in the partition of Poland, and as her family in Europe would be again. The war did bring about changes in the life of the Peplau family. The German families in the 1200 block on Church Street quit speaking German, even at home. The German-language day school that Clara and Hilda attended was closed forever. The girls continued to attend the Lutheran Sunday school, but the language of instruction there was changed to English. Ottylie lived in fear that someone would harm her children because the family was German. She was not one to show emotions, but in this period she cried often and unexpectedly when letters arrived from Russia with news that the Elgert family had again been displaced by the war. Flour, sugar, salt, coffee, and other staples were bundled with clothing and tightly sewn into burlap bags for shipment to family relocated to Russia.[34] At least some of these packages got through. Twenty years later, during World War II, the nightmare would be repeated. The children were sheltered from the details of family distress during World War I, but the tension in the home was pervasive and Ottylie's fierce determination to shield her own family from catastrophe was palpable. Hilda did not understand then how a generations-deep memory of forcible relocation in Europe fed Ottylie's anxiety. She did understand somehow, however, that her mother wanted to protect her.

TEENAGE YEARS

In 1920 Hilda was 11 years old. It was a time when the world was changing rapidly. World War I was over, and the United States had emerged an undisputed world power. Trade and industry expanded, stock markets boomed, jazz blared, and bathtubs overflowed with bootleg gin. The Roaring Twenties were characterized by continued urbanization, the emergence of the country's first youth culture, newfound freedom for women, and unprecedented technological advances. The 19th Amendment passed, and women voted in their first presidential election in 1920.

A tall and lanky child with a great deal of energy, Hilda seemed never to be still. She hiked up the hills, played furiously in the streets and in the parks, and concentrated with fearsome intensity on her studies. Although she was always healthy, Hilda was very thin. She had grown tall quickly. While still in grade school she reached 5 eet, 7 inches and was by far the tallest student in her class. Because she was so thin, her mother feared "consumption," and took her to a doctor who prescribed lots of ice cream, milk shakes, and eggnog, which Hilda thoroughly enjoyed—and olive oil in grape juice, which she definitely did not. Throughout her childhood and teenage years, her mother and her friends would worry that Hilda was too thin and urge her to eat. She enjoyed food and had a healthy appetite, but did not gain weight. Her next-door neighbor, Paul Kinsey, worked as a "soda jerk" at Pomeroy's Department Store on Penn Street, and added extra ice cream to Hilda's sodas whenever she came in. Nothing worked, however. Hilda remained exceedingly thin well into her adult life.

Hilda was 12 years old and in junior high school before a history teacher took the interest and the time to tell her that she was smart. Helen Kaiser found great pleasure in discovering and encouraging a truly bright student, particularly a girl. She understood such children would have a hard road ahead, and therefore made sure to take a personal interest by showing her appreciation for their intelligence and encouraging them to use their minds. She also visited their homes to urge parents to encourage their daughters. In Hilda's case, this was not a good idea. The immediate consequence of Mrs. Kaiser's first visit was another whipping, administered after Ottylie had chased the teacher from the house. "Encouragement" was not a word used in relation to daughters. With unrelenting consistency her parents attempted to teach her that people did not want to be "annoyed" by her questions, and that adults did not like children who asked them questions.[35] These admonitions and the corporal punishment that accompanied them continued into Hilda's teenage years. The message they imprinted was that adults did not like her and that she must be lacking in some essential qualities that adults required. These feelings led to great reticence in personal relationships that lasted well into her own adulthood.

Hilda was not only bright, but was also a good athlete with a healthy, if somewhat repressed, competitive spirit. Athletics afforded her the opportunity to focus her energy and work out her anger and the frustration she felt but did not understand. She was a runner and even when walking was always in a hurry. She was so good in sports that her physical education teacher, Bessie Mason (whose windblown hair and breathless appearance inspired the children to refer to her as "Messy Basin") called at the Peplau home, accompanied by an undaunted Mrs. Kaiser. Their mission was to encourage the Peplaus to point Hilda toward the college track in high school in order that she might go on to the local junior college to study to become a physical education teacher. Again, their visit was not welcomed. Gustav was furious and Ottylie frightened. Gustav made it clear that no daughter of his was going to college. Absolutely not. He ordered the teachers to leave, and made it quite clear they were not welcome to return. Mrs. Kaiser and Miss Mason later assured Hilda that they would personally loan her the money to go to college. The young girl feared, though, that this would lead to an irrevocable break with her parents. This was a consequence she was not yet ready to contemplate, although she continued to dream of getting away from Reading.[36]

Hilda's athletic pursuits, even outside of school, provoked Ottylie's wrath, at least on one occasion. The sons of the Peplau's next-door neighbors, Paul and Raymond Kinsey, decided to introduce Hilda to a new sport. Up the hill they went to Hamden Park at the top of Spring Street, where racquets and balls were produced. Hilda loved the game called tennis—the rhythmic twang of the ball, and the focus and concentration required, a concentration that forced all else out of her mind. Tennis became almost an addiction. Impressed with both her skill and her dedication, the Kinsey brothers' father went next door to 1232 in order to present the Peplaus with a gift for Hilda, a tennis racquet all her own. Ottylie was appalled and very upset. She was opposed to anyone giving her children gifts, perhaps because she would feel a need to reciprocate or perhaps because she felt the children did not deserve presents. (Hilda remembered a similar occasion when her Uncle Karl gave her a silver dollar, and Ottylie made her return the gift immediately.) When Ottylie expressed her displeasure over the tennis racquet, Mr. Kinsey tried to argue with her. Ottylie became so agitated that she picked up the tennis racquet and hit him over the head. Mr. Kinsey was infuriated by this hostile reception to his act of generosity and took Mrs. Peplau to court. She was found guilty of disorderly conduct and fined $3.[37]

While the block was friendly and congenial and her home was secure, Hilda recalled that as a child she was always fighting a feeling of loneliness, a loneliness so painful that she felt she must always strive to hide it, disguise it, defend against it. Although her parents often spoke German or Russian with each other, the children were permitted to speak only English at home, thus emphasizing their exclusion from the intimacy of family life. Hilda's early experiences in school and the anger she seemed to provoke in her mother, even as she grew into her teens, reinforced her feeling that she must try harder than her siblings to succeed, to win approval. Although from the outside a family might appear to be a homogeneous unit, from a child's perspective the family does not provide a monolithic experience. Each child experiences it differently. The family is a collection of niches among which each child tries to find his or her place. Niches provide distinct vantage points from which siblings experience the same events in very different ways. Although her younger sister

Bertha remembered an enchanted childhood, Hilda did not. In this family, the three sisters, Clara, Hilda, and Bertha, were very different from one another and each had strikingly different memories of the family environment and their childhood.[38]

Until Hilda was 14, she and Clara slept in the double bed in the front bedroom. Her mother made all the girls' clothes, and Hilda and Clara were dressed alike until they went to high school. But the two sisters could not have been more unlike. The torture for Hilda of sharing a room with Clara came to an end when a woman for whom Ottylie occasionally cleaned house gave her a white, stenciled bedroom set. This bedroom set would greatly change Hilda's life at home. With help from her brothers, Hilda moved the furniture up the stairs to the unheated third floor. The attic room was dark and cold, but was private and it was hers. And, it had a great view over Church Street, over the railroad yards, and up the hills and away from Reading. It was the perfect place for a teenage girl to spin her dreams. At last, she was free of Clara.

MAKING HER OWN WAY

Hilda wryly acknowledged in later life that she was a "pretty snotty kid" who "had problems with authority" in school. There was also something of a pattern to her occasional problems at school. For example, in the co-ed junior high school she attended, she was once caught making faces in class at a fellow student. She was sent to the principal, Mr. Klinger, who told her that if she had been a boy he would have caned and beaten her. He said, however, since she was a girl, she would receive only a stern lecture, to which Hilda replied, "Go ahead, I'm used to being beaten." Years later, after Hilda finished nurses' training, she cared for Mr. Klinger's dying mother. Remembering her misbehavior in junior high school, Mr. Klinger commented, "You turned out pretty well anyway."[39]

Hilda had a run-in with the Girls High School principal when she was 15. This was an incident that would have more far-reaching consequences and that would, in fact, change the course of her life. A teacher reported that Hilda and her friends were talking in the classroom while their teacher was out of the room. Others of the accused students "confessed" when the teacher demanded that they do so and accepted extra homework assignments as punishment. Hilda, however, protested that she was innocent, that she was not among those who were talking. The teacher was incensed that a student would dare to argue with her, and banished Hilda to the principal's office. There she protested the unjust treatment. The principal was not interested in denials. She decreed that the tall, thin, rigidly angry girl would sit in front of her desk until she confessed and apologized. Hilda was to sit there from the time school opened in the morning until it closed in the afternoon, with her hands folded in her lap. She was neither to read nor talk, and she would stay for as long as the principal deemed necessary. Hilda sat and seethed, and by the end of the day had made up her mind that she would never confess to something she did not do, that she would not apologize when she was right, and that she would not return to school the next morning. When she was allowed to go home at the end of the day, she marched straight to the W. T. Grant five-and-dime variety store where she worked on Saturdays. She asked the manager, Sam Wolfson, for full-time work. Mr. Wolfson was delighted to give the serious, hardworking Hilda Peplau a regular job in the store but insisted that she complete her education. She would be forever grateful to Mr. Wolfson for his support and for his interest in her and in her future. Before going home that afternoon to inform her parents of her decision, Hilda checked on how to enroll in the evening high school.

Ottylie was upset because she truly wanted her children to finish high school, and Hilda, in fact, was first in her class. Hilda assured her mother she intended to finish high school in the evening. Gustav was not so upset, particularly since Hilda had gone to work full time and would be bringing home her earnings. In fact, Hilda's first pay envelope was the source of another confrontation at 1232 Church Street. Gustav demanded that all the cash be turned over to him. Hilda insisted this was "unjust" since it was she who had worked to earn the money. By this time, Hilda and Walter had outgrown the strap. The war of words raged fast and furious until Ottylie took charge. She divided the money and decreed that Hilda would contribute two thirds of her paycheck for "board," an amount that satisfied Gustav and left Hilda's dignity intact.

Hilda, now a "working girl," realized that she would need to gain skills to qualify her for higher paid employment. She decided to study first at the McCann Business School before going on to evening high school. After a few months at W. T. Grant, and with Mr. Wolfson's blessing, Hilda accepted a more challenging position as the payroll clerk at a men's pants factory. On Saturdays she earned extra money working at Sears Roebuck. After 3 months, a small recession caused the pants factory to lay off all the men, but, knowing a good thing when he saw it, the owner kept Hilda on the job. This was a godsend as she could bring her homework from McCann to the pants factory and get it all completed during working hours. With this luxury of time, she sped through McCann, earning all As. After a few month's lay-off, the pants factory went back into production. Hilda was sent out, mostly to the Italian section of town south of Penn Street, to inform the men they could come back to work. There was much rejoicing, much wine was shared, and the payroll clerk was loaded down with gifts of spaghetti, lasagne, and meatballs. Thus began a lifelong appreciation for wine and pasta. But for

Hilda, it was also time to move on. She started classes at the evening high school, and found an even better paying position as a bookkeeper with the Eaches Coal Company.

When she went to work at Eaches Coal, the world began to open up. Lester B. Eaches came into the office every day. He loved to talk politics, and he found a curious and avid listener in his new bookkeeper. Soon he began encouraging her in her ambition to move out into the world. He brought in a radio so she could listen to the news, and then newspapers, which she read avidly. It was in these newspapers that she saw advertisements for nurses' training schools and began to envision the nursing career first suggested by the Koehler sisters years earlier. Once a month Spencer B. Roland, a lawyer, would come from Philadelphia to go over the books. He soon discovered the books were just fine, and he too began to encourage the precocious bookkeeper to use her mind and her talents. At Eaches Coal, Hilda gradually expanded her area of responsibilities. She kept the books, took the orders, kept the money, paid the men, cleaned the office, and assumed day-to-day operating responsibilities.

Reading evening high school turned out to be a true blessing. The students were older and more mature, and were treated as adults. Hildegard found the raised level of discussion made even the dullest course more interesting. She joined the debate team, and found a mentor in the debate coach, Hayes K. McClelland, who complimented her intelligence and urged her to think about how she could use it to fashion a future for herself. Through debate, she gained an appreciation for direct, succinct, and clear communication—traits she would develop and use for the rest of her life. And through debate her horizons began to expand. She began to add news magazines and the *Saturday Evening Post* to her reading at the library. Her friend Peg Mlodoch lived near the library south of Penn Street and agreed to take books out for Hilda. Although she objected to Hilda going to the library, Ottylie did not object to her going to her friend Peg's home. With Peg available to get the books, Hilda's reading began to get serious. In May 1928, Hilda graduated from Reading's Girls Evening High School as class valedictorian and winner of the literature medal.

All through her teenage years, Hilda sought but could not find a spiritually comfortable place. In addition to Sunday school and church services at St. John's, Hilda and her friends managed at one time or another to attend Sunday afternoon and evening services in virtually every church in Reading. They discussed religion endlessly.[40] With her friend Peg Mlodoch, she read Nietzsche through her last 2 years at the evening high school and her years at the Pottstown Hospital Training School. The two young, untutored girls argued endlessly about what he meant.[41] Her several readings of *Beyond Good and Evil* gave her much to think about and in the end an understanding of where she stood when it came to religion. Perspective, Nietzsche wrote, is the essence of what we call values in life. Nietzsche's view that there is no true world independent of individual perspective suggests that there is no one way we ought to think and act—that we alone are responsible for what we choose to do. Hilda was comfortable with this philosophy, and in later years, when asked in interviews for faculty positions about her faith, she would explain that she believed in values, but not necessarily in a particular God, or religion.[42] This was not the answer that interviewers were looking for.

When Hilda entered McCann Business School and became a full-time working girl, her younger sister, Bertha, was just emerging from infancy to childhood. With Bertha, who was 10 years younger than Hilda, Ottylie began to relax. By this time, Ottylie had begun to understand that she was safe in America and that this land encouraged, rather than punished, the bright and ambitious. She felt the desperate pressures to protect and provide begin to lift. Bertha was a lovely, engaging, and lively child whose dimpled smiles and abundant good humor were hard to resist. Bertha loved plants and flowers, and Ottylie discovered that she did too. Together they would go to pick dandelions, and then lilacs when they were in bloom. Ottylie began to enjoy growing things not just for their utilitarian value, but also for their beauty. Unlike her four siblings, however, Bertha was often sick and seemed to fall victim to every childhood illness. Partly because of her frailty, there was a major bonding between Bertha and her mother. In 1927 Bertha, who was then 8 years old, experienced a year of very serious illnesses: mumps, measles, chicken pox, pneumonia, scarlet fever, diphtheria. The house was quarantined, and everyone except Bertha and her parents moved out. Ottylie slept in the room with Bertha, tending to all her needs and praying that her youngest daughter would survive. Bertha recalled,

> When I was sick, she would sleep at the foot of my bed. But she was not warm and cuddly. She had a hard, hard life. She was very resourceful. She could cook up a storm with no money. Warm and cuddly was not what it took. Grit was what it took. She had major talents—they showed up in her sewing and cooking. She was deeply religious. She read the whole Bible every year in German.[43]

Probably because she was so sick for so long, Bertha did not have many childhood friends. Instead, she formed an intense relationship to the land, to growing things. In later years, Bertha would become to herbs what Hilda would become to nursing—a major figure and world-renowned expert.[44]

For Hilda, the year of Bertha's illness became a year of growth and freedom. She was 17 when she moved to the home of her good friends Betty and Natalie Kreiger who lived on West Douglass Street. The three girls were very close, almost sisters. It was a year to work, to visit the library, and to read as much as she wanted in her spare time, a year to explore dating relationships, and a year free from the tensions at home. Because for all practical purposes Hilda had left home, she missed the experience of her mother's mellowing.

Because she was fun-loving and quick witted, Hilda was a popular and sought after friend. She was creative and energetic, and she had true friends from whom she received positive reinforcement. Hilda was a natural leader. In junior high school she and two of her friends, Kit Yeager and Mim Hoover, organized their group into the "Combined Athletic Club," which they called the CAC. The group met in the afternoons and evenings and on weekends to play, to party, to hike. While living with the Kreigers, Hilda was always up by 5:30 in the morning, and, weather permitting, she would pick up a friend, usually Joyce Zerbe, and walk up to the park for a quick game of tennis before going to work at W. T. Grant and later at Eaches Coal. After work, she walked home to help "Pop" Kreiger with the chores.[45] Dinner was served promptly at 5:00 p.m., and it was off to walk to evening high school, and then a brisk walk back home again. It was a long and full day, but one that Hilda found exhilarating. She did not know for sure where she was headed, but she was sure that she was going somewhere.

Many young men would gather during that year on the Kreiger's front porch where Hilda, Natalie, Betty, and Peg held court. Friday nights "out with the girls" almost always ended up in the Pennsylvania Diner for a hot roast beef sandwich before going home. Saturday nights were date nights and were often spent in nightclubs around Reading where Betty Kreiger sang. Betty had a rich lyrical voice, and was very popular. Soon, she was earning money with her singing and bought a car. She was very generous, and soon taught Hilda to drive. While Betty sang for her living, Hilda smoked, and Peg Mlodoch danced.[46] Judging by the photos in the archived albums, there were many romances. Even late in life, however, Peplau was reluctant to talk much about them:

> Oh, well, yes—I had lots of romances. I would just as soon not talk about those . . . every girl has romances . . . I was engaged a couple of times, and I think that, fortunately for me, it became self-evident that there were intellectual incompatibilities between the men I was attracted to and the men I was interested in and knew. I would say there were two men I might have married, and looking back, it never would have worked . . . I had lots of male friends along the way, but I don't think marriage was ever a viable goal. In my neighborhood, marriages were not great. There was never a great competition between marriage and a career for me . . . I think there is much merit in finding someone to spend the rest of your life with, with whom there's sufficient compatibility . . . but it just didn't happen with me.[47]

Although popular with men, Hilda's close and lasting relationships were with her girlfriends. An archive photograph from 1927 shows a group of young women perched on the porch of a house in the country.[48] The house was owned by the mother of a friend who let the CAC girls use it for a week. Boys visited, and the girls smoked cigarettes, swam in the river, talked all night, fished, played cards, and had a grand old time. A year after the country house excursion with school girlfriends, Hilda took a canoe trip up the Schuylkill River with Joyce Zerbe. They were gone a week. Because she wasn't living at home, Hilda had a newfound freedom of movement. For their week's adventure, the girls packed up cans of beans, tuna, and peanut butter; bread and fruit; a couple of blankets; and a change of shirts, and took off. They would row and drift until it got dark, and then pull up to the bank, disembark, and sleep beside the canal. Joyce, who was a good swimmer, often took a swim before supper while Hilda, who never learned to swim, watched from the shore.[49] In this way, many a happy day was spent, plotting her future, daydreaming, and enjoying days of quiet pleasure. Betty and Natalie Kreiger, Peg Mlodoch, and Joyce Zerbe would remain lifelong friends. These friendships went a long way toward mitigating the sense of isolation and loneliness she had felt in her childhood home.

LEAVING READING

One Friday night, instead of going to the Pennsylvania Diner, the group of friends chose a Chinese restaurant for dinner. A serendipitous observation turned out to be uncannily predictive of the powerful personality that was emerging as the strong-willed little girl born into an immigrant family in Reading grew into adulthood. Moving her plate and looking at the wheel displayed on the paper place mat, Hilda was delighted to discover that the year of her birth, 1909, was the Chinese year of the cock. She read the accompanying character profile:

> Hard working and a deep thinker, with much ability and talent, you hate to fail. You would rather work by yourself than with others and your futures can swing high or low. A knowledge seeking pioneer who tends to be selfish and lonely.[50]

"The Chinese got it right!" she noted in the margin. Indeed, much of her future *was* foretold on this Chinese place mat. From this time onward, Hilda paid attention also to her astrological sign, Virgo. It was an apt sign for her. According to the charts, Virgos may appear diffident, but tensile strength and sharp intelligence make them a worthy ally—and a formidable adversary. Hilda often would be mistakenly depicted as prudish or a relentless perfectionist. It would be more accurate to say that she was a purist. Throughout her life, both personal and professional, Hildegard Peplau would adhere scrupulously to the facts as she observed them. She would tell unvarnished truth when she thought it important. She would not needlessly hurt another person, but nor would she flatter or hide her considered judgment, particularly when asked for an opinion. Although she never understood why, the impact of her candor was more often negative than positive. While willing to give others the benefit of the doubt, when there was no doubt there would be no benefit. Throughout her life, Hildegard Peplau would provoke strong feelings in others and precipitate explosive situations. Virgos, the perfectionists of the zodiac, it is said, may also tend to be agonizingly tuned in to their own imperfections and shortcomings. It was often as difficult for Hilda to accept her own limits as it was for her to recognize and accept them in others. Wisdom lies in accepting that one cannot control everything and that knowing that forbearance and forgiveness will go a long way. Hilda tried mightily to achieve that peace with her parents, and to a large extent succeeded. She remembered that her remote and authoritarian father had great talent in his hands and she remembered the beauty of the work he did around the house. Later in life she recognized that her mother's sternness and anger were more an expression of fear than of dismay at her second daughter's need to excel and escape.[51] Hilda would always have a sharp wit and a love of parties, but she would never lose her seriousness of purpose.

Hilda's separation from the emotional bonds that had clouded her childhood may have been eased by the arrival in the family of little Johnny Forster. Ottylie was 50 when she became a foster mother in 1931. Her life had always revolved around *kirche*, *küche*, and *kinder*, and her self-appointed guardianship of baby Johnny was to assure this would continue even after her own children had grown and left the home. Ottylie's Wednesday baking day was well known, and one result was a rather eclectic group of visitors for a woman so staid and home centered. The insurance man timed his weekly pickup of 25-cent payments on policies for Wednesdays on Church Street when he could be sure of finding fresh-baked goods at the Peplau house. Gawky Bill Koehler from next door always came over on Wednesday; Mrs. Bauscher, who lived diagonally across the street from 1232 always managed to get over; and finally, old Rosie Forster would scuffle up from Wunder Street. Rumor had it that she had come to America on the same boat as Ottylie. It always seemed a strange relationship, but when Rosie came by, the work would stop, the coffee would be put on (always boiled with an eggshell for greater clarity), and the cake would be cut. One day Rosie lamented that her unmarried daughter was going to have a baby. Ottylie immediately began sewing little things from fabric scraps. About 6 weeks after the birth of the infant, Rosie's young daughter assessed the situation, wrapped him in a blanket, put him in a basket, and left him on Ottylie

Peplau's kitchen table. Rosie threw up her hands, claiming she could not possibly raise another child as she had been so unsuccessful with the first two. The baby was so tiny. He didn't cry or move. He couldn't hold up his head. He seemed so sweet, though. Ottylie marched down to the baby welfare center to find out what to do and immediately began feeding him condensed milk laced with Karo syrup. Soon she had a well and happy baby, Johnny Forster, who was to become the joy of her last years.[52]

After receiving her high school diploma, Hildegard Peplau had only one goal: to get out of Reading as soon as possible. She had been speaking for some time with the Koehler sisters who had become private-duty nurses in New York City. Hilda thought them to be the most sophisticated ladies the neighborhood had produced. She was determined to join them. She began investigating nurses' training by responding to newspaper announcements of hospital training school programs. Her first choice was the Church Home and Hospital Training School in Baltimore, across the street from Johns Hopkins University. Although Johns Hopkins had a university-based school of nursing, it never occurred to Hilda that she herself might be admitted to a university. Instead, she reasoned, the hospital training school across from Johns Hopkins might be a good place for her because perhaps she could slip in and use the Johns Hopkins library. Ottylie was appalled by Hilda's interest in nursing. She could not understand why anyone would want to clean up "other people's filth and dirt." She certainly didn't want her daughter going to the big, dirty, dangerous city of Baltimore. Hilda compromised to the extent that she agreed to go to Pottstown Hospital Training School for Nurses just 20 miles east of Reading. She applied and was admitted. Hilda was on her way out of Reading at last, if only down the road to Pottstown.

No matter your age, childhood really ends when your mother dies. For Hildegard, it was fausnacht day, a Tuesday, in February 1944. Hilda, Walter, and Harold then were all serving in the military. Bertha was at work and only 13-year-old Johnny was at home. Ottylie was in the kitchen kneading the mountain of dough to make her famous fausnachts. Johnny grated the nutmeg into powdered sugar in a big brown paper bag. Ottylie made a small dent in the rising donuts covering every table top. The board on top of the refrigerator, the sideboard in the dining room, and even the ironing board was filled with beautiful, fluffy, pre-Lenten treats. Ottylie carefully guided them into fresh lard that was heated exactly right, turning out golden-brown perfection, one after another. That night, Johnny and Bertha took turns shaking them in the bag of spiced sugar, then running them, a dozen at a time, to the lucky neighbors. First the Kinseys on the left and the Koehlers on the right got theirs. Then a boxful went across the street to the Fichthorns, and more down that side of the street to the Bauschers. The Kochs and Sieferts got theirs, then on to the Schumachers. Let the fasts of Lent begin: Church Street was donut-ed to the hilt.[53]

The next day, Bertha received a call from Johnny at the pediatrician's office where she worked: "Mother's sick, you'd better come home." Ottylie was indeed sick, sick enough to summon the doctor, which very seldom if ever had happened. She was given pills and put to bed. Although she apparently slept peacefully, she woke up in great pain the next morning. Her house was in order, the bills had been paid. There was no sign of the massive baking of 2 days before. She called Bertha and Gustav to her side and said simply, "I am going home. Take care of Johnny." The doctor was summoned again, but before he arrived, she was dead. Bertha searched high and low for that magical donut recipe, but never found it. Church Street would never again know such fausnachts.[54]

ENDNOTES

1. Reading was a working-class town—for both men and women. The women worked in sewing machine factories, stocking mills, linen mills, underwear mills, cotton mills, glove factories, and dress shops. Vanity Fair, Nolde's, and Berkshire were Reading brands. See *Official Program of the 150th Anniversary of the Reading Voluntary Fire Department*, Box 8, #261, in the Hildegard E. Peplau Collection in the Schlesinger Library, Radcliffe College, Cambridge, Massachusetts.
2. *The Official Program*, op cit.
3. All those enormous factories are now outlet stores, and Reading, once known for its railroad yards and sewing factories, is now the "Factory Outlet Capital of the World."
4. Ottylie Peplau gave birth to five children, and would later foster a sixth child.
5. These facts are recorded by Christian Prill's grandson, Gustav Prill (Hildegard Peplau's mother's cousin), in "How Our Fathers Created A Homeland For Us" printed in 1938 in the *Volkskalender* and translated from the German by Ida Gordon in 1990, and then reproduced in a large genealogical study completed by Hildegard Peplau in 1992. This *Peplau Genealogy* is now deposited in the Peplau Collection in the Schlesinger Library.
6. Life for both Gustav Peplau and Ottylie Elgert in Europe had been traumatic. Neither would ever discuss life before meeting and marrying in America, but diligent work at the historical record by Hildegard Peplau, after her retirement from Rutgers, allow us to piece it together.
7. Interview, Hildegard Peplau, January 28, 1992, in Sherman Oaks, California.
8. *Peplau Genealogy*.
9. Document #70, *Peplau Genealogy*.
10. Marriage license in Box 2, #51, Peplau collection.
11. See Mortgage Book, Berks County, Pennsylvania, Mortgage 458, Mortgage Book Volume 221, 634. Soon after Ottylie died in 1944, Gustav conveyed the property to his son Harold, who apparently continued this somewhat haphazard business transaction for a few years. By 1949, however, Harold had decided "enough of this" and sought a regular mortgage with the Reading Trust Company, which had a difficult time deciding what was left to pay. So they negotiated a price. On June 29, 1949, a mortgage of $2,800 was recorded! Harold paid this off in November, 1953, and in May, 1960, sold the house to his young foster brother, John Forster and his wife, Dorothy, for $5,700.

12. As was the norm in those days, all the Peplau children were born at home with the help of a midwife, in this case Mrs. Felix Winterhalter.

13. This description of her mother is found in a story written by Hildegard Peplau located in Box 2, #50, in the Schlesinger collection.

14. Interview, Bertha Reppert, October 19, 1994, in Mechanicsburg, Pennsylvania.

15. Interview, Hildegard Peplau, January 28, 1992.

16. Interview, Hildegard Peplau, March 28, 1992, in Sherman Oaks.

17. Interview, Bertha Reppert, October 19, 1994.

18. Ibid.

19. Notes from an oral interview with Hildegard Peplau found in Box 2, #45, Peplau collection, Schlesinger Library.

20. Interview, Hildegard Peplau, April 22, 1992.

21. Interviews, Hildegard Peplau and Bertha Reppert, February/March 1994, in Jim Thorpe, Pennsylvania.

22. See Hildegard E. Peplau, *Cultural Conditioning and Growth: Some Factors in the Development of a Second-Generation Immigrant,* a final term project written at Bennington College in November, 1945, p. 3. Found in Box 2 in the Peplau collection at the Schlesinger Library.

23. See Hildegard E. Peplau, *Cultural Conditioning,* 3.

24. Interview, Hildegard Peplau, January 28, 1992.

25. In a highly provocative book Frank Sulloway suggests that across the centuries birth order is the best predictor of revolutionary creativity—that laterborns are much more likely to be free-thinking iconoclasts, to be the engines that drive history. He contends that birth order is predictive of behavior in religion, science, and politics, that "history is biography writ large" and that laterborns are consistently overrepresented among champions of social and conceptual change. Frank Sulloway, *Born to Rebel* (New York: Pantheon, 1996).

26. Walter Peplau eventually lied about his age and joined the army while still in high school. He took advantage of whatever courses were available in the army, and rose steadily through the ranks, concluding his career in Livorno, Italy, where he ran the port.

27. And it was not only her granddaughter who felt the impact of Grossmutter's disapproval. Her own seventh child, Emil, was slight of build and intelligence. In about 1927, when he was 26 years old, Emil suffered a stroke and was taken to St. Joseph's Hospital in Reading. When he was discharged, on a very hot day, his mother refused to send taxi fare. While dragging himself home, Emil had another stroke that left him paralyzed on one side. Since he could not work, Grossmutter kicked him out of her house. He wandered the streets of Reading for the rest of his life, one of its first homeless citizens. He died in 1951.

28. Interview, Hildegard Peplau, January 28, 1992.

29. These remembrances are taken from a typewritten biography, "Hildegard Peplau and Psychodynamic Nursing," 1964, no name, found in Box 2, #38, Peplau collection, Schlesinger Library.

30. David Brown, "Scientists and Flu Vaccines," *The Washington Post National Weekly Edition,* March 23–29, 1992.

31. This account is given in *Cultural Conditioning,* 3 (found in Box 2, #52).

32. Ibid.

33. These descriptions are found in notations on the back of photographs in the small photo album in Box 1, Peplau collection.

34. Just prior to the outbreak of the second World War, Ottylie's parents and other Germans who had homesteaded in what was then Poland, were rounded up by the Russians and marched on foot to Samara, near Kiev, on the Volga, where they

were to work as virtual serfs while in Russia for the duration of the war. The Russians feared these Germans would side with Germany as Germany and Russia approached war. The three daughters in the United States—Ottylie, Olga, and Amalia—did what they could in sending supplies and money to their parents and their families. It wasn't until near the end of World War II, in 1944, that the Elgerts made the trek back to Poland. They got only as far as Vienna, however. Ottylie's 84-year-old mother who had made the 350-mile trip, mostly in the rain, in a horse-drawn cart, finally announced she was "too tired to eat," went to bed, and died quietly in her sleep in Vienna on November 14, 1944. Recounted in the *Peplau Genealogy*.

35. Hildegard E. Peplau, an autobiographical term paper written for a psychology class at Bennington College in 1945, found in Box 7, #123, in the Schlesinger Library collection.

36. Interview, Hildegard Peplau, January 28, 1992, in Sherman Oaks.

37. Interview, Hildegard Peplau, January 30, 1992, in Sherman Oaks.

38. Hilda's younger sister, Bertha Reppert, experienced her home as a warm and supportive one. In contrast to Hildegard, her memories are longingly nostalgic. Interview, Bertha Reppert, October 19, 1994.

39. This account was found in a handwritten undated autobiography found by Anne Peplau in Hilda Peplau's closet after her death. This document is now in the Schlesinger collection.

40. Written correspondence, Hildegard Peplau to Barbara Callaway, March 14, 1993.

41. Interview, Hildegard Peplau, May 1994, in Newark, New Jersey.

42. Interview, Hildegard Peplau, March 14, 1992, in Sherman Oaks.

43. Interview, Bertha Reppert, October 19, 1999.

44. Unlike Hildegard, Bertha always knew she wanted to get married and have children. During World War II, she met a tall and extremely kind man, Byron Reppert. They were married on May 25, 1945 and began a family. After their four daughters were in school or away from home, Bertha allowed her mind and talents to soar. She was the proprietress of Rosemary House in Mechanicsburg (where Byron was the mayor during the 1970s), and became one of the best known herbalists in the United States, widely recognized as a leader in her field. "I've had a good life. I have no regrets. Not one." (Interview, Bertha Reppert, February/March 1994, in Jim Thorpe, Pennsylvania). Bertha Reppert died shortly after her sister, Hilda, on June 8, 1999. She had written eight books and hundreds of articles, and gave renowned and memorable gardening talks around the country. Bertha Reppert's name has become synonymous with herbs to the people attracted to their study, and there is now a memorial to her in the National Herb Garden in the United States Arboretum in Washington, D.C.

45. According to Peplau's handwritten and undated autobiography (cited above), Betty Kreiger's mother had died when she was 8 years old, and "Pop" Kreiger was raising his daughters as a single parent when Hilda lived with Betty and Natalie.

46. Written correspondence, Hildegard Peplau to Barbara Callaway, July 29, 1995.

47. Interview, Hildegard Peplau, April 22, 1992, in Sherman Oaks.

48. Peplau Papers, Schlesinger Library, Carton One, little photo album.

49. Interview, Hildegard Peplau, April 22, 1992.

50. This place mat is found in Box 2 of the Schlesinger Library collection. Throughout the archival collection astrological observations, clipped through the years from magazines and newspapers, are inserted.

51. Interview, Hildegard Peplau, January 22, 1992, in Sherman Oaks.

52. Ibid.

53. Bertha Reppert, untitled remembrances, Spring 1987.

54. Bertha Reppert, 1987.

Becoming a Nurse

2

I have no regrets about Pottstown Hospital Training School, none whatsoever. It provided the entre to my field, the work was challenging, it was right for me at the time.

—Hildegard Peplau
January 28, 1992

Hildegard Peplau arrived at the Pottstown Hospital Training School (PHTS) on a Sunday, the 1st of September 1928. It was her 19th birthday. Pottstown was just 20 miles from Reading, down Highway 100; but it *was* out of Reading, and that was good enough for Hilda. The Borough of Pottstown was named after its founder, John Potts, a wealthy Quaker ironmaster and associate of William Penn. The town was smaller than Reading, but it was equally attractive with its red brick houses and lovely town square. The Hill School, an exclusive private academy, located just down the street from Pottstown Hospital, lent a graceful dignity to the town.

Hilda was met by a member of the staff and shown to her room in the nurses' home, a pleasant red brick building set back from the road, a few hundred yards from the hospital. Treading fearfully, not quite knowing what to expect, Hilda walked hesitantly up the stairs and into the beginning of a new life, one that would give her independence, a career, and recognition beyond anything she could have imagined. It never occurred to her then that she might go on to college, let alone become an honored professor and nationally recognized leader in the field of psychiatric nursing. Hilda knew only that when it came to making career choices, there were few options for women of the working class. Nursing was hard, physical work, but it seemed a reasonable, if not the only, choice for her. Hilda was content to pursue it.

She was very pleased with the room assigned to her in the nurses' home. It was a corner room with windows on two sides. After unpacking and getting acquainted with one another, the seven new Pottstown Hospital Training School students met for dinner that first Sunday evening with Superintendent Pearl Edith Parker. Miss Parker advised them to get their rest because their days as students would begin early. They were told to report to the front steps of the hospital at 6:30 in the morning to join the other student nurses for the daily hymn singing. It was a cold September morning when they gathered for the first time on the steps of the hospital, facing Miss Parker, and earnestly singing "Rock of Ages, Cleft for Me," and "Holy, Holy, Holy, Glory Be to Thee." The hymns were the wake-up call for the patients, but new patients sometimes asked if the Salvation Army always came that early in the m orning.[1]

POTTSTOWN HOSPITAL TRAINING SCHOOL

That first day the anesthesiologist, Mrs. Irene Oberholzer, took the new students upstairs to a private room and put seven chairs around a bed. On the bed were mounds of cotton. Hilda's first assignment at Pottstown Hospital Training School (PHTS) was to learn how to make cotton balls. (You pinch some off the mound, add a little water, mold the ball, and put it in a pillowcase.) Every day for 2 weeks, all day long, this was the assignment. While sitting around the bed making cotton balls, the students were not allowed to speak; but they managed to communicate using gestures and body language. After cotton ball making, the students went on to bed-making, then on to bathing patients. When these basics had been mastered, the students began rotating on and off the floors, and in and out of the units. A week on the medical ward was followed by a week on the pediatric ward, then the surgical ward. On these wards, they learned to scour bedpans; scrub floors; clean the rooms using Lysol, brushes, and mops; and organize the utility room, putting everything in its place. Training was not only hard work, it was also strict. Students were not allowed to speak to either the patients or the doctors; they could respond only if spoken to.

The daily routine did not often vary. After morning hymns, it was upstairs for the large breakfasts prepared by staff under the direction of Elizabeth Bick, the dietician. Miss Bick made sure there was plenty of food, all of it fresh. At 5 feet 10 inches, Hilda was still model-slender, and, as in Reading, there was much concern that she was too thin. She was given diet supplements, such as Blaud's Pills and green elixir pills, and permitted second helpings of French toast, eggs, juice, bacon, homemade Pennsylvania Dutch sausage, or scrapple. Still she did not gain weight. Then, to work. Scrub the floors, change the sheets, wash the patients, wash and sterilize the bedpans and return them to the patients, wash the sheets, take the temperatures, observe and record notes for the doctors.

Insofar as hospital staff nursing scarcely existed in the late 1920s and early 1930s, student nurses constituted a vital labor force. For the students, it was a very long and hard day.

In this period, a nurse-training school aimed to be a total institution. Student nurses lived, studied, and worked in the hospital. Nurse training reflected the social assumptions and power relationships that characterized the times. In training, the emphasis was on womanly demeanor, submission to authority, and practical, hard labor. Absolute cleanliness, in the tradition of the Florence Nightingale model for nursing, was the standard for performance. Ward work superseded every other pedagogic goal. The labor demands of the hospital, rather than the educational needs of the young women entering nursing, were the driving force. Rigid and paternalistic discipline shaped every aspect of the students' day. Few, including Hildegard Peplau, challenged the structured subordination within which students' manual work was performed. Training was essentially 2 years of hard work, plus a third year on staff under supervision, after which a diploma would be granted. What the hospital offered the students was on-the-job training. In most respects, then, nurse training was an apprenticeship. Most physicians believed nurses were not capable of assimilating complex material, certainly nothing more than basic anatomy or physiology.[2] Nurse training emphasized character and internal discipline and ignored the problematic relationship between those attributes and intellect.

Classes at PHTS generally were conducted in the late afternoons, and the students were tired after a full day's work on the wards. The physicians lectured, the students listened. No questions were allowed, nor was there discussion. To ensure that the students did not bother the instructors with silly questions, a supervisor always sat in. Lectures varied from 1 to 2 hours each and covered elementary anatomy, physiology, disease processes, and operating room techniques. In the second year there were 1-hour lectures on communicable diseases such as scarlet fever, diphtheria, syphilis, and tuberculosis, and on medical/surgical procedures. When they could be fitted in, there would be lectures in chemistry and biology given by teachers from the Hill School. For the convenience of these visiting lecturers, or of the physicians, a few classes were held in the afternoon. In this event, second-year students often had to do a double shift in order to release their upper or lower classmates to go to class. Hilda never minded that. The only break from the routine was that the students were allowed to observe operations and other procedures when they were off duty, provided they stayed to clean up the dirty linen.

Hilda's first-year class at PHTS numbered only 7 students, but the two classes ahead of hers were a little larger, providing a fairly substantial work force of some 30 student nurses for the 60-bed hospital. The students worked, in effect, for room and board. In addition, they were given

$5 a month for incidental expenses in their first year and $10 a month in their second year. In their third year, students were put in charge of a ward, or a floor, or the kitchen, or the operating room, and were to be paid $20 a month. Hilda Peplau, not surprisingly, was made operating room supervisor in her last year at Pottstown, but this was 1931, in the depth of the Great Depression. That year Hilda and the other members of her class would work without compensation.

At Pottstown, Pearl Edith Parker wore every hat. She was the hospital superintendent as well as the director of the training school. Pictures at the time show an attractive, tall, impeccably dressed woman whom Hilda remembered fondly as "absolutely fair," about as high a compliment as she could give.[3] Insofar as the hospital nursing service was, for all practical purposes, the student nurse corps, the jobs of hospital superintendent and director of the nurse training school were intricately connected.

Most of the teaching at Pottstown was done by physicians, offering a watered-down version of entry-level medical courses. In the absence of a medical training program in the hospital, however, the doctors tended to treat student nurses as though they were physician's assistants. For Hilda, this opportunity more than compensated for the dreary work on the wards that was the students' primary responsibility. It provided what she considered to be excellent training, as well as a good education for her chosen field. She helped deliver babies, assisted in common surgical operations, and participated in the setting of fractures. Ever curious, very serious, and genuinely intellectually alert, she sought access whenever possible to the physicians' lounge and its small library of medical texts, seeking answers to questions. The physicians seldom used their library so it was hers alone. There were only 25 to 30 books in the lone bookcase, and she read them all.

AN UNUSUAL STUDENT

In the first 2 years, students learned by rote everything they were required to know. Every activity was thoroughly supervised to ensure that exact procedures were followed. Unlike her peers, Hilda did nothing by rote. She always wanted to understand the why of things. Thus she began to think conceptually, to try out hypotheses, to search for knowledge. Although she learned much, she could not find answers to all her questions in the books she found in the physicians' library. Why did some patients mend quickly and others not, when there seemed to be little medical reason for this to be so? Why were some of the sickest the most optimistic, and why were some of the least medically ill the most difficult? Why did appendixes burst? Why did hearts stop? Why were so many of the female patients so clearly depressed, particularly after the birth of a child? Why could the nurses not talk to the doctors, and vice versa? Such curiosity was not encouraged in 1928.[4] As she cleaned and scrubbed and tended to her patients, Hilda was full of observations and questions, but there was no one with whom she could discuss them. Her fellow students were not curious in the way that she was and teased her for spending most of what little spare time the hard schedule afforded in the physicians' library.

The nurse instructors, similarly, were not comfortable around the assertive and bright Hilda Peplau. Her intense curiosity and quest for knowledge made them uncomfortable. Mrs. McElfatrick, one of the instructors, was, like Hilda's mother, always looking for something wrong in her behavior in order that she might be reprimanded.[5] Pearl Edith Parker, however, recognized and encouraged her intelligence. Hilda treasured an elaborately carved ashtray, a souvenir of a trip that Miss Parker and Miss Bick made to Egypt. This memento symbolized for Hilda the possibilities—opportunities far beyond marriage and a life in Reading—that could open up to an independent woman with a career of her own.

In those days, there were no residents or interns at a hospital as small as that at Pottstown. In the summer, sons of physicians on staff, pre-med students home from college for the summer, sometimes appeared to "play doctor." Because nursing students had more direct experience with patients, the intervention of these summertime "interns" sometimes caused tension. Hilda took advantage of the situation, however, to engage the medical students in discussions of patient illnesses. At PHTS, as in most nurse-training programs, there was often a fatherly physician who took particular interest in the nurses' training. In Pottstown, it was "Daddy Bushong," memorable to Hilda because he talked baby talk to her. At the time, she had no objection. How that would change in the years ahead! During these years, though, baby talk was illustrative of the relationship between doctors and nurses.

There were, however, two other men on the medical staff who were so impressed with the inquisitive young student nurse that they offered to send her to medical school, telling her that she was too bright to be "just a nurse." Hilda declined. She was sure she liked what nurses did, and not at all sure she liked what she saw of what doctors did. To her mind, it was the nurses who actually took care of patients, who were directly involved in helping sick people get well. And, in fact, it was the daily care by nurses that saved many lives. Doctors were experienced diagnosticians, but actual medical practice was limited at this time to the skill of the surgeon's hand and the pharmacopoeia available to the general physician. The great advances in drugs, vaccines, and medical technologies were yet to come.

In her second year, Hilda found an affirmation of her intuitive sense of the critical role that a relationship between nurse and patient—forbidden in the catechism of the training school—might play in the healing process. Instructed not to ask questions of the physicians, Hilda nonetheless decided on her own that one might be allowed to speak to a lecturer who was not a physician. Thus, when an instructor from the Hill School came to lecture, she asked what was the most important thing a nurse could do for a patient. He replied, "Sit at the bedside, listen to the patient, and try to understand the patient." This was to be immensely important advice, advice around which she would later build her reputation as a pioneer in the field of psychiatric nursing. "I never forgot that. That was something we *never* did at Pottstown," she stated.[6]

In 1928 psychiatric nursing was not a typical part of the curriculum in nurse-training programs. If it was offered at all, there was usually only one lecture on the subject. But in Hilda's second year something extraordinary happened. Several of the student nurses were offered a 4-day "course" at the Norristown State Hospital in eastern Pennsylvania. Dr. Arthur Noyes, the chief psychiatrist, whom Peplau identified as "a great friend of nursing," made the arrangement and accepted full responsibility for the students' safety. The five students electing this rotation were sent to the hospital in a limousine. Dr. Noyes did the teaching himself and there was no nurse supervisor present. Unlike other physicians and in violation of the rules of the hospital and its nurse-training school, Noyes went out of his way to encourage questions. Hilda asked plenty.[7] What causes this? What do you know about that? Dr. Noyes engaged her in conversation and encouraged her independent thinking. That openness to inquiry, so out of the ordinary in that time and place, suggested to her that psychiatric nursing might allow for greater flexibility and more opportunity for innovation than other areas of nursing. She could not have known then that her own future would be to develop the field of psychiatric nursing. It was while at Norristown that Hilda understood for the first time the circumstances of her Uncle Emil's condition. Emil, Hilda's grandmother's seventh child, had suffered what was said to have been a series of strokes and subsequently had been expelled by Grossmutter from her home in Reading because he could not work. Hilda had befriended the homeless young man and helped him with food and money when she worked at Eaches Coal. She now realized that Emil clearly suffered from brain damage. She began to comprehend that such damage could be caused by repeated beatings around the head, something of which Grossmutter was almost certainly guilty.[8]

Although the religious influence was strong at PHTS, as evidenced by the singing of hymns in the morning, Sunday was a free day. Church was not required, and on Sundays Hilda's class often went out to classmate Pat Allen's farm. Pat's father loved having the nurses visit. With him they watched the birthing of calves and goats and learned where the country stills and speakeasies were—these were the days of Prohibition.[9] Hilda in her third year became a tutor to Pat Allen and other students, and was at times frustrated that her classmates, most of whom, like Pat, had been raised on farms, used colloquial rather than scientific terms when describing patients' problems. For instance, Pat would say a patient "yorked" or "pitched up his lunch." In the interest of helping her to graduate, Hilda suggested she use the correct scientific term: patient emesis. Pat looked Hilda straight in the eye and said, "You think you're so smart, I'll bet you don't know the difference between a pitch fork and a hay fork." She was right. It was a lesson in humility Hilda would not forget.

Other than the unusual Norristown rotation and trips to the Allen farm, there were a few other additions to the normal curriculum. The hospital had a silver tea service, and before they graduated all the students learned the proper way to serve tea. It was unlikely any of them would ever own such a service, but Pearl Edith Parker felt it an important skill to acquire. Once they completed training, most of the student nurses would be employed in private-duty nursing, and in private duty they very likely would need to know what to do with a tea service. A few years later, when doing private-duty nursing in wealthy homes, Hilda would discover that it was indeed an advantage to have had this experience.[10]

In her last year at PHTS, while serving as operating room supervisor, an event occurred that again underscored Peplau's determination to become master of her own fate. A patient with a ruptured kidney came into the emergency room after a terrible accident. His condition was beyond the capability of the local surgeons, so a doctor was called in from Philadelphia. In anticipation of the arrival of this specialist, Hilda had carefully set up the operating room, placing all the equipment exactly where she thought it should be. She had found time to go to the library to look at the physiology books and conceptualize how the operation would proceed. The specialist arrived, and as he was scrubbing up Mrs. Oberholzer, the anesthesiologist, whisked into the room and turned the patient around, thus reversing the position of the patient in relation to Hilda's arrangement of the instruments. When the doctor came in, he went into a rage which continued as he operated, all the while throwing things, including bloody sponges, around the room. Hilda understood his anger. She too was doing a slow boil, and wished she could throw things, specifically at Mrs. Oberholzer. When the doctor left, Hilda turned on her superior, demanding to know why she did not speak up and take responsibility for her action. Why would she let the doctor think that it was the nurse, Hildegard Peplau, who had caused the disarray? Mrs. Oberholzer told her to mind her place, adding that the physician was simply difficult. Right then Hilda resolved she would someday be responsible only for her own mistakes and that as soon as she could she would find a job in New York City and leave not only Reading but also Pottstown behind her.

While Hilda experienced frustration with what she perceived to be the ineptitude of others (as she would throughout her career), at PHTS she also found satisfaction in her talent for teaching. In addition to supervising the operating room, Hilda found time to tutor two of her classmates who had done poorly and flunked the operating room rotation. They were sent to Hilda by the superintendent because of her demonstrated skill in the operating room. Her first students! Not surprisingly, after a few months of tutoring they passed their operating room rotation with flying colors and soon became RNs. Then several other student nurses who couldn't graduate were sent to Hilda for tutoring. She had enormous patience, and managed to get them all through. In later years, she would discover how very limited many of her classmates actually were. Unlike Hilda, they did not move to nursing's higher echelons and were somewhat in awe of Peplau's career. She never lost touch with them, however, always sending appropriate notes whenever she had news of their lives. Student nurses, of course, conspired to escape the ever vigilant supervisors to win moments of release from the endless toil, and in this Hilda and her peers were often successful. The resulting shared memories of hard-times-survived led to an allegiance to schools and classmates that lasted a lifetime.

The work had been hard, and the education limited, as was most nursing education at the time. Hilda, however, had no regrets about Pottstown Hospital Training School. Throughout her career, Peplau would be available to PHTS for whatever she could give. She returned whenever invited to conduct workshops, to consult, or to give graduation speeches. Pottstown was perhaps smaller than many programs and thus more limited in its offerings, but such small programs certainly were not unusual. Upon graduation each new nurse was given a sterling silver pin—Hilda's first piece of jewelry. Years later she would donate this pin to an American Nurses Association auction, at which it brought an "outlandish" sum of money.[11]

FLORENCE NIGHTINGALE AND AMERICAN NURSING

American nursing was greatly influenced by the ideas of Florence Nightingale and the theories of sanitary nursing and care of the injured she introduced to the world during the mid-19th century Crimean War.[12] Nightingale's work and the principles she introduced in the nursing school she founded became a model for American nursing education in the late 19th and early 20th centuries. Florence Nightingale was named for Florence, Italy, where she was born in 1820, the daughter of wealthy British parents who were then living abroad. She was raised on the two family estates in England, and tutored at home in Greek, Latin, mathematics, and philosophy by her Cambridge-educated father, William Nightingale. As a young woman, she was described as elegant and graceful, and deeply spiritual. At age 17, she heard a call from God and began to visit the sick in hospitals. Without the blessing of her parents who forbade her to work in English hospitals, she enrolled in a 3-month nursing course at the Institute for Protestant Deaconesses in Kaiserswerth, Germany, and later traveled in Europe studying methods of nursing. In August 1853, she was appointed superintendent of the Establishment for Gentlewomen, a women's hospital on Harley Street in London.

In 1854, Britain and France declared war on Russia in the Crimea. Conditions for British soldiers wounded in the Crimean War were deplorable and were widely reported in the British press. As a result, Secretary of War Sidney Herbert asked Miss Nightingale to supervise the introduction of female nurses into the military hospital in Turkey. She accepted the challenge and sailed for Scutari with a band of 38 nurses. There she immediately began to apply the principles of "sanitary science" she had learned in Europe to the makeshift hospital at Scutari, which was housed in an old Turkish barracks and was without medical supplies, cots, or bandages. While improving the hygiene, and urgently petitioning the British military officials for food and supplies, she reorganized the wards and established a laundry and kitchens. Within a month the mortality rates began to decline. By the end of the war, Florence Nightingale had become a legend in England. With the testimonial fund collected for her war services, in 1860 she established the Nightingale School and Home, a training school for nurses at St. Thomas Hospital in London. She was called the "Lady with a Lamp" by British soldiers when she walked the halls of their hospital at night. The lamp became a symbol of her belief that a nurse's care was never ceasing, night or day.

The whole notion of the trained nurse, with her stress on sanitary methods, as well as orderly and efficient administration of the hospital wards, originated with Florence Nightingale. Even hospital design, with pavilion wards joined by corridors, good ventilation, and limited density, is traced to Nightingale. Her ideas and example led nurse-training schools to stress the connection of good health to good care and a clean environment. Nightingale saw the world in terms of polarities: purity as opposed to filth, order versus disorder, health versus disease. In her own training, the focus on cleanliness was something Hilda Peplau could relate to. Her mother's house had been spotless and was cleaned relentlessly. Thus, when Hilda cleaned a room, she cleaned *everything*. She remembered well cleaning, waxing, and polishing until rooms at Pottstown Hospital gleamed. She even commandeered the hospital's ladder in order to clean the ceiling lights.

While Nightingale's contribution to the organization of the hospital and to an appreciation of the importance of good nursing care to patient health goes without question, her incorporation of prevailing Victorian attitudes toward gender, class, and human nature does not.[13] Her own high social class and extraordinary energy influenced the nature and structure of nursing for nearly a century. In the Nightingale tradition, acceptance of crippling paternalism, abnegation of self, and the belief that nurses are of a higher moral order because they possess idealized feminine attributes gave nursing a new legitimacy and thus allowed women of "good background" to enter the field.[14] This emphasis on the presumed attributes of femininity—good housekeeping, care for the sick, and respect for male authority—were bonded to Nightingale's advanced theories of hygienic nursing care and thus became deeply embedded in the nurse-training environment. This convenient conjunction between dominant beliefs about femininity and attitudes toward the practice of nursing would hinder the development of nursing as a profession for many decades.

At the time Peplau entered nurse training, a very few national nursing leaders were demanding increased attention to classroom work, decreased hours on hospital wards, an expanded curriculum, and the certification of hospital schools. The changes they advocated would be a long time in coming. (It was not until 1952 that both theory and clinical experience would be required for all nursing students, as a result of a resolution promoted by Hildegard Peplau and adopted by the National League for Nurses.) Recent nurse historians construe the attitudes rooted in the Nightingale tradition not as the moral basis for the nursing profession but as constraints that long limited nursing's professional aspirations.[15] It was this tradition that Hildegard Peplau would challenge.

WOMEN'S WORK

As Peplau would eventually understand, nurse-training schools in the early part of the 20th century offered women qualifications for a *job*. They did not provide entry into a *profession* requiring specialized knowledge and advanced study in a professional school. Hospitals needed a workforce, and nurse-training schools provided it. If she were truly bright, an occasional student nurse might be encouraged to pursue a medical career. Peplau was one of these, but she had no such aspirations. She already intuitively understood that nursing and medicine were separate occupations, with different and separate missions, and therefore requiring separate knowledge bases in meeting the health needs of people. There was no uncertainty in her own identification with nursing as a profession, rather than a job, and throughout her career she would seek to push nursing's growth to its full potential.

As the daughter of immigrant parents, Hilda was not atypical of young women entering nursing in the early part of the 20th century. Certainly the nursing profession grew in response to the needs of the more than 25 million immigrants who entered the country between 1870 and 1921. Professional nursing's birth, with the establishment of three hospital training programs in 1873, occurred in part as a result of the influx of immigrants. City hospitals in Boston, New Haven, and New York established nursing programs to train a workforce of women to care for patients in crowded wards, most of them immigrants. As the European-born population of cities and towns increased, new municipal and private hospitals appeared. Of the almost 2,000 general hospitals in 1904, many were designed to care for specific religious and cultural groups. Catholic, Protestant, Jewish, Polish, German, and Swedish communities established hospitals to care for their own;[16] and it was from these immigrant communities that many young women entered nursing.

It was not yet the age of medicine, so most of the drugs available were those to be found in the old-fashioned apothecary shops. The apothecary shop sold vegetable and flower seeds, farm and garden equipment, dental equipment, false teeth, and window glass along with Seidlitz powders, elixirs, and tinctures. The late 19th century was a time of few doctors, no general anesthetics or antibiotics, and no prescription medicines as we know them today. Early remedies were made from roots, seeds, barks, and minerals. Medicines were not standardized, and each immigrant group had its own folk remedies for most illnesses. Patients went to hospitals to die. After the turn of the century, hospitals began to be seen by more middle-class patrons as places of care and healing rather than the last stop in the life of indigents.[17] Growing urbanization meant fewer people were able to provide full-time care for the sick in their family homes, and advances in medicine meant that people actually could get well in hospitals. The need for hospital nursing staffs grew accordingly, and the young women of immigrant families provided a pool of willing labor.

Nursing education, too, was directly and powerfully influenced by the large number of immigrant women entering its ranks. Although U.S. immigration laws in the 1920s drastically curtailed the influx of immigrants, the influence of their members on nursing practice and education would be felt for decades to come. In fact, three of the most important figures in early nursing history in this country were of immigrant origin and came to the United States by way of Canada: Isabel Hampton, superintendent of the Johns Hopkins School of Nursing; Adelaide Nutting, director of the Division of Nursing Education at Columbia University's Teachers College and America's first professor of nursing; and Isabel Stewart, successor to Miss Nutting. All were early leaders in the effort to move nursing from a vocation to a profession.

Nurses are essential to the smooth functioning of the health care system, but historically they have not been held in high regard. Nursing is the most female of professions: In the collective imagination every nurse is a woman and every woman can take care of the sick. The image of the nurse in the popular imagination is that of the mother-nurturer. To be a successful nurse, it was thought, one simply had to enlarge upon God-given female characteristics. Nurses were self-sacrificing, dutiful, warm, caring—the ultimate mother figures. They were helpmates to doctors, they fended off disorder, disaster, and chaos in the hospital wards, just as they did in the perfect imagined home. Reflecting the Nightingale tradition, most nursing schools, like Pottstown Hospital Training School, emphasized moral rectitude, order, cleanliness, proper diet, and deference to, and respect for, authority, be that to the nursing superintendent or the attending physician, who almost always was a man.[18] While nurses were popularly characterized as responding to a higher calling in keeping with their natural maternal natures, in fact, at the turn of the century nursing provided low-paid, low-status jobs for the daughters of the new immigrant working class in America. Few middle- or upper-class women went into nursing. The 12-hour days tending to the patients' physical needs and the heavy domestic work on the wards had little appeal to them. Conversely, many poor and working-class women, seeking to escape the confines of their class, chose nursing as a means to better their station in life. To achieve this, they were willing to endure the paternalism and regimentation of the typical hospital training school.[19] In this Hildegard Peplau was no exception.

In the 1930s, when nursing leaders began the long struggle to move beyond hospital diploma schools and elevate nursing education to the college level, they encountered strong opposition from hospital administrators and physicians. Nursing reform was particularly threatening to community hospitals with fragile budgets dependent on cheap student labor. Upgrading nursing curricula clashed with hospitals' labor requirements.[20] If students were in the classroom they were not available to make beds, empty bedpans, or clean the floors. Moreover, it was believed that most nursing skills could and should be learned at the bedside, not in the classroom.

As nursing leaders increasingly saw the need to sever the link between hospital work and nursing education, they developed strategies to upgrade training through an academic curriculum, the development of national standards and licensure, and a movement away from hospital and physician domination. The women in the ranks themselves, however, felt threatened by change. Hence, education was resisted, not only by small hospitals and the medical establishment but also by trained nurses. Hospitals and physicians were able to unite the fears of nursing's ranks with the self-interest of its hospital nursing administrators to frustrate the efforts of nursing's educational leaders.[21] There was no need to upset the status quo, it was claimed. Physicians cared for their patients, and nurses helped. This was important work and both physicians and nursing staff demanded "respect" for the relationship. Feminism and conscious-ness-raising about the disadvantages of carrying traditional gender roles into the workplace would develop later, and in response to different issues. The effort to upgrade standards for nursing education, together with and linked to the struggle to move nursing from the ranks of a voca-tion to those of a profession would become constant themes in Peplau's career. It was a battle to which she would devote a major part of her tal-ents and energies, and it was a battle that she could not win.

Nurse's training, unlike college education, discouraged rather than encouraged independent thinking. It would take an extraordinarily strong will, such as that possessed by Hildegard Peplau, to resist the pressure to conform. The effect of nurses' training was to stifle initiative and discour-age change while reinforcing ritualistic behavior.[22] It is not surprising that later feminist messages concerning autonomy and gender roles were lost on nurses, for, as one of American nursing's early founders stated, "implicit unquestioning obedience must be the foundation of the nurse's work."[23] With this kind of thinking ingrained in the overwhelming majority of the country's nurses early in the 20th century, it could be pre-dicted that Peplau and other reformers would have a hard time.

There were two kinds of students in the early nurse-training programs. A small minority were middle-class women who desired an acceptable career outside the family. The vast majority, however, needed the housing and the few dollars in income that came with nurse-training programs. There was no way Hilda Peplau, for instance, could have comfortably left her home in Reading if she had had to support herself completely. Her options were few. The future nurse contributed her labor as the cost of entering a credentialed vocation that would give her a foundation for independent living. Hilda, like her classmates, understood implicitly that after 3 years of exhausting "training" and work, there was the potential for a lifetime of respectable self-employment. For this and other reasons, nursing was overwhelmingly a single women's profession. In 1928, a demo-graphically disproportionate majority of students in the nurse-training schools came from small towns, rural areas, and farms where, for large families of moderate means, hard physical labor for small reward was expected. For such women, the opportunity to get off the farm and go to a training school without a need to lay out much money was very attrac-tive.[24] For the first 50 years of the 20th century, the majority of nurses were native-born, White, working-class women.[25] Until the 1930s, the average age of a trainee was 23, suggesting a few years at home helping to support their families before setting out for nurse training. Educational prerequisites were lax. In the 1930s, 25% of all nurses had 1 year, or less, of high school.[26] It was not until after Peplau's retirement in 1974 that a majority of nursing's new recruits would be urban-born, middle-class, and married.[27]

Although the overwhelming majority of nursing students, even at the most selective schools, were not of middle-class origin until mid-century, there was a small minority of solidly middle-class young women attracted to the profession. These women, such as Pearl Edith Parker and Elizabeth Bick in the case of the Pottstown Hospital Training School, became supervisors and administrators. Thus, a de facto two-track system came into existence in which the less educated or less ambitious were consigned to hospital work and private duty, and the better prepared and more ambitious advanced to administrative positions. In this respect, nursing offered one of the few executive careers open to women. As an occupation, however, nursing remained in an ambiguous status. It was women's work in a field dominated by male physicians, and as such represented subordinate labor. As women's work, nursing was expected to demand self-sacrifice and self-denial. As work for a woman in the first half of the century, however, nursing provided independence and mobility, freedom, comfort, and self-worth.

HOSPITALS AND THE NURSE'S ROLE

The advent of the modern hospital itself reinforced the traditional system of nurse training and, until World War II, militated against the heightened educational standards advocated by the nurse reformers. By the end of the 1920s, the hospital had assumed its basic shape and had to a large extent replaced the family home as the place to treat illness and manage death. Physicians were an even more dominant force as care for critically ill patients was moved out of the home and into the hospital. The hospital became central to every aspect of medicine, and physicians became tightly organized, uniformly trained, and systematically licensed. The system of interns and residents served to reinforce the hospital experience as an accepted part of medical training. The experience of the doctor-in-training, though, was very different from that of the hospital-trained nurse. During the Great Depression many families could no longer afford private nursing in their homes and the sick were of necessity sent to hospitals. Consequently, nurses who formerly worked in private homes were pushed into hospital staff duty. The hospital staff was organized in a fashion that implied the accepted division of authority between hospital boards and physicians, on the one hand, and employees, primarily nurses and attendants, on the other. The nurses, who were not professional in the sense that we understand the term today—that is, were not the products of advanced degrees given by accredited professional schools—represented social stratum and social experience very different from that of the lay trustees and physicians who essentially controlled the institution. The unquestioning acceptance of paternalism was assumed, just as it had always been.

The hospital nurse-training schools continued to perpetuate gender attitudes that included the belief that men did not have the right instincts for nursing and that women's innate sympathies brought warmth and reassurance to patients, just as their domestic instincts brought cleanliness and order to the ward. These stereotypical beliefs were further reinforced by the dominant evangelisms of the day that stressed that lives were not to be wasted but rather dedicated to morally appropriate vocations. For women, such vocations were, first, wife and mother, then teacher and nurse. An appropriate vocation was particularly important to that minority of women who sought acceptable activity outside the home.[28] Such a paternalistic belief system gave hospital trustees hope for a stable, relatively inexpensive labor force imbued with the moral attitudes and understanding of responsibility that would lead to lowered mortality rates and hence increased hospital utilization and greater profits. This package of convenience and belief enhanced public support for hospital-based nurse training. The system did lead to the justification of a more or less autonomous female role in the hospital, one that wedded intuitive moral capacity, intellect, and piety to efficiency and cleanliness.[29] The belief that nursing was particularly suited for women and key to controlling hospital internal order and patient care, however, remained inconsistent with fostering professional aspirations for nurses. Although early on a cause for Hildegard Peplau, it would be a long time before most rank-and-file nurses understood this contradiction.

After World War II, hospitals themselves became more interesting. As the health care system changed and hospitals could recoup the cost of nursing from insurance companies, the opposition to more and better education for nurses began to dissipate. The postwar hospital grew out of the complex interaction between technological innovation, changing social attitudes, and demographic and economic change. Following World War II, most physicians and even hospital boards conceded that the tremendous increase in medical knowledge demanded parallel upgrading in nursing education. By then, the beginnings of specialization in nursing itself were discernible, as advanced skills became more important in the operating room and in public health, as well as on the floors of the hospital. Even with that, the status of the trained nurse reflected but could not rival the growing influence of a male-dominated medical profession. The central emphasis of "trained" nursing remained its relentless focus on discipline and efficiency, paralleling medicine's newly scientific self-image. Nursing administration added a layer to hospital management, but this enhanced rather than undermined the growing power of scientific medicine and provided additional allies for those within nursing who proposed reforms.

PRIVATE DUTY

Well into the 1930s new nurses entered private duty after completing
training school, unlike physicians who, when they completed medical
school, entered private practice. The terminology alone—private *duty* versus private *practice*—reveals something of the respective roles of nurse
and doctor and the relationship of each to the patient. Upon completing
their training, new nurses took a state examination to be licensed as registered nurses (RNs). Generally, new RNs waited for private cases, visiting and leaving cards at doctors' offices, or registering with directories or
registries, significantly called "services." In service to wealthy patients
who employed them on a private basis, nurses were relatively well paid
compared to other women workers. After World War I, as middle- and
upper-class patients entered hospitals, they brought their private-duty
nurses in with them as "specials." Specials worked for the patient. They
earned income in the hospital but were not employed by the hospital.
Graduates of the hospital training schools were referred to as "graduate
nurses," and until the mid-1940s "graduate" nursing was, for all practical
purposes, private-duty nursing. Hospitals were staffed by student nurses. Senior students were the head nurses and entering students were the
ward nurses. In the senior, or third, year of training, there was an informal arrangement between the students and the doctors. If she did well,
the doctors more or less guaranteed the new nurse her first patient.
Hildegard Peplau had no worries in this regard, since it was clear the
physicians recognized her intelligence and diligence and were all too
willing to give her cases.

Peplau's first patient was the daughter of Dr. Paul Hanley, one of the
Pottstown Hospital physicians. The child was recovering from acute
appendicitis. The prescribed protocol was to wear a tight binder after
surgery, which this girl refused to do. Hilda's assignment was to sit by
her side to make sure the wound was clean. The child healed with no
trouble, and after 10 days Hilda was ready for her second case, a new
mother who had come down with acute migratory pneumonia in her
lungs. This case was more memorable. Peplau was to be on duty for 20
hours, then have 4 hours off to sleep. The first night she had just gone to
sleep when she was awakened by a scream. Peplau rushed into her
patient's room, and found the husband in effect raping the ill new mother. Peplau yanked him off the woman, ordering him to "Get the hell out
of here!" and pushed him from the room. She bathed the woman, whose
temperature had gone up to 106°, and called the doctor. The doctor
recommitted the woman to the hospital, but her spirit had been broken.
The patient did not respond to treatment. She was listless and despondent,
suffering from what is known today as postpartum depression. That,
together with her illness and the attack by an obviously brutal husband,

had robbed her of her desire to live. The doctor revived her by giving her shots of adrenalin, but she kept talking about how peaceful death seemed. The patient remained in the hospital and died there some weeks later. Although it was clear the patient did not want to live, Hilda took the loss personally. She felt there was no excuse for losing a young patient to pneumonia. She had yet to learn about depression and its devastating ability to rob one of the desire to live. This would be the only patient she ever lost.

These first cases were followed by a series of work-related cases for which the employers hired Hilda to care for their employees in the Pottstown hospital—a man badly burned in an accident at a steel mill, a man with a fractured pelvis, and a man with advanced tuberculosis. In each case, Peplau would spend several weeks with the patient in the hospital, and then go home with the patient to continue the 20-hour-a-day duty regimen. After this, several later cases stand out in her memory. One was the Jewish patient with whom she stayed for 4 months, living in his gracious home in Philadelphia with his family and learning a great deal about Jewish family life and culture. Their son would later drive Hilda to take her RN licensure test.[30]

By then, Hilda felt rich, for she'd saved almost all the money she'd earned. Hence, when that case was over, she could afford to buy herself a car, and she did—a used black Ford Roadster. With its chrome wire wheels, tire mounted on the running board, top down, and snazzy genuine leather rumble seat open, it was definitely a conversation-stopper in Reading. Hilda Peplau's roadster was the first car on Church Street, and it caused quite a stir. The automobile, one of the most coveted possessions of 1920s life, brought about vast changes in the United States, including the development of a national highway system; roadside restaurants, motels, and gas stations; and the nuisance of outdoor advertising. Offering mobility, freedom, and prestige, nearly 23 million cars were owned by Americans in 1929. Hilda's roadster provided her a new freedom and a definite urge for mobility. Once she had her little car she could run back and forth between cases. She was immensely popular during this period of her life, with a lively group of friends who knew all the clubs and nightspots. With the gang piled in the roadster, weekends were always fun. Bertha remembered well her older sister's first car:

> It was a Model A. It was a racy little number. It was stinking hot on Church Street in the summer . . . Hilda would come zooming into town and barreling down Church Street. She had the only car in sight! . . . All the kids would pile in and she'd take us all swimming. What a neat big sister![31]

Meanwhile, Hilda's private-duty practice continued to flourish. A newborn baby provided her with her first experience of the Philadelphia

Main Line, the fashionable suburb and center of Philadelphia society that grew up along the railroad's "main line" west of the city. The birth had gone fine, but the baby cried a lot, so the family requested that Nurse Hilda go home with them to help care for the infant. The prevailing wisdom at that time was to let the baby cry, but Peplau felt strongly that something was wrong, so she would pick up the crying baby, against the wishes of the imperious father. Hilda dared to argue with him, insisting that something more than temper was wrong with the baby, who continued to whimper even when held. After many days of this discussion, the family agreed to return to the hospital. The baby had a hernia, which was successfully operated upon. Returning to Pottstown, Peplau also worked with Dr. Bushong on a home delivery for a wealthy three-generation family all living together—parents, grandparents, and great-grandparents. It was important to the family that the new baby and male heir be born in the same bed as his grandfather and great grandfather. It was a low, wooden sleigh bed. Constantly bending over that bed was not easy. "It would have been easier to take this damn bed to the hospital," said Dr. Bushong. After the birth, the doctor left and the nurse stayed. The mother was not permitted to arise from her bed until after the baby was baptized, and that would not be for 2 weeks. On the appointed day, the Episcopal Bishop of Philadelphia arrived, and many items of symbolic value—such as salt, the family Bible, silver, and money—were placed in a basket with the baby. The entire entourage trekked to the highest point in the three-story house, a turret above the attic. At the appropriate time, a $1 gold coin was placed in the baby's hand, and Nurse Hilda was instructed to sit with her hand under the baby's fist until he released the coin, thus assuring that he would be generous. The tightfisted child took 2 hours to release the coin. Not until then was the mother allowed to get up. Except she couldn't. After so much bed rest, she was weak and unstable. Thus, Hilda stayed another month helping the mother to get back on her feet. At the end of the month, she was given the gold coin, which she kept for her lifetime.

Soon after this her friend Ann Kerr, a classmate at PHTS who had married a physician and moved to New York City, began to write to Hilda about how exciting the big city was. Ann assured her there were great opportunities for nurses in the city, and urged her to write to Grace Warman, the nurse superintendent at Mount Sinai Hospital. For Hilda, New York was the goal, but she could not see it as an immediate possibility. This would change, however, as events in her private life unfolded.

A PRIVATE LIFE, TOO

As she had been in high school, Hilda was popular during her years in nurse-training school and private-duty nursing. At first, she was particularly attracted to boys on motorcycles. She and her friend Peg Mlodoch were having quite a good time meeting boyfriends from Allbright Junior College in Reading who had motorcycles. It was "great good clean fun" to race up and down the hills and take the gently curving roads out in the countryside at high speed. One day word must have gotten back to Superintendent Parker at PHTS, because she posted a notice in the nurses' quarters stating, "Any student found on a motorcycle will be automatically dismissed."[32] Such activity did not fit with the image the hospital expected nurses to maintain.

There were many boyfriends, several of them serious. When she arrived at Pottstown, Hilda was officially engaged to Bill Bannon, who taught bookkeeping at the Reading Evening High School. Hilda's mother, Ottylie, had been delighted at the engagement, and was dismayed at Hilda's decision to go to Pottstown for nurses' training instead of getting married right away. Although she accepted Bill's ring and wore it, at least initially, in Pottstown, Hilda knew in her heart of hearts that she really did not want to get married. "I could see that I wasn't the marrying kind, I was a free spirit. I didn't see any happy marriages. My parents liked each other well enough, but I could see that they were really mismatched."[33] Marriage to her meant exactly what her mother told her it meant: "settling down, having children, serving your husband." Hilda, on the other hand, wanted to be off seeing the world, finding something useful and significant to do, never "settling down," and certainly not subjugating her interests and talents to someone else's demands. Thus, although engaged to Bill Bannon, she arrived in Pottstown knowing she had to give back the ring. He was a nice man, and she agonized for many weeks about how to explain how she felt so that he would not feel rejected but would understand that it was impossible. In the end, she decided that "It was nonsense to prolong the agony," so she wrote suggesting that he meet her at the train station in Reading. Bill arrived full of expectations and excitement about this uncharacteristic gesture on Hilda's part, and was dismayed beyond description when she handed him back the ring and explained that she simply "was not the marrying kind." The scene was so excruciating that Hilda jumped back on the next train without realizing that it was an express train that went straight through to Philadelphia without stopping in Pottstown. She got off in Philadelphia and made the return trip to Reading where she furtively waited for a train that would, in fact, take her to Pottstown. Bill Bannon continued to make the trip to Pottstown for many weeks in a vain attempt to change her mind.

Soon her social life was in full swing again. For Hilda this meant plenty of singing, dancing away the evening, and sharing cigarettes and whiskey every Saturday night with her friends from Reading. Her very close high school friend Betty Kreiger had married her high school sweetheart, Ted Price. After high school, Betty continued to sing in nightclubs and was very good at it and well known in the area. Ted played in a band. This was the tail end of the Roaring Twenties, and Betty and Ted were very popular. Hilda was included in their circle and was always meeting new men, many of whom were very interested in the tall, serious but fun-loving nurse-to-be. There were several more marriage proposals, and one taken seriously enough that she actually bought a dress and a hope chest. His name was Walter Wurster. She met him in 1930, and the next year, when it looked as though this might be serious, Hilda took Walter home to meet her parents. She arrived at the house on Church Street to find her mother in tears. There was no food in the house, and Hilda's 12-year-old sister Bertha and the baby, Johnny, were hungry.

Hilda discovered that her father, Gustav, like so many others in 1931, was unemployed. He had been laid off the job in the railroad yards that he had held for nearly 25 years. With the town out of work there were no housecleaning jobs for Ottylie, and no buyers for her baked goods, even had she the means to buy the flour, sugar, eggs, and lard that were her staples. On Black Thursday, October 24, 1929, the stock market had crashed, sending tremors from Wall Street to the West Coast. Reading was not spared. Gustav was sinking into a depression and his family was hungry. During this time, Hilda had been fully employed and blithely unaware of the impact of the depression on her family. She was appalled by the desperate circumstances in which she found them and felt she had no choice but to move home and to work out of Reading in order to provide for them. Her intended was not supportive, in part because Hilda had related to him the favoritism shown her older sister Clara and the resultant mistreatment that Hilda experienced during their childhood. Wurster urged her to walk away from her family, leave with him, get married, and forget her ties to Reading. This discussion led to a breakup, and Hilda moved back home for a period between 1931 and 1933, after accepting a position as the operating and emergency room nurse at the Pottstown Hospital in order to live and help out at home.

Ottylie was deeply grateful, and gained a new respect for her independent daughter. She kept Hilda's uniforms washed and ironed, kept her room immaculate, and of course cooked up a storm. In return, other than gas money to keep her car on the road, Hilda turned her wages over to her family. This time, in contrast to her teenage argument with her father about wages, Gustav did not have to ask.

One day that winter, at the end of a particularly long private-duty case, Hilda drove home to Reading. It was a extraordinarily cold night, and the road was a sheet of ice. The little roadster had no heater. On arriving, Hilda sat with her feet in the oven while Ottylie was uncharacteristically very solicitous—something Hilda would never forget. From this time onward, she began to think about the strains under which Ottylie had labored and to appreciate her enormous energy and creativity, all channeled into her housekeeping, canning, and cooking.

During this time, Clara was in Philadelphia, and Hilda did not inquire of her. While her mother was grateful for Hilda's help, her father found the state of affairs much more difficult to accept. He was withdrawn and angry. Hilda was already beginning to show her mental health clinical skills, as she invested in bags of concrete and put her father to work cementing the basement. Gustav's spirits lifted somewhat once he was busy, but his total dependence on his daughter for however short a time put a strain on their relationship from which it would not recover. After 3 months out of work, Gustav was called back to the yards for part-time work, but remained uncomfortable that he could not fully support his family.

A CAMP NURSE

During Peplau's second year at PHTS, a female physician had joined the staff. Dr. Alice Shepard came from a wealthy Pottstown family and her father taught at the Hill School. It is likely the generosity of the family to the school, and most probably to the hospital as well, that assured Dr. Shepard hospital physician privileges. Privileges, however, did not extend to sociability. Dr. Shepard was a tennis player, but the mores of the time made it awkward at best for her to play with the male physicians on the staff. She approached Pearl Edith Parker to see if she could or would assign a nursing student to play tennis with her. Hilda Peplau was assigned the task of playing tennis with the only female doctor in the vicinity. During the spring, summer, and into the fall, they played every morning at 6, and often in the evening as well. A tennis match, however, did not give the student nurse license to talk with the doctor. At the appointed hour, the young student nurse met the young doctor, played two sets of tennis, and left with scarcely a word being spoken. Unbeknownst to Hilda, however, this particular assignment was to be fortuitous indeed.

While a student at Mount Holyoke College, Alice Shepard had a roommate, "Pop" Emma Frazier, who was later married to the director of the School of Physical Education at New York University (NYU), Dr. J. B. Nash. The NYU physical education program ran a summer camp on Lake Sebago in Bear Mountain State Park, near Sloatsburg, New York. The summer of 1932 the camp was in need of both a camp nurse and a tennis instructor who could also teach archery. "Pop" asked her college roommate, now a physician, somewhat in jest, if she perhaps knew of a tennis-playing nurse who could teach archery. "Just maybe," replied Dr. Shepard. She in turn contacted Hilda, who was then a private-duty nurse working in Pottstown and Reading. Hilda quickly sized up the opportunity and determined on the spot to learn archery. This would be an easy enough feat, she decided, and with no hesitation responded "yes" in her most authoritative voice to Dr. Shepard's query. As simply as that, a new chapter in her life began.

By this time, Hilda Peplau was fast becoming aware of the advantages and disadvantages of class in America. In Reading, most of the population was working class. By now, however, Hilda was beginning to recognize that the people living in the big houses on Fifth Street belonged to a different class, as did many of her private patients. She had learned during her childhood in Reading that it was "wealthy" women in New York who employed private-duty nurses and gave them their glamorous cast-off clothing to take to Reading for little girls who dreamed. At Pottstown, the students were taught how to use the silver tea service in order that they might know how to serve tea in patients' homes once they left training school. Hilda realized that the chance to be the camp nurse would put her in touch with a different class of people, people she would not be likely to meet or know under other circumstances. Moreover, she did love tennis and the outdoors.

Set among rolling hills 50 miles north of New York City, Lake Sebago is a large and beautiful lake, long popular as a summer resort. The camp offered what was in effect a summer school for young female physical education majors from NYU. It also offered Hilda an introduction into the world of college faculty life. The instructors for the camp were professors from the Seven Sister colleges and from others such as William and Mary and Purdue. These remarkable women, in addition to their academic specialties, were experts in sports—swimming, boating, hockey, lacrosse, baseball. They were intelligent, well-educated, and world traveled. Sitting on the porch of the lodge during free periods, they talked about their work—faculty qualifications, work evaluations, teacher-student relationships—and about their foreign travel. At night, around a roaring fire inside the lodge, the women faculty gathered and had discussions of college curricula and problems and issues in education, as well as the status of women in sports. For 10 years, from 1932 through the summer of 1942, Peplau looked forward to going to "camp" in June where she enormously enjoyed the excuse to be outside, to perfect her tennis, to learn new sports, and to form close personal friendships with both college students and camp faculty members.[34] In 1937 the camp's program in Physical Education and Health, at Lake Sebago, became an official option in the NYU School of Education summer session. Hildegard Peplau was officially appointed to a 3-year term, 1937–1940, as an instructor in education, with a contract and salary of $225 a summer.[35]

There was no doctor on the staff at Lake Sebago, and Peplau had no knowledge of sports medicine. So, she bought a copy of Gray's *Anatomy* and Cecil's *Physiology* and tried to figure out as she went along the nature of the injuries brought to the camp nurse. She made friends with the doctors at the nearby Tuxedo Park Hospital and when in doubt took the injured there. Ever conscientious, and beginning the habit of a lifetime, she kept copious, accurate records. This was a good thing, because inevitably the day came when a camper's family would accuse her of malpractice. In 1935 the plaintiff, Janet Held, sued New York University, claiming that she had a skin disorder that the camp nurse, Hildegard Peplau, had misdiagnosed and treated as ringworm, thereby permanently scarring the plaintiff, who was a dancer. The scar was very visible and a distinct disadvantage in her chosen career. Peplau's notes saved the day, for they proved that the student treated for ringworm was one Sylvia Shapiro, and that Janet Held indeed had a skin disorder, but nurse Peplau had declined to treat an outbreak of her disorder and instead had referred her to Wiff Yeend Meyers, an instructor of physical education at NYU and the camp director. Her husband, Jim Meyers, then drove Miss Held to New York City to her own physician. The Zurich Insurance Company asked for Peplau's notes, and they proved decisive. The case was dismissed. The impressed Zurich insurance representatives took Hilda to lunch and gave her New York theater tickets. These tickets introduced her to the world of New York theater, a love she would never lose. The NYU lawyers were also much impressed with the thorough and conscientious nurse. In fact, Dr. George Deaver, NYU's professor of sports and rehabilitation medicine, tried to persuade her to enter the Kessler Institute in New Jersey and make physical injuries/rehabilitation her field. She had already decided that her future was in nursing, however, and she could not be dissuaded.

Although Peplau was greatly admired and well liked, her camping days were numbered. In September 1941, Wiff Yeend Meyers wrote to "Dear Peppy," warning her that NYU was pressuring them to employ the university nurse as the camp nurse. In 1942, Hilda informed them, with obvious regret, that this would probably be her last summer, since she both understood the pressure the camp was under to appoint the NYU nurse to the camp position, and "because I am probably going to join the army anyway."[36]

CLARA

As the Great Depression ended, Hilda knew her days in the Reading and Pottstown area were limited. She was anxious to move to New York City. This dream was hastened in its realization by the reappearance in her life of her sister Clara, who was 2 years older than Hilda. During Hilda's last years in Reading before going to PHTS, Clara had difficulty holding a job, but no one at the time thought there might be something actually amiss in her personality. She'd always competed with Hilda, and Hilda believed every competition was resolved in Clara's favor. Grossmutter, uncles, neighbors, and teachers, as well as Gustav and Ottylie, all seemed to favor Clara. Clara was an obedient and exemplary child who always sought to please, and seemed possessed with the necessity to search out and expose her sister Hilda's every failing. Sometime during the years that Hilda was at PHTS, Clara enrolled in the nursing program at St. Luke's and Children's Hospital in Philadelphia, from which she graduated in 1932. Hilda had graduated from Pottstown in 1931 and began her private-duty nursing. Her life was full. The doctors liked her because she was bright and worked hard. Since there were no interns or residents for them to teach, by the end of her training the doctors had begun to treat Peplau almost like a colleague. She was earning good money and the help given to her parents during the Depression had not been a hardship. She had her car, Ottylie took good care of her at home, and her lively circle of friends guaranteed good times when she was not on duty. Clara was truly out of sight and out of mind.

That was the situation when in the middle of January 1933 Ottylie received a very garbled letter from Clara informing her family that she feared threats on her life. Hilda was still living at home. Ottylie was frightened by Clara's letter and distraught. Hilda said she would go to Philadelphia to find Clara and try to get to the root of the problem. Off she went in her roadster, to the rescue of her not-missed older sister.[37] This trip would focus Hilda's interests and would play a major role in setting her on the road to a career in psychiatric nursing.

She drove straight to St. Luke's Hospital where, unexpectedly, she was greeted with hostility and a notable lack of cooperation from the hospital and training school personnel. The director of nursing at first refused to see her at all. Being assertive when she was sure she was right, Hilda refused to take "no" for an answer and went around the director by confronting student nurses in the hall, inquiring of Clara. All were evasive, but one did refer her to a staff physician whom Hilda found to be condescending and arrogant. He opined that Clara was a "dope addict," and hence not worthy of anyone's time or concern. Further questioning of nurses in the hospital produced a list of boarding houses where graduate nurses were likely to room. Armed with her list, Hilda set off in the pouring rain to begin a door-to-door search for her sister. Eventually, she found her. She had first been to several boarding houses at the better addresses near to the hospital. Now she was ranging farther from the hospital, and definitely moving down the socioeconomic ladder. This particular home looked derelict, but she knocked anyway, and the door was answered by an old and odoriferous handicapped man. Inside, the house was dark and smelled of stale dust and sour food. "Yes," he replied to her query, "Clara lives here." Hilda apprehensively fumbled her way up the dark stairs, not knowing what to expect. At this point, she knew very little about mental illness. She knocked on the designated door and called her sister's name. It took a long time for a sloven and agitated Clara to answer the door. The room was dark and filthy. Clara took a seat on the unmade bed and commenced staring at an apple on the nightstand, announcing that it was poisoned and she must divine who was trying to poison her with it. Because she understood little, Hilda said little. She simply announced that she had come to take Clara home. Clara made no objection, and began throwing her things—including an open bottle of ink—into two suitcases. Hilda intuitively knew not to interfere, to let Clara do it her way. It was still raining outside, and it continued to pour all the way from Philadelphia to Reading. Little was said in the car.

At this point, Hilda experienced a phenomenon she was to experience at other extremely stressful points in her life—amnesia. She had no memory of arriving home, or of the reception, or of how things got sorted out. The end result, however, was that Clara was moved into Hilda's room on the third floor, as Johnny and Bertha now occupied the two bedrooms on the second floor. Hilda slept on the couch in the living room that night. The next day she declined to return to the third floor and share a room once again with Clara. Instead, she moved back to Pottstown, where she stayed with her friend Ann Kerr's aunt, Ginny Robinson.[38] Before leaving, however, she did convince her anxious mother that Clara needed to be seen by a doctor, and Ottylie reluctantly agreed. Gustav made no contribution to the discussion. Several doctors were consulted and were unanimous in their recommendation that Clara be committed to the state mental hospital in Wernersville. The Peplaus at first declined these recommendations, but changed their minds as Clara continued to deteriorate.

Clara did well in the hospital. She was fortunate in that a woman physician there was particularly interested in her because she was a nurse. She spent time talking with her, and Clara responded well to the attention. Hilda regularly drove over to Reading from Pottstown to take Ottylie to Wernersville to visit. Clara showed improvement and began working in the hospital as a nurse's aide. Then Grossmutter got into the act, insisting that she, too, be taken to visit Clara. Hilda reluctantly agreed to take her, and Clara predictably was delighted. Clara, an accomplished pianist, played the piano in fine style for her grandmother. After this visit, Grossmutter was convinced that Clara was fine, and began to insist that Ottylie bring Clara home—or God, she warned, would wreak vengeance on the family. Her view was that Clara was in the hospital "only because Hilda put her there." She insisted that Hilda had never liked Clara and now had put her away. Gustav, as he always did, agreed with his mother, and over Ottylie's reservations and Hilda's objections, it was agreed that Clara would come home to Reading. Ottylie pleaded with Hilda to take her and Grossmutter to Wernersville to collect Clara and bring her home again. Hilda most definitely did not think this a good idea, but with the assertiveness and straightforward manner for which she was later to become infamous, finally declared, "All right, I'll get her and bring her home, but I'll have nothing to do with consequent interactions or the consequences." Hilda did bring Clara home on October 28, 1934, but she herself would never live at home again. She felt the family had made its choices, and she was now more determined than ever to get away and on with her life. She would phone and even visit from time to time and send money when it was needed, but she stopped thinking of Reading as "home."

It was not long before Clara began to deteriorate again—threatening people, pouring shakers of salt into the food, and generally disrupting the family, finally threatening a terrified Ottylie with a butcher's knife. By the end of the year, Ottylie was again pleading with Hilda to come home to Reading in order to take Clara back to Wernersville True to her word, Hilda refused to have anything to do with the situation or its consequences. Eventually, with the assistance of their pastor, Reverend Ischinger, and the police, the family recommitted Clara to Wernersville.

Clara would remain at Wernersville until the well-meaning but misguided de-institutionalization movement of the 1960s sent her back to Reading, where she died in a nursing home on October 28, 1984, exactly 50 years to the day from her first ill-fated return from Wernersville to Reading. As the years went by, Hilda would phone the hospital to check on her sister, and she routinely sent Christmas and birthday gifts, provided small amounts of spending money, and sent money for clothes and shoes when needed. In fact, once back in the hospital, Clara did rather well. Basically, she managed to replicate the life she lived before she left home to go into nurses' training. She became the "ward pet," keeping an eye on the other patients, cleaning up the ward for the staff, fetching coffee, and earning special privileges such as being able to sit in the nurses office, stay up late, and eating ahead of the other patients.[39]

ON TO NEW YORK CITY

Hilda lived in Pottstown from 1933 to 1936, but she had not forgotten her dreams of New York City. She contacted Ann Kerr in New York who again gave her the name of the director of Nursing at Mount Sinai Hospital, Grace Warman. Hilda wrote a formal letter to Miss Warman stating that, "I want to round out my experience and fill in some of the gaps in my nurses' training." Peplau had met her match. Grace Warman wrote back a rather salty letter, to the effect that "we are not a training institution for nurses with poor training." Peplau had strong feelings about communication and miscommunication. She could be challenged, in fact she welcomed challenge when it was based on fact, logic, or new information. When assumptions were incorrect or her motivations misinterpreted, however, she reacted decisively. In high school, it was not so much the punishment she objected to during the fateful incident that resulted in her leaving before her senior year but the fact that she had been wrongly accused, and the principal was not interested in the truth. She immediately wrote back to Miss Warman, not to challenge her decision, but to clarify the request. Hilda informed the director of nursing that her initial letter had been misunderstood, that Hilda believed her training to have been excellent but was now eager to build upon it. "Very well, I like your style, come on to New York City and we'll find something for you,"[40] Grace Warman responded.

Within the month, Peplau had accepted a staff position at Mount Sinai Hospital and moved to New York City, where she lived in the nurses' residence at 5 East 98th Street. She loved the hospital. It was there she met "a mad surgeon," known as "Daddy Blumenthal," who favored intelligent nurses and especially the one just arrived from Pottstown. He assured that she was assigned to the operating room when he was using it. She loved it all. Although she was happy with her room in the nurses' residence, Hilda was seldom to be found there. She signed up for philosophy courses at the New School for Social Research, attended lecture series at Cooper Union, and found out which concerts and museums were free and made it a point to visit as many as possible. In those days, New York was safe, clean, and definitely exciting. At the New School she heard Eric Fromm and Karen Horney speak; at Cooper Union she found out about a field called psychology and began to slip into the back of classrooms, soaking up the lectures.[41] It still did not occur to her that there might be a way she, herself, could get a college degree. She did not pursue the opportunity for a virtually free education at the City University of New York, assuming that the only additional education she could acquire would come from her independent reading and whatever free lectures she could find to attend in her spare time.[42]

Grace Warman turned out to be both a mentor and an unselfish supervisor. She encouraged Hilda to continue to spend the month of June at the NYU camp, believing that this was a very good opportunity for Hilda. She permitted Hilda to make up the time by working double shifts, the night shift in addition to the day shift, when she returned in July. During her third summer's leave from Mount Sinai to attend the NYU camp, an unexpected opportunity arose—one that again would change the course of her life. Wiff Yeend Myers, the camp director, was a personal friend of Mary Garrett, the director of admissions at a new college for women in New England: Bennington College in Bennington, Vermont. Its young new president, Dr. Robert Leigh, was assembling a college staff, and at the suggestion of Wiff Yeend, Mary Garrett recommended Hildegard Peplau to him for a position in the College Health

Service. The offer of a job at Bennington presented Peplau with a wrenching decision, for she truly enjoyed her work at Mount Sinai and life in New York City. She consulted Grace Warman, explaining, "I am in this terrible quandary. I like it here very much, I am learning so much, I love New York City, but I have this letter from the president of Bennington College and I don't know what to do about it."[43] Miss Warman read the letter, put it down, took off her glasses and rubbed her eyes, before stating unequivocally that this was a "once in a lifetime opportunity, one which must not be missed." A wise and gracious woman who put others' best interests ahead of her own, Grace Warman urged Peplau to take advantage of this opportunity, advising her also, "And while you are there, get your BA."[44] To Hildegard Peplau a college degree seemed beyond the realm of possibility, but the opportunity to be in an academic environment, and a new and experimental one at that, was clearly exciting. So, she took a deep breath, packed her bags, went back to Reading to reclaim her roadster, and headed for the green hills of southwestern Vermont to be a part of a new experiment in American higher education.

ENDNOTES

1. The reminiscences that follow were provided by Hildegard Peplau in interviews given from January–April, 1992 in Sherman Oaks, California.
2. See JoAnn Ashly, *Hospitals, Paternalism, and the Role of the Nurse* (New York: Teachers College Press, 1976).
3. Interview, Hildegard Peplau, January 28, 1992, and notes and photographs found in Schlesinger Library collection, Box 2, # 45.
4. From reflections recorded and found in the Schlesinger Library collection, Box 8, Folders #266, #267, #268.
5. In her undated autobiography, Peplau stated that Mrs. McElfatrick once reprimanded her in front of a patient for not having folded a washcloth correctly. Having no sense of burning bridges, Hilda announced that if this was what nursing was about, it wasn't for her. She went to her room, packed her bags, and was out on the steps with her bags when Mrs. McElfatrick came to get her, apologized, and helped her move back into her room.
6. Interview, Hildegard Peplau, April 6, 1992.
7. Interview, Hildegard Peplau, January 28, 1992.
8. Interview, Hildegard Peplau, January 28, 1992.
9. Interview, Hildegard Peplau, April 6, 1992. The 18th Amendment to the Constitution was adopted in 1919 and prohibited the sale of alcoholic beverages in the United States. It was repealed by the 21st Amendment in 1933. The 13 years of Prohibition were characterized by widespread violation of the law, and country speakeasies met the undiminished demands of the population for supply.
10. Interview, Hildegard Peplau, April 6, 1999.
11. Interview, Hildegard Peplau, March 28, 1992.
12. See W. J. Bishop, ed., *A Bio-Bibliography of Florence Nightingale* (London: Dawsons for the International Council of Nurses, 1962); Josephine Dolan, *A History of Nursing* (Philadelphia: W. B. Saunders Company, 1968); Sandra Holten, "Feminine Authority

and Social Order: Florence Nightingale's Conception of Nursing and Health Care," *Social Analysis* (1987); Lois A. Monteiro, "On Separate Roads: Florence Nightingale and Elizabeth Blackwell," *Signs 9* (Spring, 1984): 520–533; Jane Mottus, *New York Nightingales: The Emergence of the Nursing Profession at Bellevue and New York Hospitals, 1850–1920* (Ann Arbor: University Microfilm Books, 1981); Charles E. Rosenberg, "Florence Nightingale on Contagion: The Hospital as Moral Universe" in Charles E. Rosenberg, ed., *Healing and History: Essays for George Rosen* (New York: Science History Publications, 1979); Lucy Seymer, *Selected Writings of Florence Nightingale* (New York: Macmillan, 1954); Elaine Showalter, "Florence Nightingale's Feminist Complaint: Suggestions for Thought," *Signs 6* (Spring, 1981): 395–412; Frances Barrymore Smith, *Florence Nightingale: Reputation and Power* (New York: St. Martin's Press, 1982); Anne Summers, "Ladies and Nurses in the Crimean War," *History Workshop Journal 16* (Autumn, 1983): 33–56; and Cecil Woodham-Smith, *Florence Nightingale* (London: Constable, 1950).

13. See Eva Gamarnikov, "Sexual Division of Labor: The Case of Nursing," in Annette Kihn and Ann Marie Wolpe, eds., *Feminism and Materialism: Women and Modes of Production* (Boston: Routledge and Kegan Paul, 1978), 96–123; Sandra Holton (1987); Monteiro (1984); Showalter (1981); Smith (1982); and Summers (1983).

14. See JoAnn Ashly, *Hospitals, Paternalism and the Role of the Nurse* (New York: Teacher's College Press, 1976); N. L. Chaska, *The Nursing Profession—Turning Points* (St. Louis: Mosby, 1990); Celia Davies, *Rewriting Nursing History* (London: Croom, Helm, 1980); Barbara Harris, *Beyond Her Sphere: Women and the Professions in American History* (Westport: Greenwood, 1978); Barbara and Phillip Kalisch, *The Politics of Nursing* (Philadelphia: J. B. Lippincott and Co., 1982); Barbara Melosh, *The Physician's Hand: Work, Culture and Conflict in American Nursing* (Philadelphia: Temple University Press, 1982); and Susan Reverby, *Ordered to Care: The Dilemma of American Nursing, 1850–1945* (Cambridge: Cambridge University Press, 1987).

15. Ibid.

16. R. Stevens, *In Sickness and in Wealth* (New York: Basic Books, 1989), 17–51.

17. See Charles E. Rosenberg, *The Care of Strangers: The Rise of America's Hospital System* (New York: Basic Books, 1987), 215–235.

18. See Reverby.

19. The development of nursing is also closely tied to the development of hospitals in this country. Clearly the economics of hospitals are such that early hospitals could not have survived without the long hours of free labor provided by student nurses in the hospital training schools. This also explains why hospitals were reluctant to give up their schools, and why even the smallest community hospitals sponsored such a school. In 1909 there were 4,359 hospitals in the United States; by 1923 there were 6,830. About a quarter of these sponsored nurse-training schools.

From the beginning, the American Medical Association was most concerned about the nature and quality of nursing schools, and in 1920 offered the following recommendations concerning what sort of candidates they should seek, the skills students should possess, and the essentials of their training. The student nurses should be

> Of sound constitution, of good muscular strength, of great power of endurance, capable of bearing up manfully under fatigue and loss of sleep . . . literate, courageous, patient, temperate, punctual, cheerful, discreet, honest, sympathetic, refined, selfless, and devoted . . . they should be able to notice the character of secretions and excretions, changes in patients' physical countenance . . . be proficient in making up beds, changing sheets, and handling patients exhausted by disease and injury. [Quoted by Darlene Clark Hine, *Black Women in White* (Bloomington: Indiana University Press, 1989), 4]

Certainly the Pottstown Hospital Training School followed these guidelines. Like the first three schools founded in 1873 at the Massachusetts General Hospital in Boston, Bellevue Hospital in New York City, and the New Haven Hospital in Connecticut, the Pottstown Hospital Training School adhered rather closely to the Florence Nightingale model, emphasizing cleanliness, discipline, and regimentation, including the wearing of starched, clean uniforms. For an excellent discussion of these and related issues, see Hine and Reverby, op cit.

20. Rosenberg (1987), 223-224.
21. Rosenberg (1987) and Reverby.
22. See Nancy Cott, *The Bonds of Womanhood* (New Haven: Yale University Press, 1977), for example. Some women did make the transition from "women's sphere" to "women's rights"—but they are found more frequently in Quakerism or Unitarianism rather than in nursing.
23. Lavinia Dock, "The Relation of Training Schools to Hospitals," in Isabel Hampton, Ed., *Nursing of the Sick* (New York: McGraw Hill Book Company, 1949), 16.
24. Dorothy Sheahan, *The Social Origins of American Nursing and Its Movement into the University* (PhD Dissertation; Ann Arbor: University Microfilms, 1980), 60–75.
25. Reverby, 84.
26. Reverby, 85.
27. Sheahan, 60–75.
28. Rosenberg (1987), "Pietism," 16–35.
29. Nightingale, "Notes on Nursing," in Rosenberg, *Healing and History*, 5.
30. Interview, Hildegard Peplau, April 6, 1992, in Sherman Oaks.
31. Interview, Bertha Reppert, October 19, 1994, in Mechanicsburg, Pennsylvania.
32. Interview, Hildegard Peplau, January 28, 1992, in Sherman Oaks.
33. Ibid.
34. Letter from Hildegard Peplau to Barbara Callaway, August 9, 1998.
35. Letter of appointment in Schlesinger Library collection, Box 8, Folder #270.
36. Letter from Hildegard Peplau to Wiff Yeend Myers, January 10, 1942, Schlesinger Library, Box 8, #271.
37. The following account was found in Hildegard Peplau's Diary, recorded December 6, 1972, and found in the Schlesinger Library collection, Box 8, #242.
38. Ann Kerr, who was a year ahead of Hilda at Pottstown Hospital Training School, was a longtime friend. Her aunt, Ginny Robinson and her husband had a large house in Pottstown with several guest rooms, and enjoyed having Hilda stay with them.
39. Interview, Hildegard Peplau, March 28, 1992. Other materials relating to Clara and her life may be found in the Peplau Genealogy, p. 99 and Documents 75–76.
40. Letters to and from Miss Grace Warman may be found in the Schlesinger Library collection, Box 2, #45.
41. Interview, Hildegard Peplau, January 28, 1992.
42. Interview, Hildegard Peplau, January 30, 1992.
43. Ibid.
44. Ibid.

A Nurse Goes to College

3

Every one of my Bennington friends and classmates wanted to contribute something concrete to the world they lived in . . . They taught, they acted, they wrote, they painted, or designed houses or gardens. Bennington started the whole trend of women doing something with their lives as well as just living good women's lives.

—Hildegard Peplau
January 10, 1992

D riving contentedly through the quiet New England countryside, Hilda Peplau tried to imagine what the new world she was about to enter might hold. The drive up the Hudson River at first seemed familiar, although the farther north she went the more she was aware that she was leaving the world she knew. When she finally turned east, crossed the river, and came into Vermont, she knew she was in a very different place. Vermont's Route 9 gently meanders a short 3 miles from the New York border into the town of Bennington. The lush green mountains that give the state its name surround the valley. Tinges of fall color were just beginning to touch the leaves—crimson, gold, coral, and orange. The sky was a deep Vermont blue, and the air seemed purified.

The New England simplicity of the town, dominated by Bennington's Old First Church gracing the town green, and the Bennington Monument, a 300-foot shaft of blue-grey limestone commemorating the Battle of Bennington in the Revolutionary War, was about as far as one could get from the heat and bustle of New York City at this time of year. Bennington and Vermont were old in a way that the rest of the country was not. The Bennington Historical District consists of nearly 100 Georgian and Federal structures dating from 1761–1830. In January 1777, Vermont declared itself an independent republic, adopting a constitution and the name Vermont the following July. George Washington and the Continental Congress briefly considered sending troops to fight against the "Green Mountain Boys," but Vermont remained independent until rejoining the union on March 4, 1791.

BENNINGTON COLLEGE

In 1937 Bennington College was unlike like any other U.S. women's college at the time. The campus spread over 150 acres on the hills to the north of the town, with views of the Green Mountains to the east and the Palisade Mountains of New York State to the west. The campus, which was once a farm, still has many of the original buildings and an appealing New England village serenity. The great red barn remains to this day the main administration building.

Bennington College owed its beginnings to Vincent Ravi Booth, the pastor of the Congregational Church in Old Bennington, who, in 1923, launched the campaign that led to the opening of the college 9 years later.[1] As pastor of a church in Cambridge, Massachusetts, Reverend Booth had come to know many of the Harvard faculty, and in the summers visited them in their summer homes in the southwestern corner of Vermont. He fell in love with Bennington—which he found to be small, quaint, and lovely. When the opportunity came he accepted the call to pastor the Congregational Church there. He soon discovered, however, that once the summer people left in the early fall, Bennington was lonely. Booth decided that what Bennington needed was a college. He broached the idea to some of the town's more influential summer people and found significant support for it. Booth then consulted with Rev. Paul D. Moody, the president of nearby Middlebury College, and then with William A. Nilson, the president of Smith College, who had been a member of Booth's church in Cambridge. Nilson urged Booth to champion a different kind of women's college, not patterned after men's colleges, but "designed to meet the needs of women . . . art, music, literature."[2] Booth went on to enlist the support of the presidents of six of the Seven Sister Colleges (Radcliffe, Wellesley, Smith, Mount Holyoke, Barnard, and Vassar), as well as that of the presidents of Middlebury, Cornell, and Swarthmore. These college presidents had been increasingly concerned by the fact that while demand for women's education was growing, many bright young women had been denied college entrance, in part because of limited space but, more painfully, because they scored too low on the required mathematics entrance exams.[3]

Unlike other colleges with grand buildings built by wealthy donors, the onset of the Depression ensured that Bennington would have simple structures fitted to the essentials of education. According to its first president, Robert Devore Leigh, Bennington's campus came to symbolize "simplicity, directness, and relation to the function."[4] Eventually there would be 12 identical wood-frame student houses built exactly alike and finished with white clapboard and green shutters. The sturdy red barn was converted for use as classrooms, laboratories, a library, and offices. The only building built to the architects' original neo-Gothic specifications was the hall known as the Commons. Featuring white columns and a cupola, the Commons was a handsome edifice, containing a dining hall, the infirmary where Hilda was to work, the college store, post office, art studios, and the campus theater. Economic constraints had by accident or serendipity created a distinctive campus for the new college. Bennington's Spartan simplicity suggested a small New England town, with tasteful, white houses surrounding a village green, at the head of which stood a white columned town hall. It was as though Bennington, the ultimate progressive college for women, had consciously broken from the traditional Gothic architecture to offer students a campus where they could learn about the arts and themselves undistracted by the artificial grandness characteristic of colleges elsewhere.

This was the scene that greeted Hilda Peplau as she steered her little green roadster, a successor to her first car, up the hill toward the Commons in August of 1937. Although she came in the role of college nurse, not student, she nonetheless could not have found an environment more suited to her own individualistic temperament and her intense intellectual curiosity. Bennington's "New England village," the college on the hill, was the utopian community where intellectual adventure and intense personal relationships flourished. Leigh's vision was to create a college where students would learn the classics, acquire knowledge of themselves and their talents, and be challenged to make real contributions to their communities and their world.[5] Once a student had a solid foundation, Leigh envisioned encouragement on campus of what was new and cutting edge in art, dance, and literature.

President Leigh was creative and innovative, and Bennington had a faculty, a student body, and a curriculum that reflected these qualities. In his search for faculty, Leigh had sought scholars and practitioners who had an "understanding and enthusiastic interest in" their own fields, in undergraduate students, and in the "principles and problems of modern education."[6] Taking advantage of the Great Depression, Bennington had recruited a truly outstanding faculty of highly individualistic but dedicated teachers who set their stamp on the new college. They created an intense intellectual atmosphere that shaped undergraduate experiences. Early alumnae remember Bennington not so much for its student pranks and student life, but for its faculty—Ben Bellitt, Genevieve Taggard, Julian deGray, Catharine ("Kit") Osgood Foster, and Martha Hill among others. Bennington is one of the places where Martha Graham helped invent modern dance. It is where Kenneth Burke, the noted critic and man of letters, taught for many years, as did Erich Fromm, the great psychologist/philosopher. So, too, in later years did Stanley Kunitz, Howard Nemerov, Stanley Edgar Hyman, Theodore Roethke, W. H. Auden, Bernard Malamud—and the list goes on. Bennington was an early home to major composers such as Henry Brent and Vivian Fine. At Bennington,

Buckminster Fuller built one of his first geodesic domes. The school pioneered workshop approaches to writing and set the arts on a par with the academic disciplines before other colleges and universities were willing to do so. In lieu of generous salaries, faculty were given housing on campus, faculty privileges such as health care and long vacations, and the promise of intellectual challenge and an unusual degree of academic freedom and autonomy.

From the beginning, a Bennington education was expensive. Because it was established in the first years of the Depression, Bennington never was able to build a substantial endowment such as those that sustained the Seven Sister Colleges through the Depression and on into better times. Bennington's sponsors were able to launch the college by providing the land and minimal physical facilities, but student tuition had to pay for the daily operating expenses, including salaries. For this reason, there was something unique and privileged about the Bennington College community. By and large, its students were from wealthy families—young women with a strong streak of independence, often highly creative, who did not fit the mold or who had not been admitted to the more traditional colleges.

Each of the student residences was a two-storied house with an attic where trunks and suitcases could be stored. On the first floor there were 8 student rooms, bathrooms, a large living room elegantly furnished with donated antiques, and a faculty apartment with a private entrance. On the second floor were 12 student rooms, bathrooms, a kitchenette, and washtub and ironing board. There were few surprises as the 20 or so students in each house made the acquaintance of their house mates. All were White, most had come from New England or New York, most had attended private schools, most were Protestant—and three quarters of these were Episcopalian. Many were nonconformists, often also idiosyncratic or artistic. All were distinctly at least upper-middle class.[7] Hilda Peplau, in contrast—working class, Lutheran, evening-high-school graduate—felt herself to be a distinct outsider.[8] But she was eager to derive everything she could from the experience. She recognized before she arrived at Bennington that she was entering a unique milieu, and she was determined she would find a place in it for herself. At first, that place was in the student health service where she was to be the college nurse.

Unlike the underlying motif of other women's colleges, Bennington students were encouraged to be ambitious for personal success on their own terms rather than to enhance the status of presumed future husbands. In the public's mind, however, it was the social freedom given Bennington students that distinguished the college from other women's colleges. At other women's colleges of the time, strict dress codes were enforced both on and off campus, dormitory doors were locked early in the evening, off-campus visitors were allowed only on special occasions, male students were never allowed in bedrooms, and young women were taught social graces such as how to set a proper table and pour tea. There were no arbitrary rules such as these governing behavior at Bennington because President Leigh believed that rules stressing "thou-shalt-nots" were invitations to evasion and thus hypocrisy.[9] Students were free to come and go and live their own lives. There were no housemothers, and the faculty living in apartments in the student houses had no custodial or disciplinary duties. Students who had spent their high school years in highly supervised boarding schools had never known such freedom.[10] Hilda Peplau had never experienced such intense commitment to learning and experimentation. She was both awed and thrilled. Altogether, Bennington College was about as far from a hospital training school as could be imagined.

At Bennington there would be no required courses. Each student planned a program of study in consultation with a faculty member charged with assuring that the student's study plan afforded sufficient content to assure a liberal learning experience and that it accorded with her interests and needs, based on summaries of her school record, professed interests, characteristics, and hobbies. Each professor, in turn, was challenged *not* to develop a course syllabus until after having met with his or her students. The content of courses must evolve in light of students' needs, interests, and aptitudes. As student interests emerged, tutorials were developed covering subjects never listed in the catalogue.[11] For a serious young woman with an adventuresome, independent streak, Bennington was the perfect place. When Hilda arrived in 1937, the college was in its fifth year. There were 300 undergraduates, and all were women. They had a great deal to say about their own educations—in fact, they were *required* to have a great deal to say about their own educations. Although there were no specific requirements, there were guidelines, expectations, and, most important, there were counselors. All faculty members served as counselors. Each was assigned about 10 students whom he or she would guide through the Bennington experience. Each student met with her counselor for an hour each week. Questions were asked: "What makes you think that? Where's your evidence? What do you want to learn? What do you think you need to do to learn it?" This was good training for a future educator and these were questions that Peplau in the future would ask her own students over and over again. Examinations were optional as students and faculty worked together to develop the term's work, and written work was stressed. Students were evaluated in writing in each course and told whether or not they had passed or failed, but no grades as such were given. The written comments would be made a part of the student's personal file. Toward the end of her second year, a student was promoted to the senior division if her counselor could certify she was capable of "sustained and independent work." At the end of the fourth year, the counselor certified that both her total record and her senior project were of sufficient quality to merit a Bennington degree.

Bennington's governance structure reflected the innovative spirit its president was determined to impart. There were neither departments nor department chairs. Community participation was stressed, and students were full members of the community. Students had the majority of members on the Community Council, which set standards and disciplined students and faculty alike. Students advised on everything from educational policy to landscaping. The college store was a consumer cooperative run by faculty and students. One of the radical innovations at Bennington was the process by which students evaluated the instructors. At least twice during the term students met without the instructor, discussed the course, and selected a spokesperson to give the instructor feedback on behalf of the group.[12] Something of the spirit of Bennington is captured by the poet and long-time Bennington faculty member, Ben Bellitt, who would become one of Hilda's first teachers:

> My reasons for teaching at Bennington have to be retrospective, at this point, since they were long ago absorbed into a way of life and an identity that I can no longer interpret as a set of academic premises. Putting aside all pastoral reflections on scenery, ecology, and seasonal dividends of the Good Life on the Bennington campus . . . I think it was the atmosphere of optimistic risk that intrigued me most . . . I taught in a constant atmosphere of human and intellectual hazard. Bennington made everything tentative, scary, vulnerable. Courses were planted and plowed under annually . . . Therefore the risk. Risk was laid upon me in every act of counseling, where the outcome was always in doubt, as two human beings tried to improvise a regimen of intellectual exchanges by which the teacher could test the uses to which the learning of the classroom was being put at the discretion of the student.[13]

Bennington students were the first to wear blue jeans to class; the first to be allowed to have men in their rooms (from 10:00 a.m. to 6:00 p.m.); the first to go around with Flat Fifties (a small tin box of cigarettes) in their pockets; certainly the first to be able to study, as regular courses, dance, painting, drama, music, photography; and the first to be required to take internships in the outside world each year as a part of their academic program.[14] Unlike other women's colleges, Bennington had no chapel. The lack of a chapel together with the unorthodox academic program, and the great emphasis on counseling and mental health, gave Bennington early on the reputation of being both godless and "arty."

Most colleges provide a minimum of health services for their students. In this too, Bennington would prove to be less conventional than its sister colleges. At a time when other colleges hardly acknowledged the importance of mental health, Robert Leigh announced that Bennington would avoid the "fumbling and inexpert efforts of the traditional college dean" in dealing with the wide range of student problems by appointing a psychiatrist to be director of the college health service. The director then would combine the roles of college physician and psychotherapist.[15] He convinced Dr. Wilmoth Osborne, a graduate of the University of Oregon Medical School, to come to Bennington. Dr. Osborne had worked as physician and adviser to women students at the University of Oregon. Dealing with the medical problems of young adult students had failed to challenge her, as it seemed clear to her that the problems of her students could not be adequately resolved by medical means alone. She decided to enter psychiatry, and moved to New York City to enter the Psychiatric Institute of the New York Medical Center. She went on to work at Yale before Robert Leigh convinced her to come to Bennington.[16] It was a good match. To students, Dr. Osborne often appeared formidable. As was said of Hilda in later life, she was not known to suffer fools easily, but she willingly went out of her way when she could help another human being. She met students with great directness and gave them loyalty. She was the acknowledged counselor of counselors, and many at Bennington agreed with Hilda who said, "I would trust her with my life."[17] Like Hilda Peplau she was tall, with a mop of unruly, curly hair— in her case, red.

HEALTH SERVICE NURSE

Peplau's letter of appointment from Robert D. Leigh, dated June 24, 1937, stated: "I am happy to offer you an appointment as head nurse at Bennington College for the next academic year. Your salary will be $1,500 per year, plus room and board."[18] In 1939, her salary increased to $1,600. Upon arriving at Bennington, Hilda reported first to the health service on the first floor of the imposing Commons building. There she met Mrs. Lavina Kelly, her predecessor as the college nurse, who showed her to her room, a large, sunny studio room immediately behind the infirmary. Peplau would live and work in this space for her first 2 years at Bennington College. Before the two women could become acquainted and before Mrs. Kelly could go over her responsibilities with the new nurse, Dr. Osborne phoned and said to send Miss Peplau right on over to her private office, which was on the other side of the building. Hilda walked down the hall and across the building, knocked, and was told to enter. She was taken aback when she opened the door, looked straight across the office into the door of an open bathroom and saw Dr. Osborne sitting on the toilet. The bathroom door was *never* left open in the Peplau home. In fact, not only were the doors to bathrooms always closed, but no one ever even so much as mentioned the necessity to use a toilet. Dr. Osborne blithely waved Hilda in, telling her to come on through the entryway and find a seat in the office. She'd be right with her, Dr. Osborne said.[19] At this moment, Hilda knew for sure that Bennington College was to be far different from any place she had been up to this time in her life. Hilda's initial shock turned to profound respect:

> Then she came into the room where I sat in stunned disbelief, and acted totally matter of fact and professionally. She made it very clear that she was the doctor and that she set the rules, but that I was the nurse and she respected me as a professional. And that was that. I could call her anytime. It was really quite simple. Her matter of factness, lack of pretense, and straightforwardness made a big impression.[20]

Ever after, Peplau would seek to make the same first impression. She decided she would model herself professionally after Dr. Osborne. Most importantly, she had met someone she trusted absolutely, one of the few people in her life about whom she would say this.[21]

The next morning, when the doctor entered the health service, Hilda jumped up and said, "Good morning, Doctor." After jumping up like a robot several times as the doctor came and went, Osborne, who at 6 feet was a couple of inches taller than the 5-foot 10-inch nurse, pointed her finger at Hilda, looked her straight in the eye, and said, "Don't ever do that again. We are equals, you in your field and I in mine. I will not jump up when you come in the room, and please spare me when I come into the room."[22] After that, Hilda made it a point to teach her students not to stand up for doctors unless the doctor requested it, explaining that the gesture was to be made, if at all, not because the woman was a nurse, but because the doctor required such deference "to know who he was."[23]

Dr. Osborne began almost immediately to reorient Peplau's thinking about health care, about how to treat patients, and about how to do things in student health as distinct from other kinds of health care. Hilda already showed an inclination toward academic life. The nurse and the doctor spent many hours discussing the goals and practices of an ideal health service, and Hilda did all she could to implement these ideas at Bennington. When she discovered the periodical *Public Health Nursing*, she decided to send this journal her first article, "The College Health Service." It was published in 1942. The article presented a visionary view of how the ideal college health service might function. According to Hilda, it really focused on Dr. Osborne's philosophy—"I just implemented it, and then wrote about it."[24] Basically, Dr. Osborne impressed upon her that in student health, any student who said that she was ill was to be taken at her word. The nurse should listen intently, take everything seriously, and, if indicated, put the student to bed immediately. In student health, at least at Bennington College, there would be no assumption of malingering. The soundness of this advice was soon dramatically demonstrated when a student came into the infirmary saying she "felt sorta sick," although she couldn't verbalize any actual physical symptoms. Peplau took her at her word, put her to bed, and kept an eye on her during the night. The next morning, although the student still had no fever, Peplau called the doctor. The student was later diagnosed with polio.

Bennington had a near monopoly on gifted students who failed to meet one or more of the conventional requirements for admission to college. Very bright, precocious, and independent-minded young women made for a most unconventional student body. Free spirits were encouraged. Peplau thought that things might have gone too far when on a snowy morning in the middle of winter a barefooted student wearing an evening gown walked into the infirmary and asked Peplau to watch her books while she went to class to take an exam. Peplau did not know whether to detain her, go with her to class, give her own shoes to her, loan her a coat, or call the professor. The student insisted she had to go to class, so Peplau simply gave the student a coat, and asked her to come back after class. The student left, promising to return. Peplau was at a loss as to what course of action to take: "I honestly didn't know what to do, and that was the first time that had happened to me. That was the first time I was totally stymied. Usually, if I didn't know anything, I would look it up. Here I didn't even know what to look up where."[25] Always before, at least in a health care setting, she had felt entirely confident that if she did not know what to do, she would know how to find out. This time, however, she was at a loss. She called Dr. Osborne who advised her that when the student returned, Hilda should put her to bed, keep her warm, talk to her, and see what she had to say. She asked Hilda to call back when that had been done. The doctor did come over, and later the student was taken to Albany and then flown to a private psychiatric hospital in Chicago. The next year, this student was back and had resumed her normal college life. Unlike the situation with her sister Clara, Hilda now had an example of a person with mental illness able to return in a relatively short time to a normal life. This incident became a catalyst for her life's work. She knew now that a nurse, encouraged to act on her own, could make a difference.[26]

Because the infirmary was at the foot of the stairs, faculty, students, and even visiting lecturers and artists would stop by the infirmary on their way upstairs to lectures or performances. In this way, Hilda began to meet not only students, but faculty members, and even some rather famous guests. The president, Dr. Robert Leigh, began to stop by on a regular basis, dancer Martha Graham came in to put her feet under the heat lamps, and other members of the faculty would stop by just to see what the nurse was reading, what she was thinking.

Although enjoying her work and thrilled to be at Bennington, Peplau knew she had entered a world she did not know, but she could not anticipate just how overwhelmed and out of place she would feel. She had learned about social class and sophistication in New York City, and she had learned something of the culture of the young and educated at the New York University camp. She had not yet experienced, however, the world of genteel money, Yankee reticence, or focused intellectual exuberance. Acutely conscious of the small and constrained world of her childhood in Reading, she felt the limitations of her formal education at the Pottstown Hospital Training School, and she was painfully mindful of her working-class background. She proceeded cautiously. At first she felt her difference keenly, and, although she had many social interactions, at times she experienced feelings of profound psychological loneliness.

> I doubt that anyone can fully appreciate my private terrors on first being at Bennington. Such enormous contrasts: I'd come from a secretive family with large anti-education elements; Bennington was open and hell-bent on educating its students. I was from a small, constricted, training school governed at every turn by rules; Bennington's community was almost anti-rules. I was born poor and in a poor paying occupation; Bennington dripped with rich people. I was reared and educated with non-risk takers; Bennington folk had expansive visions and courage to forge ahead . . . Challenges to my ignorance were everywhere at Bennington while its other members extended their well-ingrained knowledge.[27]

In spite of her insecurities, Hilda was determined to take advantage of every opportunity this beautiful school could offer her. She spent many evenings on the second floor of the Commons, where college events were held right above her room. Dr. Osborne had told her she was expected to take part in any activities that interested her, so Hilda began to go upstairs whenever anything was going on. She was thrilled at the seemingly never-ending schedule of activities that took place there, including musicals, plays, and dances. It was indeed a new world. Soon, Hilda's social life at Bennington became anything but bleak. Hilda and fellow staff members Martha LeVeck, Natalie Disston, and the college dietician cooked meals together as often as two or three times a week, and Hilda's apartment often became the scene for Saturday night dinner parties. Friday nights were movie nights and Ben Bellitt, Bill Bales, Gene Lundberg, Natalie Disston, and Hilda went to the movies, sitting in the balcony eating peanuts, and afterward adjourning to Gene's apartment to talk. Sundays in the fall and spring were days to drive out into the Vermont countryside to hike and explore. There were occasional dinners at a country inn, or a weekend trip to New York where she still had friends. Hilda often attended faculty meetings, and eventually was asked to serve as a member of the administrative subcommittee of the college executive committee.[28] On this committee, she kept the most complete records imaginable, recording every word and every action.[29]

She soon found that the word that best described the feeling at Bennington was "exhilaration." Like so many of the students, Hilda was excited to find a place where ideas were taken very seriously. Peplau had always taken ideas seriously, but in her formative years she had been made to feel that intellectual interests were somehow unacceptable. At Bennington, it was as though she had at last come home. Bennington, as Hilda often said, had the feel of a "magical place," where other people cared about knowledge and ideas the way she did.

Hilda's parents showed a total lack of curiosity about what she was doing. Perhaps the idea of college was simply beyond them. In any event, neither her parents nor her friends in Reading seemed interested in the nature of her new life. Hilda, however, was very curious about the foster brother, Johnny Forster, who had come into her parents' home as an infant in 1931, while Hilda was living in Pottstown. When Johnny was 8 or 9 years old, Hilda drove to Reading and brought him back to Bennington to spend some time with her. Johnny, however, was young and totally lacking in experience that might prepare him for a summer on a college campus. He was far too reticent to play with the other children, electing to sit quietly in the infirmary waiting for Hilda to take him outside onto the campus grounds. One evening the young boy heard music coming from somewhere beyond the Commons. The sound was irresistible. Taking Hilda's hand, he led her outside, following the sound of the music to a dormitory window across the campus green. Johnny was too shy to go in. So, the tall nurse and the little boy stood outside enraptured, listening intently to the music of a harpsichord. Johnny Forster knew then that music would be his life—and so it was.[30]

THE STUDENT

Early in her second year at Bennington, Dr. Leigh asked Peplau to come to his office. Not knowing what to expect, Hilda immediately began to develop a severe migraine headache. She feared she had done something wrong, even that she would be asked to leave—a fear that echoed childhood punishments in Reading. She was still her mother's child, after all; but the visit proved to be another turning point. "You are clearly bright," the president said, "Have you ever thought of being a student?"[31] Hilda was floored. She was a good 10 years older than the typical Bennington student, she had no money, and she certainly could not afford Bennington's high tuition. By now she knew, too, that Reading Evening High School and Pottstown Hospital Training School had not given her a sound foundation for pursuing a liberal arts college education. Dr. Leigh, however, was not a conventional president. He immediately reassured Hilda, and informed her that the college would offer her a "paper scholarship." There would be no money involved from either side, but she was being invited to begin to take classes for credit.[32] Peplau, as college nurse, was also a full-time professional, and thus would become the only student at Bennington on full salary.

Her new status as a student coincided with a major change in the health service. Dr. Osborne took a leave in the fall of 1939 in order to enter psychoanalysis with Dr. Clara Thompson at the William Alanson White Institute in New York. Upon her return to Bennington, Dr. Osborne felt increasingly exhausted. She resigned to take up private practice in New York, but died of cancer in September 1940. President Leigh appointed Mrs. Leigh's brother-in-law, Dr. Joseph Chassell, to succeed Dr. Osborne as director of the college health service. Chassell, like Osborne, had been trained in medicine and psychiatry, and for 7 years had been the senior physician and psychoanalyst at the Sheppard Pratt Hospital in Towson, Maryland. Almost immediately, Dr. Chassell appointed Peplau his "executive officer." Her efficiency and competence allowed him to spend most of his time either in the classroom or advising and counseling students. Later that year, a second physician, Dr. Elizabeth McCullough, was employed, and Dr. Chassell was able to devote more time to teaching. In this role he became Hilda Peplau's academic adviser.

In the fall of 1939 Peplau started to take courses officially. As a student, she was intense to say the least. Volumes and volumes of densely handwritten notes of lectures given in her Bennington classes indicate a student hungry for intellectual input and deeply impressed with her teachers and their knowledge. It was not easy going, but she was exceedingly hard-working. Hilda at first thought she would be a science major, but she found her lack of foundation too serious an obstacle to overcome. In her first term as a student, Hilda took a psychology course with Eric Fromm, one of the foremost post-Freudian psychologists in the United States at that time, who in his work drew substantially on insights gained from anthropology and sociology to emphasize the ethical core of psychology.[33] It was immediately clear that Peplau's interests were more attuned to psychology than to natural science.

The strain of feeling slightly misfit, uneasy about her economic and educational background, her overwhelming desire to do well, and her driving passion to learn all she could, took a toll. Hilda's Bennington years, while truly "exhilarating," were also marred by serious, though not quite debilitating, stress reactions. She broke out in rashes and had severe anxiety attacks. Although intensified at Bennington, these signs of physical reaction to psychic stress were not new. As a child Hilda had been an anxious nail-biter, and had suffered from rashes and migraine headaches while at Pottstown. In her own words, "I was a walking text-book of psychosomatic ailments."[34] Although she functioned well in her role as nurse, in her role as student she felt under enormous stress and was wracked by insecurity.[35] Once she started taking classes for credit, she again began to suffer nearly unbearable migraines. Dr. Chassell, a kindly man, recognized some of the signs and suggested Hilda try psychoanalysis with him. But Peplau at that time was not a good candidate for analysis. She later claimed she gained few insights from the experience—she already knew her limitations and understood the challenges she was accepting for herself. In fact, when asked about how she explained her migraines to her analyst, she replied, "Well, I don't remember actually talking about migraines with him. But, I did notice these contrasts, and of course I could put two plus two together."[36]

Her teachers, while not ignoring her lack of academic background, also recorded that Peplau was "energetic, patient, understanding, well-organized, and has great powers of concentration."[37] It was clear to Hilda that in situations where she was unsure of herself, or in situations when she knew she would be judged—as in the operating room in Pottstown or in the classroom at Bennington—the rashes and other psychosomatic symptoms would appear. However, when she was in her own element, when she was sure of herself, when she felt confident, there were no migraines or blemishes. While she never felt excluded, she was nonetheless always conscious that her background was working class, not middle or upper class, that she was not a "paying" student but rather a lower level staff person, and that her fellow students were much younger and presumably better educated than she. She acknowledged that students often made an effort to include her, but she was reticent to join in. "At Bennington, I was always treated absolutely as an equal, but I was painfully aware of major differences," she recalled. "So there were constraints, but they were of my own doing."[38]

She found security in the fact that what she truly did know was nursing. "But let me tell you, there wasn't much to know," she later remarked.[39] This security about her professional responsibilities gave her the self-assurance to know that she *could* succeed as a student. In all her courses she kept meticulous notes, worked very hard, and began to feel that she could do it: that she, Hildegard Peplau, could earn a college degree, with a major in psychology, at a progressive, upper-class, New England women's college. This was indeed a giant jump from her Church Street home near the railroad yards in Reading, Pennsylvania. The fact that she could, and did, earn a degree at Bennington as a working student instilled the confidence that was to become central to Hilda Peplau's nature. After Bennington, she seldom suffered stress-related illnesses. Extremely trying and stressful service during the World War II tested her endurance beyond anything she had previously experienced, and she was not found wanting.

Once she became a student, Hilda moved from her room behind the health service into an apartment in one of the student houses. She shared the room briefly with Natalie Disston, a college secretary, before having it to herself. The bedroom was furnished with a desk, bed, and bureau, but the living room was empty. Ever industrious, Hilda took a course in interior design with two members of the drama faculty in order to meet a distribution credit in art. She selected peach and blue as her colors, and from her friend, Helen Cummings, whose father owned a wool factory, she got wool and learned to braid herself a wool rug. To go with the hand-braided wool rug she sent to Reading for a Victorian love seat she had bought on Church Street during the Depression. It was her first effort at interior decoration, and she was quite proud of herself.[40]

In spite of all the encouragement and special concessions, the path to a bachelor's degree was not an easy journey for Hilda. She had to be tutored in English and had trouble with the minimum science distribution requirement. She managed to get some science credit for her work on laboratory techniques at Pottstown Hospital and at Bellevue, and she had a tiny lab at Bennington where she could do urinalyses and simple blood tests. For this, the college waived half of her science requirement. Without having a name for it, what Bennington in effect was doing was allowing Hilda experiential credit. The absence of any science preparation in high school left her feeling handicapped, but more importantly, it made her acutely aware that nurse-training's scientific foundation, to that date, was narrow to the point of being nonexistent.

She tried to take German to meet her foreign language distribution and signed up for a tutorial with Mrs. Wunderlich. To her horror she found she simply could not do it, the fact that German was spoken in her home and that she had attended a German-language primary school notwithstanding. Every time she walked into Mrs. Wunderlich's apartment she literally froze. She felt she was back in her grandmother's house, although, in fact, the only time she remembers being within the walls of Grossmutter's house was at the time of her final illness. That one time, Hilda remembered, she had been overwhelmed with the overstuffed furniture and overcome by a feeling of claustrophobia. Hilda herself was basically a minimalist: a rug, a sofa, a lamp. Something deep in her subconscious mind reacted viscerally to both Mrs. Wunderlich and her apartment. German was dropped. There were other emotional blocks as well. For instance, Hilda wanted to take a music course and elected piano. As a child in Reading, she had taken piano lessons. She remembered that the teacher come to the house at 1232 Church Street to teach the Peplau children to play. This teacher was not a sympathetic soul, nor an empathetic one. To learn proper hand position and movement, quarters were placed on top of the Hilda's hands. If she made a mistake, the teacher would strike her hand and the quarters would fall off. Such was not the case with her sister Clara, who showed considerable musical aptitude. As an adult, Hilda assumed that her feelings about the piano would be different. Yet she found herself physically blocked, precluded from learning the piano just as she had been from learning German. The problem may have been a simple lack of natural talent, but then too it may have been an unconscious reaction to the pain of being forced to take piano lessons in Reading compounded by the psychic pain of being the nonmusical child of a gifted mother and sister of a talented older sibling. Hilda could not overcome these feelings and was never comfortable when seated at the piano—although a few years later she would use the publisher's advance on her first book to purchase a fine baby grand.[41]

Although she worked very hard, Peplau was not an outstanding student. Her lack of preparation precluded that. Little by little, however, she overcame her feelings of academic inadequacy and began to do relatively well in her courses. She never quite hit her full stride at Bennington, but she did begin to feel as though she was not such an outsider or, at least, not so inferior an outsider. Her evident analytic abilities began to emerge in her classes, and her teachers were encouraging. As Hilda put it, ". . . from the time I arrived, I never heard a discouraging word."[42]

Her most exciting courses were with Eric Fromm. While still in high school, she had tried to understand and interpret Nietzsche with her friend Peg Mlodoch, but she had yet to encounter an intellect such as Fromm's. Not only did he clearly know and understand Nietzsche, but he quoted liberally and without notes from the Bible and the Talmud, as well as from Kafka and a wide range of European and American literature. Hilda always made a beeline to the library after a Fromm lecture, trying to track down all the citations. Gradually she began to find her way, began to think analytically, and began to find themes on her own. Fromm was her ideal of a professor—brilliant, slightly confused, always rushing, always carrying books and papers, speaking extemporaneously and learnedly about an infinite variety of themes and topics. She knew him as a teacher, not the famous psychoanalyst. In fact, she knew him in the years before he became famous. In the future she would make a few feeble attempts to maintain contact with Fromm and other persons she knew at Bennington, but eventually her efforts petered out. In later years she would explain that she was afraid to ruin the memories, so she carefully protected them from any retrospective reassessment.

Her memories of Bennington are of a lovely interlude, an extra special time in her life. Self-conscious and realistic, she felt she was not good enough in any subject to consider a change of career. She simply felt that as a nurse, she was extremely fortunate to have the opportunity to earn a college degree. She had little understanding that her relentless intellectual hunger, her love of knowledge, and her respect for brilliance, revealed something about herself, and no idea at all that these drives presaged an extraordinary career of her own. By this time, she was fairly certain that she would never marry and would have to be solely responsible for her own well-being.[43] The Bennington experience, however, was bringing about a sea change in her thinking. She was beginning to see herself as a professional, not as a subordinate. She began to see that nursing could be coequal with medicine in health care and began to think about what changes in nursing education would be necessary to bring this about. In later years, she would regard the creation of pride of profession and professional self-confidence in nursing students as one of her most significant challenges.[44]

WINTER RECESSES:
NEW YORK CITY AND CHESTNUT LODGE

Because of the severity of the Vermont winters, the cost of heating buildings, and Bennington's slender financial base, the college closed each winter between Christmas and Washington's birthday. During this "nonresident term," students were expected to engage in fieldwork experiences related to their interests or course of studies. Students apprenticed themselves to artists, to writers, to editors, or to their fathers' businesses. Under the guidance of Joseph Chassell, psychology students had an opportunity to take their winter field experiences in some of the leading private and public psychiatric clinics in the country. Hilda's first experience was to return to New York City to work on the child and adolescent units of Bellevue Hospital under the direction of the nurse supervisor of the psychiatric division. She worked closely with Dr. Benjamin Wortis and Dr. Sylvan Kaiser. The physicians were impressed with the Bennington student, and urged her to switch her major to "pre-med." Ever self-conscious, however, Hilda feared she could not repair her deficiencies in science and thus never seriously considered the suggestion. With prescience of what was to come, however, they cautioned her that she would have a difficult time in nursing precisely because she was bright and intellectually curious as well as committed to building nursing's professional foundations by changing its educational requirements. Such dedication and interest in the work for its own sake would make her a pariah in nursing, they predicted.[45]

The second winter she returned to New York again. Hilda considered this a real treat. This time she would work as a research assistant to Dr. David M. Levy, a well-known child psychiatrist whose office was in the Sherry Netherland Hotel on Park Avenue. Under Dr. Levy's direction, she looked at the issues of foster care, orphanages, and adoption in New York City. Her 1943 Bennington senior thesis, "The Problem of Juvenile Delinquency and Child Care in New York City," based on this fieldwork, is a very dense and detailed review of the literature and an effort to apply its major concepts to her work in the city.[46] In the course of this work, she often attended Justine Wise Polier's children's court and was most impressed with this remarkable, just, and wise woman. Although Hilda had no personal interaction with Judge Polier, she regarded her as a mentor. As she had a few years earlier, she again found time to go downtown to the New School of Social Research and slip into Judge Polier's seminar on juvenile delinquency. On Sundays she ventured over to Union Theological Seminary and the Riverside Church to listen to Reinhold Niebuhr or Harry Emerson Fosdick, two of America's foremost theologians.

Peplau's third work-experience session, which took place in the 1941–1942 winter term, would set the direction for her future work. This time Chassell's connections and endorsement sent her to Chestnut Lodge, a private psychiatric hospital in Rockville, Maryland. There she met Frieda Fromm Reichman and came into contact with the work of Harry Stack Sullivan. Sullivan's theories would become the primary intellectual influence in Peplau's own later work. By this time, she had begun to feel professionally confident and knew with certainty that her interest lay in what was to become the field of psychiatric nursing. The early 1940s were decisive years in the development of American psychiatry, and it was at Chestnut Lodge that the genesis of a new psychotherapeutic school based on Sullivanian principles was taking form. Clara Thompson, Frieda Fromm Reichman, Eric Fromm, Harry Stack Sullivan, and Janet Rioch were already the nucleus of a new and important branch of American psychiatry. These key players were all at Chestnut Lodge when Peplau arrived for her Bennington field experience. Their work was to lead to the founding of the Washington School of Psychiatry, with a branch in New York.[47] The New York branch became the William Alanson White Institute, and it too would play a most important role in Hilda's life just a few years hence. The director at Chestnut Lodge, Dr. Dexter Bullard, provided the physical and intellectual space for these innovative therapists, and Peplau had walked right into it. Never one to miss an opportunity, she immediately began attending Sullivan's weekly lectures for junior and senior staff that had begun the previous October.

This was a time of considerable personal and professional frustration for Sullivan, and Chestnut Lodge provided the leisure and the space for him to press on with the development of his theories on schizophrenia and new techniques of psychotherapy. He related these new ideas through a series of lectures and subsequent discussion groups that winter at Chestnut Lodge. During December and February, these lectures were held in Bethesda Golf and Country Club with those in attendance sitting around the fire. Sullivan sat in a comfortable chair next to the fire, with the Bullards' Great Dane at his feet. In this comfortable and informal setting, Sullivan began to pull together his life work and cumulative observations. Hilda sat behind everyone else, listening intently, but never speaking.[48] Sullivan promoted an optimistic view of serious mental disorder, believing that deterioration was not inevitable and that, through appropriate treatment, mental health could be regained.[49] His emphasis on the underlying emotional and cognitive factors that motivate an individual's withdrawal from interpersonal relationships made him the first major theorist to develop psychological interventions in schizophrenia.

Peplau almost immediately fit into life at Chestnut Lodge, reading in the library, attending lectures, seeing patients, and consulting with Frieda Fromm Reichman. On the nights when there were no lectures she generally stayed in her room reading. Unlike the other student interns, she was a woman of some experience, having worked in private-duty nursing in Pennsylvania and at Bellevue and Mount Sinai hospitals in New York before becoming a Bennington student. In fact, her great capacity for overwork was clearly evident. She went far beyond what was required of a student intern.[50]

Once a week Peplau had a 1-hour conference with Bullard to review her work and share her observations. Dr. Bullard also agreed that Hilda could attend the seminars held for physicians. One of the patients she heard about was a medical doctor who had found his wife in bed with another man. He became very agitated, suffered a nervous breakdown, and was brought to Chestnut Lodge in a suicidal state. He was placed in isolation in a room with only a mattress and his pajama bottoms. A full-time attendant sat outside his door. Peplau had the temerity when meeting with Dr. Bullard to suggest that she thought she could help this patient. Bullard leaned back, put his feet on his desk, and asked, "In your now vast knowledge and experience, what do you recommend?" Peplau replied, "Just common sense, take him on walks, let him talk, do that until he winds down, and the hurt and the anger begin to diminish." Bullard said, "Very well," and gave his permission. The next day Peplau went to the isolation ward and explained to both the patient and the attendant what they were going to do. The patient responded by throwing soapy water in her face. She did not give up, however, and every day went to see the patient. Eventually he accepted the invitation to walk. He talked obsessively, but in time the walking and talking took on their own comforting rhythm. He began to get better. Soon he was given his clothes and gradually became stronger. Years later, Peplau saw him again. It was in a hospital where he was supervising medical residents. Peplau believed he did not recognize her and she did not remind him.[51]

At Chestnut Lodge she was next assigned floor duty on a locked ward, a ward on which Frieda Fromm Reichman had several schizophrenic patients. It was agreed that Hilda would work closely with one young male schizophrenic patient and confer over Wednesday lunch with Fromm

Reichman in her apartment. Frieda Fromm Reichman believed that the aloofness of patients with schizophrenia represented a wish to avoid repetition of rebuffs suffered in childhood. She emphasized the need for patience and optimism and, together with Harry Stack Sullivan, helped establish psychoanalysis in the psychotherapeutic treatment of schizophrenia.[52] In addition to listening to and reading about Sullivan's work with schizophrenics, Hilda read everything she could find written by Frieda Fromm Reichman.[53]

Hilda was daring, courageous, and convinced she could help with some of the most disturbed patients on this ward. One patient was deathly afraid to go outside. Peplau kept talking to him, and, as in the case of the suicidal doctor, the young man eventually responded to the attention—but in the classic way that men respond to attention from women. Peplau tried to ignore this, without discouraging opportunities for conversation. She was able to persuade him to leave the building by offering to take him for a ride in her car. They went sightseeing in the countryside, and eventually she was able to coax him into museums. At first he tried to hold her hand and kiss her, but "I drew the line there, even though Chestnut Lodge was pretty touchy-feely," she recalled.[54] It was most gratifying, however, to see such visible change in such a short period of time.

Not all contacts with patients on this ward were so successful. Frieda Fromm Reichman was not always as observant as her student intern. One patient was a very disturbed young girl who was locked in a room with an iron gate and who clearly had an obsessive fascination with Frieda Fromm Reichman. Once, when Hilda was walking through the ward with the therapist, they stopped in front of the iron-gated room, and Fromm Reichman commented, "By the way, our lunch will be on Thursday this week instead of Wednesday." The patient heard the remark. Later in the day, the patient called for the nurse saying she did not feel well and asked that Peplau come in to check on her. As Hilda unlocked the gate and entered the room, she sensed the patient getting ready to pounce and jumped back out, slamming and locking the gate. The patient immediately began to have a full-scale temper tantrum, screaming and screaming at the top of her lungs. Frieda Fromm Reichman never acknowledged any connection between her comment and the patient's subsequent reaction, instead suggesting to Hilda that she had exercised poor judgment in opening the gate. Hilda, however, had formed her own opinion: "I thought *she* had exercised poor judgment."[55]

Occasionally Hilda found herself in over her head. One patient, a very intelligent young man diagnosed with paranoia, kept talking with the nurse and the nurse did not observe any pathology. When the patient pleaded earnestly and repeatedly to take a walk outdoors, Hilda finally agreed and received the appropriate permission. The only condition was that he not be allowed to mail any letters. While passing a post office, the patient suddenly dashed inside, maniacally asking for a stamp so that he could mail a letter. He had to notify the President of the United States of the "atrocities" at Chestnut Lodge! Peplau convinced him to give her the letter, promising to put a stamp on it and mail it for him. Patient and nurse whispered conspiratorially about plans for the letter all the way back to Chestnut Lodge and the ward. That day she learned something about paranoia. When she recounted the story to Dr. Bullard, he responded, "Well, now you know."

In coming to Chestnut Lodge, Peplau found herself in the right place at the right time. She seized the moment and the opportunity. During her 8 weeks there, December 15, 1941 through February 10, 1942, her weekly lunches with Frieda Fromm Reichman became a one-on-one teaching seminar, an experience Peplau would treasure for the rest of her life. On the other hand, although always impressed, Peplau was never comfortable with Harry Stack Sullivan. She quickly learned that Sullivan was not particularly impressed with women in general and nurses in particular. "He was very much antiwomen," she recalled. "At Sheppard Pratt Hospital, where he worked with schizophrenic patients, he found nurses seriously wanting in providing him with usable observational data. Unfortunately, he was correct."[56]

At Chestnut Lodge, Peplau was assigned to live in a small house shared with other attendants. Sullivan was noted for the close personal relationships he formed with a number of male assistants, including Ray Pope, one of Hilda's housemates during the time she was at Chestnut Lodge.[57] Pope sensed a kindred soul in Hilda, and many an evening he would come to her room bearing hot chocolate, sit on her bed, and tell her "endless" stories about Sullivan and the going's-on at Chestnut Lodge.[58] So, although she had no direct contact with him, Peplau felt vicariously close to Sullivan and his work. Chestnut Lodge was the finest, most avant-garde psychiatric clinic in the country, but in those days it was a rather free and easy place. There were many pairings off and frequent switches of affections and partners among the staff. Peplau noted, "You had to keep your common sense about you, or you would be sucked into the endless intrigue."[59] She greatly appreciated Ray Pope's friendship, and loved the stories he told, but Hilda was diligent in keeping her distance from the staff foibles and entanglements. She would retain her connections at Chestnut Lodge for another decade, and was careful to maintain a professional detachment. Many years later she would write an article on loneliness, drawn from both her own feelings and observations of others' experiences while at Chestnut Lodge.[60] This article was a kind of catharsis—something she had to do—but she went through real agony before she published it. Although she knew much and had much to tell, Chestnut Lodge was not explicitly mentioned in the article. She felt the staff there had been good to her, that they had given her many privileges, and she put great store in loyalty and confidentiality.[61]

That she was determined to take every opportunity to learn all there was to learn during her winter field experiences can be seen in the very detailed notes she took during her field placements at Bellevue and at Chestnut Lodge.[62] At the end of her 8-week Chestnut Lodge placement, she wrote Bullard a very detailed seven-page, single-spaced, typed summary of her experience, asking for corrections of "my errors in thinking." Bullard apparently had none to offer for he responded simply, merely thanking Hilda for her thoughts.[63] He did, however, write Joseph Chassell, saying, "Thanks for sending Miss Peplau to us. She was a real asset and I am hopeful she will return to us this summer," adding that Chestnut Lodge would welcome more students like her.[64] The benefit was mutual. In her career ahead, Peplau would build on the foundation laid over that winter term at Chestnut Lodge. It would provide the intellectual framework for all her subsequent work. Her work on interpersonal relations in nursing, developed from this foundation, has been described as having had as great an influence on contemporary nursing curriculums as any subsequent nursing theory.[65]

SUMMER SCHOOL FOR THE ARTS

On February 1, 1940, Peplau was invited to join the staff of the Bennington School Summer for the Arts as nurse in charge of all regular medical services, at a salary of $35 a week for the 7-week period from June 29 to August 17.[66] It was here she met Martha Graham, one of the most richly gifted and personally vivid artists in the history of classical modern dance.[67] For Graham, dance was a physical expression of passionate feeling and was seen as a means to explore and illuminate human life and emotions. Martha Graham first came to Bennington the summer of 1935 at the invitation of Martha Hill, a former student of Graham who was then director of the College Dance Division. Some of Graham's most daring early dances were created during the summers when the Bennington School of the Arts was in session. Through Graham, Peplau learned something about near fanatic dedication to one's work. More significantly, Martha Graham exposed Peplau to a range of emotions that Hilda had not acknowledged up to this time in her life. For example, Martha Graham arrived at Bennington with her lover, Louis Horst, a much older, married man, who was also Graham's pianist. The way the two walked around the campus arm in arm, and the looks that passed between them left no doubt as to the nature of their relationship.[68] To the relatively naive, but curious, Hilda Peplau, this was high drama indeed.

Horst and Graham gave witness to passions that were hidden (if they were present at all) in the prim and proper, Bible-reading environment in which Hilda was raised. In Reading, lovers married, and marriage quickly became utilitarian. Great passion and great love were not evident, at least not in view of others. Physically, this particular match—that between Graham and Horst—seemed unlikely. Graham was elegant and graceful. Her dark hair generally was worn knotted low on the nape of her neck, except when she danced and wore it loose and flowing around her supple body. Her neck was truly swanlike, and her head was always lifted—usually looking deeply into someone's eyes, emotion pouring from her own. Horst was also tall, but in contrast to Graham's elegance, Horst was rumpled, with a tummy tending toward the rotund, thinning white hair, and a generally paternal appearance. Yet the passion between the two was not to be denied. Hilda was mesmerized.[69]

She also watched in wonder during the day as young dancers, in their bolero tops and white diaphanous skirts, contorted their bodies in unimaginable but eerily beautiful ways, and she treated their sore feet with pans of hot water and heat lamps into the evenings. When she walked to her residence hall, she invariably passed Martha Graham and Louis Horst lying together on the lawn gazing up at the stars, lost in intense conversation and oblivious to passersby.

At the end of the summer session, Hilda dutifully made her annual visit to Reading, staying with Betty Kreiger (now married to Ted Price), buying what was needed for the family, and checking up to be sure all was well on Church Street. She would also visit Betty's sister Natalie, having her hair done in Natalie's beauty parlor in her home. Emotionally, though, Hilda's home was now in Bennington. While the years at Bennington were vital and critically important for Hilda, the excitement and sense of possibility they engendered were not shared by her family. Her older brother Walter did visit the campus several times before leaving for armed service in Europe in World War II, and Johnny had come to stay the summer before. Her parents, Ottylie and Gustav, however, had no idea what Hilda's life at Bennington was like and never inquired.[70] Once she left Reading they cared only that she supported herself and made no demands on them. By this time, Ottylie's world had narrowed to her kitchen where she continued to cook up a storm, keeping Church Street supplied with donuts, cakes, jams, and rich Pennsylvania Dutch pastries. She had even stopped going to church. She had no good friends in the neighborhood other than Mrs. Koehler next door and Rose Forster, Johnny's grandmother. Because her mother never asked about her work or about Bennington College, Hilda kept her excitement to herself when she visited the house on Church Street, and made her plans without sharing them with her parents.[71] Clara's continued absence was not remarked upon, and Hilda seldom inquired about her older sister. "Home" in Reading was an emotionally lonely place, one she eagerly left behind.

THE MIDDLE YEARS

In the late spring of 1941, Robert Leigh resigned the presidency of Bennington and was succeeded by Louis Webster Jones, a member of the faculty. With the outset of World War II, Dr. Jones thought it might be a good idea if Bennington started a nursing program in conjunction with Putnam Hospital in Bennington. This would be one of the few college-based nursing education programs in the country. Dr. Chassell and Hilda Peplau were enthusiastic supporters of the idea, as were the Bennington board and the hospital physicians. After some preliminary work, Dr. Jones contacted the National League for Nursing Education requesting that they send a representative to explore the possibilities at Bennington. The NLNE dispatched Blanche Pfefferkorn, a prominent nurse educator.[72]

On the appointed day early in the spring of 1942, Mrs. Pfefferkorn arrived, already dubious about this proposal, coming as it did from "outside nursing." The idea was probably derailed at the very first meeting, which had been arranged for her visit in President Jones's office. Introductions were made, and Mrs. Pfefferkorn was visibly annoyed when Miss Peplau, the "executive officer" of the college health service, was introduced. As Hilda extended her hand, Mrs. Pfefferkorn backed away saying, "What are *you* doing here?" She then turned to Dr. Jones and suggested that Hilda leave, as *she* would speak for nursing. Louis Webster Jones, always the gentleman, asked Peplau for her opinion, and, as was typical for her, she stated straightforwardly and unflinchingly that she wished to remain. From that point on, the idea was jinxed.[73] What could have become an innovative jewel in nursing's crown was lost.

Although failing to establish a nursing program at Bennington, the college nurse and executive officer of the health service was making progress in earning her undergraduate degree. A memorandum for the file noted that "Under special arrangement with the President of the College, Hilda Peplau . . . completed one full year's work in June 1942, and was sent a regular June letter."[74] Her four courses taken with Dr. Chassell were all rated as "outstanding." In his report as her counselor, Dr. Chassell recorded that in his course on Psychiatric Concepts her "grasp of material and its implications compares favorably with that of graduate physicians with whom I have done corresponding tutorial work." In Abnormal Psychology, her "paper on 'Shock' shows a distinctly original attack, out of which she might develop a genuine contribution."[75] At this time, the college hired a second nurse with the result that Hilda would no longer have to be on call 24 hours a day, allowing her to take classes more comfortably. On June 18, 1942, she wrote Dr. Jones to thank him and to assure him that "this will not interfere and may improve the performance of my duties, other than the rearrangement of some of my working time which should be a distinct advantage for the second nurse."[76] That summer she took three courses in summer school. In addition to a course taught by Eric Fromm, she took statistics and politics—not an easy load for her.[77] At the conclusion of the politics course, Dr. Robert Lyndenberg wrote:

> Easily the star of the class, through she didn't twinkle as much . . . as I wish, or believe that she could. Exceedingly mature in her approach, she got at the heart of problems quickly, asked intelligent questions, and did far more than enough work. Maybe she should get an outstanding, clearly so in relation to the rest of the class, but I don't feel that in the short time we had, she showed quite the complete grasp that one would demand for that.[78]

Her memory that her statistics course was a "disaster" is not borne out by her file at Bennington. In summarizing her work in Elementary Statistical Methods, the instructor, Eugene Lundberg, wrote: "Unusual conscientiousness, carefulness, and neatness. Work habits of the finest type. Except for the unfamiliarity of the subject, the result would have been outstanding."[79] Finally, Erich Fromm wrote that "she has been responsible and conscientious; has shown great understanding and actively participated in the work. The paper and her work in general were excellent." Fromm rated her "outstanding."[80]

That fall, her English professor, Yvette Hardman, always a hard taskmaster and critic, rated Peplau's academic performance "above average," noting that her limited vocabulary and inability to write about abstract concepts "is often the result of her profound immersion in the words and wisdom of one area of knowledge, not to the exclusion but to the neglect of ways of thinking alien to that one . . . Perhaps the years will broaden her outlook."[81] Something of Hilda's drive and single-mindedness is also captured in this comment: "Other than this she should look for lightness and grace in writing, and these she will acquire when the problems of the war and her own personality have been lifted from her shoulders."[82] Catharine Osgood, who taught Literature and the Humanities, also commented on Peplau's deep interest in psychology and single-minded seriousness: "Her viewpoint is so largely determined by what she has already got from her work with Dr. Fromm . . . She's done all the assignments faithfully, and has obviously dealt seriously with each problem that came up. My recommendation is that she needs to think about 'the tragic sense of life.'"[83] In later years, Peplau would reveal a great sense of humor, a deep sense of the absurdity of things, and a caustic wit. At this point, though, before the maturing experiences of World War II, she was still very much the child of 1232 Church Street in Reading. She had to work too hard to get as far as she had and could not yet relax. She certainly could not play the role of the naive, impressionable college student. She was on a mission, and she had a way to go yet.

Time to Leave

In the spring of 1942, as Dr. Chassell was preparing for his retirement, a new young physician, Dr. Dorothy Hager, was appointed director of the college health service. Although her relationship with Dr. Hager was cordial, Hilda missed the easy comradeship and deep mutual respect that characterized her relationships with Wilmoth Osborne and Joseph Chassell. Perhaps more pertinently, her two brothers, Harold and Walter, had joined the U.S. Army. By January of 1943 Hilda began to think concretely about completing her degree requirements early and joining the Army Nurse Corps.

On May 25, 1943, Peplau wrote to the registrar, Mary Garrett, officially requesting senior status and asking that she be certified for early graduation. In the letter she stated that although she was a "special student" and although her educational profile was nontraditional, she had effectively completed all Bennington requirements. In addition to her work in psychology, and her nursing background, she had taken classes in anthropology, genetics, American government, American political thought, and "Non-rational Expressions of Human Nature."[84] Mary Garrett responded almost immediately, informing Hilda that her work taken to date was "well above senior quality," but urged her in the future to branch out more, insofar as so much of her work was in psychology.[85] She was, however, promoted from junior to senior status. Although her distribution requirements were limited (no foreign language, no history, and no philosophy), Bennington agreed that, under the direction of Joe Chassell, Hildegard Peplau should proceed to write her senior thesis and thus become eligible to graduate at the end of June 1943—because, as she had informed the college, at the beginning of August she was to be inducted into the United States Army Nurse Corps.

In a separate handwritten note to Yvette Hardman, Hilda acknowledged her limitations and let it be known that she was thinking ahead to the years after the war. Clearly, her sense of the ironic was taking form when she wrote, "I *do not want* a degree that this college cannot honestly award to me, but if I decide to work for an MA after the war, gaps could be filled in elsewhere. This would be preferable to being a student here again at the tender age of 38."[86] In June 1943, Mary Garrett wrote to Warren F. Gish, principal of the Evening High School in Reading, Pennsylvania, requesting confirmation that Peplau had received a high school diploma. Mr. Gish's reply contained information of which Hilda was completely unaware, and in fact did not learn until this biography was initiated. To wit: "Unfortunately for her, the school she attended was not an accredited institution. Only in July 1928 was the Evening High School standardized to meet the requirements of the Pennsylvania State Department for Certification. Nonetheless, I can vouch for her graduation in 1928 . . . It was my happy privilege to be one of this young lady's instructors."[87] The ambiguity of the Reading school's credentials notwithstanding, Hildegard Peplau did complete all her college requirements, early, as she had promised. She was awarded a Bennington BA degree in June of 1943, and thus earned the distinction of being numbered among Bennington's pioneer alumnae—those women who graduated in the college's first decade, 1933 to 1943.

Although she left the college behind, Peplau's view of her time at Bennington never changed. During the years she lived there, Bennington took on a special aura, a special pull, a magic and a charm. It was here she began to test the limits and feel the possibilities of life, to sense where her drive, determination, and ambition might take her. Her interest in psychology and psychiatry took on definite dimensions, and her exposure to two great men, Eric Fromm and Joseph Chassell, drove her to aspire to win their notice, if not admiration. One was an almost mythical influence, kind, encouraging, but removed, a man of growing international stature. The other was a daily source of encouragement, a genteel mentor who would continue to open doors for her until she found her footing.

At the same time, however, she had been intensely aware of the social and economic differences between herself and the younger students. Because she felt so different, she did not easily make friends among the students. Rather, her closest friends were fellow staff members and a few faculty members she had come to know in her role at the college health service. So, while the Bennington years are remembered as "magical," her diaries at the time also record acute loneliness—a feeling, perhaps, of being alone in a crowd.[88] In later years, she was nonetheless certain that Bennington College helped her in a major way: It gave her the confidence that she could and would make a mark in her profession. Whether she had gone to Bennington or not, she undoubtedly would have done well, perhaps even as well, but because of Bennington College she went forth armed with the knowledge, insight, hope, and energy that Bennington had awakened, endorsed, and supported.

Years later she was to feel an intellectual loneliness she had not anticipated. After Bennington, she would not again live and work in such a vital and vigorous intellectual community, where truly bright people cared about ideas and valued true creativity. "I have never been able to share or recreate that interplay that went on at Bennington," she said.[89] Despairing of ever finding such interactions or intellectual content in nursing meetings, in later years she would find herself attending meetings of the American Psychiatric Association seeking the stimulation of ideas and original thought. The lack of creative challenge evident in the hierarchies of nursing education was a factor that would contribute to Peplau's sense of professional loneliness through most of her active career.

In fact, the memories of Bennington were so special and so poignant that in future years she was reluctant to return to the Bennington campus for fear the beautiful memories would be challenged.[90]

Bennington was Hilda's gateway to another life, to a new way of thinking, to a world she had never imagined she might be a part of. With the exception of motherhood, no other experience would assume the importance of Bennington College in her life. Peplau was ready for what Bennington had to offer. She relished every minute of it and felt it a privilege just to be there. The college provided her with a stimulating and solid education, an appreciation for the full range of what a liberal education could and should be. It introduced her to upper-middle-class women and their easy acceptance of privilege. It did not overtly encourage feminism, as the term later came to be understood, but at Bennington, Hilda learned that women could be truly professional in their own fields, and could be respected for it.[91] Bennington graduates wanted to contribute something concrete to the world they lived in. Hilda noted that, "Every one of my Bennington friends and classmates had done this; they taught, they acted, they wrote, they painted, or designed houses or gardens. Bennington started the whole trend of women doing something with their lives as well as just living good women's lives."[92]

Bennington nurtured Hilda while she matured. It expanded her horizons and taught her she could do almost anything she wanted to do. Most importantly, though, it allowed her to escape spiritually as well as physically from Reading, Pennsylvania.

ENDNOTES

1. Thomas P. Brockway, *Bennington College: In the Beginning* (Bennington, Vermont: Bennington College Press, 1981). Unless otherwise noted, facts concerning the founding of Bennington College are as presented in Brockway's charming and very readable book.
2. Brockway, 4–5.
3. Helen Lefkowitz Horowitz, *Alma Mater: Design and Experience in the Women's Colleges from Their Nineteenth-Century Beginnings to the 1930s* (New York: Alfred A. Knopf, 1984), 330.
4. Horowitz, 338.
5. Ibid.
6. Brockway, 52.
7. In 1941, the Trustees, with funding from the Rockefeller and Whitney Foundations, commissioned a 2-year outside evaluation of Bennington College and student performance. The study revealed that the first classes (1932–1940) of Bennington students came from conspicuously high socioeconomic backgrounds, over 70% had attended private schools, nearly half had traveled to Europe, 40% were Episcopalian, and in 1940 all but seven students scored higher than "upper-middle-class" on the Chapin Social Status Scale. See Alvin C. Eurich, "An Evaluation of Bennington College," in the Bennington College Archives in the Bennington College Library.

8. Interview, Hildegard Peplau, January 30, 1992.
9. Brockway, 63.
10. Interview, Rebecca Strickney, Bennington College, June 15, 1993.
11. Ibid.
12. Ibid.
13. Interview, Ben Bellitt, Bennington, Vermont, May, 1991.
14. Brockway, 67.
15. Brockway, 108.
16. See clippings about Wilmoth Osborne found in the Schlesinger Library collection, Box 2, #40.
17. Interview, Hildegard Peplau, February 6, 1992.
18. Letter from Robert D. Leigh to Hilda Peplau, June 24, 1937, in the Schlesinger Library collection, Box 8, #270.
19. Interview, Hildegard Peplau, February 6, 1992.
20. Ibid.
21. Ibid.
22. Ibid.
23. Ibid.
24. Interview notes and article found in Box 2, File #45 in the Schlesinger Library collection.
25. Interview notes found in Box 2, File #43.
26. Handwritten autobiography, now deposited in the Schlesinger collection 165.
27. Ibid, 148.
28. See letter of appointment to this committee in Box 8, #271.
29. See Executive Committee notes in Box 8, #271.
30. Interview, Hildegard Peplau, February 6, 1992.
31. Ibid.
32. Ibid.
33. Complete transcripts of notes taken in Erich Fromm's lectures at Bennington College during the years Peplau was there are in Box 9 of the Schlesinger collection.
34. Ibid.
35. Peplau herself acknowledged her insecurities when she remarked in 1992 that "some of the social graces had rubbed off onto me while I was in New York doing private-duty nursing in wealthy homes through the Adele Posten Registry. I was moving out of the working class, into the middle class. At Bennington, I was always treated absolutely as an equal, but I was painfully aware of major differences then." Interview, February 6, 1992.
36. Ibid.
37. Ben Bellitt note to the file, Peplau personal file, Bennington College archives.
38. Interview, Hildegard Peplau, February 6, 1992.
39. Interview, Hildegard Peplau, January 30, 1992.
40. A photograph of the living room art project survives and may found in the Schlesinger collection, Box 9.
41. Interview, Hildegard Peplau, January 30, 1992.
42. Ibid.
43. Ibid.
44. Ibid.
45. Interview, Hildegard Peplau, January 28, 1992.
46. See Box 9 in the Schlesinger Library for a collection of notebooks, case studies, the thesis, and correspondence related to her course work and field experiences.
47. Helen Swick Perry, *Psychiatrist of America: The Life of Harry Stack Sullivan* (Cambridge: Harvard University Press, 1992), 390–395.

48. Interview, Hildegard Peplau, January 30, 1992.
49. Harry Stack Sullivan, *The Interpersonal Theory of Psychiatry* (New York: Norton, 1953).
50. Interview, Dr. Otto Will, September 22, 1993, in Denver, Colorado.
51. Interview, Hildegard Peplau, February 11, 1992.
52. Frieda Fromm Reichman, "Notes on the Treatment of Schizophrenia by Psychoanalytic Psychotherapy," *Psychiatry 11,* (1948): 263-273.
53. Interview, Hildegard Peplau, February 11, 1992, and autobiography, 158.
54. Ibid.
55. Ibid.
56. Ibid.
57. Perry, *Psychiatrist of America,* 197.
58. Interview, Hildegard Peplau, February 11, 1992.
59. Ibid.
60. Hilda E. Peplau, "Loneliness," *American Journal of Nursing* (December, 1955): 1476–1481.
61. Interview, Hildegard Peplau, February 11, 1992.
62. These voluminous notebooks are found in Box 9 in the Schlesinger collection.
63. Letter from Dexter M. Bullard to Hilda Peplau, February 15, 1942, unnumbered file, Box 9, Schlesinger Library collection.
64. Letter from Dexter M. Bullard to Joseph O. Chassell, February 23, 1942, ibid.
65. See Phil Barker, "Reflections on Peplau's Legacy," *Journal of Psychiatric and Mental Health Nursing 5* (June 1998): 213–221. The entire issue of this journal is devoted to an overview of the Peplau legacy to nursing. "It is a legacy that will survive and continue to serve the profession well into the 21st century." Grace Sills, in this same issue, 171.
66. Letter of appointment, Box 8, #272.
67. On Martha Graham see: Agnes de Mille, *The Life and Work of Martha Graham* (New York: Random House, 1991); Martha Graham, *Blood Memory* (New York: Doubleday, 1992); Marian Horosko, ed., *Martha Graham: The Evolution of Her Dance Theory and Training* (Chicago: Review Press, 1990). Graham was but one of a number of famous dancers who were attracted to Bennington and the Summer Arts program. These included Hanya Holm, Jose Limon, Eric Hawkens (who later married Graham), and others.
68. Interview, Hildegard Peplau, February 11, 1952.
69. Ibid.
70. Interview, Hildegard Peplau, January 30, 1992.
71. Ibid.
72. Correspondence between Louis Webster Jones and the National League for Nursing Education, Files, Office of the President, Bennington College Archives.
73. Interview, Hildegard Peplau, January 10, 1992.
74. Memorandum for File Re: Hilda Peplau, July 30, 1942, in Peplau Personal File at Bennington College.
75. Ibid.
76. Note found in her Bennington Personal File.
77. Bennington College records, 1941–1942.
78. Dr. Robert Lyndenberg, July 23, 1942, Memorandum for Peplau Personal File, Bennington College.
79. Dr. Eugene Lundberg, ibid.
80. Erich Fromm, ibid.
81. Yvette Hardman, ibid.
82. Ibid.

83. Kit (Catharine) Osgood, ibid.
84. Letter from Hilda Peplau to Mary Garrett, May 25, 1943, Bennington Personal File.
85. Letter from Mary Garrett to Hilda Peplau, May 27, 1943, in Box 8, #271, Schlesinger Library collection.
86. Undated handwritten note from Hilda Peplau to Yvette Hardman, in Bennington Personal File.
87. Letter to Mrs. Mary Garrett, Director of Admissions, Bennington College, from Warren P. Gish, Principal, Standard Evening High School, Reading, Pennsylvania, June 10, 1942, found in Bennington College Personal File for Hilda Peplau.
88. Personal diary, Box 2, #38, Schlesinger Library collection.
89. Interview, Hildegard Peplau, January 30, 1992.
90. Ibid. Peplau did return to Bennington on at least two occasions: when her daughter Letitia Anne applied to Bennington, which she attended for a year, and for Hilda's own 50th class reunion, when, as she anticipated, she found the experience disappointing.
91. Interview, Hildegard Peplau, January 10, 1992.
92. Ibid.

World War II: Coming Into Her Own

4

There are two cultures now. Mine and yours . . . But I and every soldier here have been exposed to a rare experience—the privilege of seeing what real stress does to people and to their relationship with others.
—Hildegard Peplau
August 17, 1944

By mid-1942 the impact of the war in Europe was being felt on campus. In June the students had been issued ration books for meat, sugar, butter, and eggs, which they turned over to the dining halls. Bennington put much of its acreage under cultivation and the college began to raise its own chickens, cattle, and hogs. Some students were planning to put their college careers on hold to join the Women's Land Army, which was dedicated to raising food crops for the war effort. Hilda Peplau, however, had decided that before the war was over she wanted to serve—not in the Women's Land Army but in the *real* army. One slow afternoon in May 1943, she drove down the long hill into the town of Bennington and, like her brothers Harold and Walter before her, enlisted in the U.S. Army. On May 25, 1943, in her letter requesting early graduation, Hilda informed the college that "on August 5, 1943, I shall be inducted into the Army Nurse Corps."[1]

Hilda left Bennington in July of 1943 and drove home to Reading to say good-bye to family. After a week in Reading, she took a train to New York City to conclude romances with two men she had dated on a casual basis throughout the Bennington years. That done, she flew to Pittsburgh (her first airplane ride) to be inducted. From there she would go by bus to Deshon General Hospital in the small town of Butler, Pennsylvania.[2]

As a recent Bennington graduate, and a fairly confident if not yet altogether poised woman of 32, Hilda was beginning to feel somewhat worldly and sophisticated. For the trip to Deshon, the designated wartime military hospital for the western Pennsylvania area, she donned her one summer dress and new white gloves and pinned a small bouquet of glass flowers, made by her sister Bertha, in her hair. When she arrived at Deshon, Hilda's newfound sense of sophistication was quickly deflated. Her commanding officer, Captain Anna Barry, was not about to give her any encouragement. Frowning, the captain's scathing opening words to the new enlistee were, "You mean, you came all this way in an airplane with glass in your hair?"[3]

World War II provided the first opportunity for women in the armed forces to become officers. These new officers, Captain Barry among them, would prove over time to be a trial to Peplau. It is hardly surprising that Hilda Peplau would have started off on the wrong foot with Anna Barry, but it was not the glass flowers that did it. Like many of her fellow nurse officers, Barry was a hospital-school graduate and a career army nurse who had found herself promoted to the rank of captain once the war was underway. There was no way that this Captain Barry was going to allow herself to be upstaged by this all-too-tall, all-too-attractive, all-too-confident *college*-educated nurse. Peplau, in turn, due to her age and specialized training, was eager to contribute to an encouraging and stimulating learning experience for the younger members of the corps. But Barry had her own ideas about the role of army nurses in general, and more particularly about Hilda Peplau. She made it unequivocally clear early on that she was not interested in Peplau's ideas—and she quickly made it clear who was in charge here. Hilda requested assignment to a special unit being given psychiatric training in preparation for immediate shipment to the war zones. Barry, in turn, assigned her to the home-front contagious disease ward at the Deshon General Hospital.

ARMY NURSE CORPS

Letters to Bertha from Deshon Hospital reflect the ups and downs of Hilda's first months in the Army Nurse Corps. At first, it seemed that Hilda clearly intended to enjoy herself. In mid-August she wrote asking Bertha to send her "the green coat, the red shoes, and *a hat*." Beginning a correspondence that would continue throughout the war, Hilda's letters, however, soon reveal instead an impatient, intense, highly motivated young woman. They are full of news and interesting observations about the military and its training and about the absurdities of military life, as well as long lists of things for Bertha—then a teenager of seventeen—to attend to at home, and requests and instructions for things to be sent to her.[4]

Captain Barry notwithstanding, Peplau's abilities were readily recognized at Deshon Hospital. Less than a month after arriving at Deshon, she wrote Bertha that on her 18th day in the Army she had become head nurse, and on her 26th day she had been recommended to the School of

Military Neuropsychiatry in Atlanta, Georgia. Hilda realized, however, that her chances of actually getting there might be slim because "it means transfer to another command which is sometimes difficult to execute."[5] She did not know just how prophetic her words were, for by September 15 she complained, "Captain Barry is trying to sabotage the opportunity because she is afraid I'll return here for life. After nine days of arguments and cold, bitter silence . . . the transfer was signed." Then, almost immediately, the School of Military Neuropsychiatry was closed. As Hilda wrote Bertha, "I must have left my lucky charms at home."[6]

After a miserable month on the Deshon Hospital contagious disease ward, where she had tried to keep her counsel and stay out of Anna Barry's way, serendipity struck. Hilda was transferred to night duty on the psychiatric unit as punishment for constantly challenging what she saw as incompetence. The patients on the psychiatric ward were actually prisoners, soldiers who had attempted to go AWOL and had then done something drastic to avoid the guard house, such as shooting themselves in the foot or attempting suicide, Hilda wrote.[7]

Her disappointment about the recommended transfer to the School of Military Neuropsychiatry was quickly left behind, as she forged ahead. Hilda's energy and ideas were appreciated. "The three medical officers on the psycho ward are overjoyed because they like my work. They are really good guys and have gone all the way with me in letting me reorganize the ward."[8] It was a busy and chaotic time. On October 2, she wrote that hundreds of new patients had arrived, casualties of the war in Europe, and "we have had to open six new wards. The usual army way—without organization, plan, or pattern."[9]

Even here, where her talent and drive were recognized, Peplau could again have been in trouble but for the good fortune of finding herself under the command of an excellent physician. The relationship began rather ominously, however. Although Hilda was where she wanted to be, she was appalled at what she found on the psychiatric ward. The hospital's chief psychiatrist, Major Robert Kemble, MD, was noted for making surprise rounds at night to assure himself all was calm and in order on the ward. It was certainly calm. The patients were nearly catatonic from boredom. There was absolutely nothing for them to do. The patients received no therapy; there were no radios, and television had not yet become part of everyday life; there were no games, no discussions, no diversion other than the patients' ever-present cigarettes.

Peplau's second night on the ward, Dr. Kemble appeared for one of his unannounced inspections. He found a cigarette butt on the floor and marched out without a word to the nurse. The next day a memo came around announcing there would be no smoking by anybody at any time on the ward. That night, the young soldiers were even more deeply depressed. When she got off duty, Hilda walked directly to the doctor's

office, knocked, marched in, saluted, and with no preliminaries asked to
be transferred. When asked for a reason, she told the doctor that he had
unjustly penalized sick young men for something more likely done by a
corpsman or a cadet nurse—a cigarette discarded on the floor rather
than in an ashtray. She stated her firm belief that this was no way to run
a mental health ward and castigated him for his lack of imagination.
"Young lady," replied Major Kemble, "do you know I could have you
court martialed for this insubordination?" "No," she replied, suddenly
shaken. The major suggested instead that she sit down and tell him
what *she* would do in these circumstances. Hilda did sit down and proceeded to tell him that first of all he should order the nurses and the corpsmen, not the patients, not to smoke. Furthermore, she said, the patients
needed things to do. They needed a program, a routine—exercise, bas-
ketball games, ping-pong. Dr. Kemble followed her suggestions, and
together they began to record the progress made by the men on the
ward.[10] Thus began a long friendship, one that was to last through the war
and well into her ensuing career. Thus too, began a pattern that would
characterize Peplau's subsequent work: tension with nurses, support
from doctors.

Hilda's relationship with Anna Barry continued to deteriorate, to the
truly petty level. The weather was turning cool, and when the nurses at
Deshon Hospital were issued overcoats Peplau did not receive one. After
a tense exchange of letters, a special order just for Peplau had to be
issued. She finally received her overcoat, but it was too small. Because
she did not have an overcoat, she missed several days of routine exercises. Hilda expressed her frustration about the captain, writing to Bertha
on October 2 that "she's senile, incompetent, impotent, and scared."[11]
Three days later she wrote,

> Big doings here!!! These new 600 patients aren't taking this mediocre
> stuff very well . . . They've gotten up a big petition . . . I am all for the
> patients too . . . [but] that 2 x 4 battleaxe must show her power. One of
> her incompetent stooges is in charge of the day shift and I, the only one
> with psychological experience, get night duty. Of course, I've more out-
> let for working directly with the patients at night—it's the principle
> that gripes me. The day charge nurse gets the patients stirred up and I
> have to quiet them down at night. She treats them like prisoners and
> criminals. I'm having a heyday writing night reports. She says "patient
> is a liar." I say "patient fantasies thus and so." She says "patient imag-
> ines he has a pain." I say "patient has a pain, which to him is real and
> supported by dreams of battle, etc." Then when she makes census mis-
> takes, etc., I write to the effect that "by actual count." Needless to say,
> we are not friends at all . . . If she's considered responsible, let her prove
> it is my game.[12]

Indeed, this was Hilda's game. Demanding the highest standards of herself, she was not tolerant of incompetence in others. She could be exceedingly kind to those who were truly handicapped—in whatever capacity, physical, mental, or emotional—but when persons around her had responsibilities, she expected them to make every effort to meet them. If they did not, her frustration quickly escalated to rage. This pattern would create difficulties throughout her professional life.

One week after writing Bertha of her disdain for Chief Nurse Barry, she wrote again, expressing puzzlement and incomprehension about the role she herself played as the target of Barry's hostility:

> My name is certainly mud around here—for some reason, unknown to me, Captain Barry has decided to focus all of her hatred of people and jealousy of young, intelligent nurses on me. Every day there is something new—she means to ruin everyone's opinion of me and so far she hasn't been able to do it . . . I'm supposed to be neglecting my work by talking to patients—for my own benefit. For my own benefit!! That's how much she knows about psychotherapy.[13]

Hilda had determined by this time that she would continue on her own to expand her knowledge of the field. The previous day she had written asking Bertha to find anything she could written by "Harry Stack Sullivan, Cantril, Maslow, Mittleman," and to order these materials for her. Classes were starting for the doctors, she explained, and perhaps, if she were up on the material, they would let her, too, attend these classes.

At this time, Hilda was writing Bertha almost daily. It seems that she was desperate for conversation, particularly about her work. With no one to talk to, she wrote Bertha a day-by-day account of her successes and frustrations. Although Bertha was 10 years younger than Hilda, the sisters clearly grew quite close through this correspondence. Their brother Walter was already overseas, and wrote warmly, affectionately and often, on tiny V-mail letters from the front. Walter, like Hilda, expressed some frustration with the army but was better able to take it in stride. He wrote Hilda from the war zone on September 14, 1943, relating that Bertha was most impressed that Hilda had graduated from Bennington (which is the only indication that any member of her family took notice). Walter continued, "But then who wouldn't be with a sister that is always outdoing herself. No kidding HEP, you have the driver's seat in the Peplau family and this little boy here is ready to take orders anytime. It was always that way though. Suggestions from you always went a long way."[14] One suggestion Hilda had not made, however, was the matter of who should purchase the coal for the house at 1232 Church Street. Walter had given instructions on this matter, and Hilda was annoyed that she had not been consulted, for in a letter sending a check to Bertha for the coal, she admonished her to "put down that Walt owes me $25 for it, since it was his idea."[15]

Peplau was fascinated with the problems brought to the hospital by the frightened and traumatized young soldiers and appalled at the treatment, or, more accurately, the lack of treatment, available to them. During October her letters are concerned with patients having "battle dreams with hysteria like convulsive seizures or suicidal intentions." She recorded her frustration at not being able either to offer or to get the help she could see the men clearly needed. She feared that if she reported the more severe cases,

> They'll be sent to psycho without treatment or worse still, they'll be put on a detail gang cleaning spittoons . . . It's a crazy business and its fine to talk about the larger issues—only the impatience bred by frustrations of a place like Deshon contributes nothing constructive to the war. No wonder these boys wonder what their comrades died for.[16]

More of Hilda's candor emerged when she wrote to Bertha on October 22 that, "The captain is actually leaving October 31 . . . They are taking up a collection . . . to buy her a farewell gift. I refuse to be a hypocrite, so I am not contributing, and furthermore I'd rather celebrate . . . They say that any nurse who has the age plus the qualifications may ask for a 1st Lt. promotion and take an exam." In the same letter, she explained that, "Patients transferred out keep coming back at night to talk or write me letters for advice. In psychiatry we call that transference—or falling in love with the person who will help you to grow up. It's a ticklish proposition."[17]

Hilda's social life at Deshon seemed to flourish. She wrote Bertha that she had just come back from a show in the auditorium after which four officers took "two of us to the PX for a *root beer*! . . . One was a colonel, one a major, and two were captains." Letters from a former boyfriend expressed his disappointment that Hilda was not around New York or Reading to join "Bert" (Bertha) and other friends in making the rounds of the clubs and bars. Apparently Hilda did not share this regret, as she wrote to Bertha that, "All in all, I manage to keep myself busy, the corpsmen on the jump, and the patients happy."[18]

ON TO ENGLAND

In early November a routine form was circulated asking nurses to list their qualifications and inquiring whether they felt they were being used to the best effect in the Army Nurse Corps. Hilda responded with her increasingly characteristic thoroughness and honesty. Not able to fit her information onto the one-page form, she attached several extra pages. On these she outlined her pre-Bennington experience as a private-duty nurse in Reading and Pottstown, her training at Mount Sinai and Bellevue in New York, her responsibilities at Bennington, and her field experiences with the well-known New York psychoanalyst Dr. David Levy and Frieda Fromm Reichman at Chestnut Lodge in Maryland. Feeling quite proud of herself, she took the form and addendums to Dr. Kemble for comment before submitting them. Dr. Kemble read Hilda's response carefully, raised an eyebrow here and there, and finally remarked that he supposed she had a duty to report all this, but added that, "It's my guess you'll be on the next boat."[19] This was precisely what Hilda wanted to hear. She hoped to be in England by Christmas. Kemble was right. Almost immediately after submitting her form and its addenda, Hilda received orders for immediate reassignment to a military hospital in England. She was given a 2-day leave to return to Reading to see her family, collect whatever she wanted to take to England with her in the single footlocker issued to her, and store her other possessions. She took a train to Reading for a quick 2-hour visit with her family and went on to New York where a former boyfriend, Bill Borman, met her for a day and a half on the town. They ate at Sardi's and saw a few shows before Bill took her to the assigned pier in a taxi.[20]

Hilda joined 75 other nurses as they began signing onto the ship. One by one they entered a large, spooky, completely empty terminal on the pier. The nurses were dwarfed by the surroundings. Far in one corner was a simulated boat where the young women were instructed on how to climb over the railing and down and up rope ladders. Many of the nurses were terrified of the height, and the young second lieutenant assigned to this teaching function let them off. Hilda, however, considered herself in reasonable shape (although she was nearly 10 years older than most of the other nurses) and quickly climbed over and down and back up again. She considered the whole exercise "stupid." She remarked, "It had nothing to do with sustenance in a cold ocean. And, this was the sum total of my army training!"[21]

As darkness fell, several thousand soldiers joined the 75 nurses and they all marched aboard a huge ship, which turned out to be the Queen Elizabeth, converted to a troop ship. Below decks, any evidence that this had been a luxury liner had been for the most part obliterated. Staterooms had been converted to bunk rooms for the nurses, with 12 to 16 women to a room, sharing one bathroom. The senior officers, two to a room, were assigned the remaining staterooms. The soldiers, on the other hand, slept all over the ship, under tent awnings pulled across the decks, in the recreation rooms, and anywhere there was space for a prone body. At midnight the ship set sail into the cold, November Atlantic.

At least 1 among the nurses carried an influenza virus aboard with her, and soon, Hilda recalls, all 75 nurses had the flu. It was cold, and raining, and rough at sea, and the soldiers too were becoming ill. As the nurses went among the troops ministering to the sick, they were of course spreading the flu virus, which added to the general misery aboard the ship. Because this was wartime, the ship zig-zagged its way across the Atlantic to avoid detection by enemy forces. By the time it arrived in Scotland, this was a shipload of truly miserable new soldiers, who were met by the Red Cross, which administered hot tea with milk, blankets, and sympathy.[22]

The debilitated nurses were put aboard a train and sent to London where they were assigned to a large house in Grosvenor Square. The house was elegant on the outside, but the inside, like most English houses of that day, was cold and drafty. One room contained an enormous bathtub on a platform, and the nurses took turns heating water and sitting in the tub. With 75 sick women sharing one tub, bathing and recouping was a slow and tedious process. Hilda, who had trouble breathing, was sent to an eye, ear, and nose clinic where the harried physician squirted pure sulfa powder up her nose. She had never felt such pain; but the drastic treatment did clear her sinuses.[23] Hilda discovered she actually did feel better and found the energy to begin an exploration of the city. In this she was accompanied by Lt. Fred Fuller, a dashing young man who wore an eye patch and whom she had first met aboard ship. Over the next 2 weeks they sought out the pubs and theaters together, dashing back to Grosvenor Square before the wartime curfew plunged the city into darkness. London was being bombed regularly, but, with Fred, Hilda quickly found herself a part of a fun-loving group, one not altogether oblivious to the fact that they were in the midst of a war.[24] They danced at Claridge's, had high tea in Grosvenor House, located favorite pubs, and became quite adept at finding the nearest shelter when the bombs began to fall.

Upon their arrival in London, the nurses were "unassigned." Hilda hoped to be assigned to a psychiatric facility, but—counting on what she had come to believe was the prevailing illogic of military orders—decided that her chances of getting the assignment she truly wanted would be improved if she requested instead the army's one eye, ear, and nose facility, which she knew was not in need of additional staff. Whether by happenstance or design, the ploy paid off. Hilda and two friends were assigned to the 312th Station Hospital for Military Neuropsychiatry, which had just been established to coordinate treatment for all cases of acute neuroses occurring on the European front.

Beginning on December 23, 1943, most of Hilda's letters home arrived on the tiny, photographically reduced V-mail ("V" for Victory) forms used in overseas correspondence during World War II. In her careful hand, Peplau began to record her experience of the war in England in letters sent home to Bertha and to Walter, who was still on the front in Italy. At first it all seemed a great adventure. Hilda was excited to be assigned to the 312th Military Hospital. The fantasies came to an end, however, when an army vehicle showed up to take Hilda and her friends north into the English Midlands—and their new duty station. The cold ride in the back of the truck was bone chilling, the rain was grey and dismal, and the countryside flat and dreary.

THE 312TH MILITARY HOSPITAL

The 312th Station hospital and School of Military Neuropsychiatry was located at Shugborough Park, near Stafford in Staffordshire, in a valley adjacent to the River Trent, on the estate of the Earl of Litchfield. It was housed for the most part in the cylindrical corrugated steel "Nissen huts" used in the First World War, and again in the Second, as military shelters. While these prefabricated huts were quick to assemble, they did little to keep out the bitter cold of the English winter. Most of the Nissen huts at the 312th had tented extensions that offered even less comfort. As the war wore on, the tent city expanded to accommodate ever larger numbers of patients.[25] It was pretty miserable, Hilda wrote, as "the area in general is damp and foggy and climatic conditions are not ideal."[26]

Once on base, the nurses were processed quickly and assigned to their quarters. After the grandeur of London, they felt cramped and cold in their Nissen huts with only small potbellied coal stoves for heat. Here, the days of gloom began. The cots were hard, the blankets not adequate for warmth, and the grey drizzle was unremitting. The one comfort, the coal stove, polluted the air and made breathing difficult. Hilda maintained that the sun shown only 2 days during the year she spent at the 312th. The six women in Hilda's hut, however, got along well, and two in particular—Anne Anton and Letitia "Tish" Towsen—became Hilda's close friends. The women quickly made the hut their home. When someone was transferred to a different location, possessions that could not be taken along were placed on a table in the officers' mess for anyone to claim. One day Tish Towsen came back with a bottle of apple blossom perfume. Just the thing to eradicate the ever-present smell of coal dust, she thought. She sprayed the hut liberally—and a swarm of bees came out of hibernation seeking apple blossoms! It was a long time before the hut was cleared of them.[27]

At 5:30 a.m. the bugle would blow, and the six hut-mates would shiver into their uniforms and appear outside for inspection—which they never passed. Something always seemed to be amiss. At first, Hilda was upset, but after a while decided to chalk up the inspection failures to the general absurdity of life in the army. For their misdeeds, however, the nurses were ordered to march. Hilda and Charlotte Stahler were the tallest women there, and hence they were always in front with the shorter women marching behind them. The sight of the two ramrod straight, tall, determined nurses marching through the marsh with most of the nurse corps behind them became commonplace at the 312th. The sergeants soon gave up trying to get them to shape up, and they were allowed to mix it up as they marched: long steps, short steps, any ol' steps. In the evenings, as the hours of daylight lengthened, the hut-mates often hiked out into the countryside. They got to know many of the neighbors, and soon were trading rations of sugar and cigarettes for fresh vegetables and especially milk.[28] Hilda truly loved milk all her life, and drank a quart a day whenever possible.

Hilda did have trouble conforming to the army routine. When things were done wrong—or when the way they were being done simply did not make sense—she complained, in writing, making suggestions for rectification. Such suggestions were not appreciated. To her chagrin, her nemesis from Deshon Military Hospital soon appeared at the 312th and admonished her in a letter shortly thereafter: "In the nurse corps we do not question the ability of our superiors, as they would not be placed in that position unless their knowledge of the work was greater than yours."[29]

The 312th Military Hospital nonetheless was a great assignment for Hilda Peplau. It had been established as a 750-bed hospital and neuropsychiatric rehabilitation center in April 1943. Lt. Col. Ernest Parsons had taken command in late December of 1943 and remained in command until August of 1944, when Lt. Col. Lewis H. Loeser took over. The regular admission of patients began at the same time that Colonel Parsons and the nurses arrived. It was a hectic time. The 312th's annual report for 1944 noted that "there was a rapid rise in the admission rate during the early months" and that the bed capacity of 824 was almost immediately expanded to 1,164. The report further noted that "only eleven of the medical officers could be classified as neuropsychiatrists on the basis of previous training experience." Of the 11 psychiatrists, 1, Major Jay L. Hoffman, served as chief of professional services and another, Major Paul V. Lemkau, was chief of neuropsychiatric services, chief medical officer, and directed the school, "leaving only nine for the actual overseeing of patients."[30]

Because there were so few psychiatrists, an outstanding faculty was drafted from among America's leading medical schools to spend time at the 312th, teaching physicians trained in other specialties to function as psychiatrists during the war. The armed services were not prepared for the emotional toll of war on young men under the stress of battle and the continuing confrontation with violent death. Thus, in crash courses ranging from 1 to 6 weeks in duration many pediatricians and gynecologists, as well as a few surgeons, became "psychiatrists." The short courses, developed for the more senior physicians, were quickly adapted to give psychiatric training to recently graduated medical students drafted as officers and shipped to the 312th to be "trained for specific tasks."[31]

Although the rain was never ending, the skies were always grey, and living conditions were rugged, there was a bright side to life at the 312th.

The nurses, physicians, and other officers gathered in the evenings around the fireplace at the officers' club. Young enlisted men kept the fire going, the officers shared rationing cards in order to keep the bar open, and visiting psychiatrists spent many an evening there discussing the day's cases, sharing their thoughts on the care of the battle scarred, or simply scared. Peplau joined the group as often as possible. It was here that she met the noted psychiatrist William Menninger, who was then chief psychiatric consultant to the Office of the Surgeon General, and other notables in the field, such as Albert Strecker from America and John Bowlby of England. For Peplau these evenings were a continuous seminar, building on the core of psychiatric theory she had first encountered in her course work at Bennington and then observed in the practice of psychotherapy at Chestnut Lodge.

In addition to the discussions, she read everything she could get her hands on. In January 1944 Hilda had asked Bertha to pay her bills promptly, as she had subscribed to the *New Yorker*, *Time*, and *Reader's Digest*, thus beginning a lifelong habit of subscribing to an ever-widening array of popular and professional publications. She was anxious for the magazines to arrive, as she clearly craved reading, the more serious the better. Huddled in her Nissen hut, as near to the little potbellied coal stove as she could get, she would read the time away. In the evenings, if not on duty, or before going on duty, she was often to be found by the fireplace in the officers' club, sipping scotch and discussing ideas with whatever group she could gather. Soon she was badgering Bertha to send the latest journal articles relevant to all she was learning and observing in England. In May she wrote impatiently asking Bertha keep her eyes open and clip newspapers and magazines, seeking "articles which pertain to psychiatry for me as few come my way." In addition, she informed Bertha that

> I have acquired the habit of writing for journals, etc. and telling them to send the bill to you. You'd better establish the policy of just sending checks to whoever asks and then let me know. It is good to get the various journals and I have just written for additional ones. As far as the more academic ones are concerned, it's the only way to sustain the intellectual spark.[32]

From this date until the end of the war, she mentioned articles of interest as she regularly read *War Medicine* and *Archives of Neurology and Psychiatry*.[33]

The hospital had many visitors, including congressmen, senators, and distinguished scientists and physicians from both the United Kingdom and the United States. Any time lectures were given and she was not on duty, Hilda was there, along with the "visiting greats," as she called them.[34] The informal discussions and general lectures were not enough for her, however. They only whet her enthusiasm for the subject. Hilda soon sought and was granted permission to audit all the classes for physicians. In these courses she came to know personally the hospital chiefs, Paul Lemkau, from Johns Hopkins, and Jay Hoffman, who after the war would direct the Veterans Administration Hospital in Bedford, Massachusetts, as well as Dr. Howard Fabing from Christ Hospital in Cincinnati who served as director of the 312th's "School of Neuropsychiatry." Dr. Hoffman, in particular, was curious about and then most supportive of the intense nurse who sat in on classes in her spare time and took everything she learned very seriously. Peplau soon became a part of the team. This was on-the-job training in every sense of the word. Hilda was learning the practice of psychotherapy from everyday experience, from lectures, reading and discussion, and from observation and interaction with the officers/physicians assigned to the unit. In the course of the war she was to meet many men who were or would become important in American psychiatry after the war.

COMBAT NEUROSIS: A LIVING LABORATORY

The army was well aware that combat exhaustion, or "battle fatigue," was a major problem at the battlefront. A field manual on the subject issued in 1945 estimated that roughly 30% of soldiers would suffer from some variation of combat exhaustion during their tour of duty and noted that prior battle experience provided "no prophylaxis against those breakdowns."[35] In one division, according to the manual, 82% of the cases were among veteran troops. The soldiers most likely to develop these "disabilities" were those pinned down by mortar fire for prolonged periods of time.

The psychiatrists tried to develop effective forms of emergency treatment on the front lines, but many young men could not go forward into battle again. These were sent, in varying degrees of shock, to units farther back. When men remained unresponsive, they were medically evacuated out to the 312th Military Hospital in Staffordshire. According to the School of Military Neuropsychiatry manual on the subject:

> The rule of treatment is that the acute neurosis must be attacked clinically in the same way that the acute abdomen must be attacked. This condition must be regarded as an emergency and treatment must be instituted immediately. The two fundamental conditions of treatment are that narcosis [drug-induced unconsciousness] will be employed and that the treatment be carried out in the forward battle area before the field medical officer who knows he must induce narcosis at the earliest possible moment . . . Combat exhaustion will be treated immediately wherever it is encountered from the battle aid station back to the evacuation hospital.[36]

Thus, the medical officers at the 312th were instructed to induce narcosis at the earliest possible moment for those soldiers who had been evacuated from the front. The sedative of choice was sodium amytal. The standard treatment was to give the soldier hot soup, then 6 grains of sodium amytal, and put him to bed.[37] If this did not produce deep sleep, further administration of the drug was advised, all the way up to 12 or even 18 grains as "enough of the sedative must be given to produce sleep quickly."[38] The hope was that the patient would sleep around the clock. At regular intervals the nurses were to awaken the patients and assist them in relieving bladder and bowels, give them fluids, and then another dose of sedatives. This procedure was continued from 48 to 72 hours.

Because it was recognized that patients coming to the hospital were suffering from "neuroses complicated by lack of sleep, exhaustion, insufficient food, loss of weight, and decreased morale," a patient who had not yet "recovered from the clinical manifestation of his combat exhaustion" after 2 to 3 days of intensive narcosis, was started on a period of sub-shock insulin therapy lasting from 5 to 7 days. In these cases high-caloric forced feedings were added to the treatment regime. According to hospital files, in this period "the average patient eats 12 lbs. (plus) food per day while under insulin and gains an average 1 lb. per day while under treatment."[39]

If, however, the patient showed signs of hysteria, such as hallucinations, more extreme measures were adopted: Intravenous pentothal or intravenous sodium amytal were to be given until the "conversion symptom is obliterated." If neither intravenous sodium amytal nor pentothal were available, the medics were instructed to use ether.[40]

The leading proponent of the drug-induced, deep sleep therapy (DST) adopted at the 312th Military Hospital was Dr. William Sargant, a psychiatrist at St. Thomas's Hospital in London. Sargant, who advocated DST as a treatment for a range of psychiatric disorders ranging from depression to schizophrenia, was a frequent visitor to the 312th and was very interested in the military uses of DST. Sargant's use of deep sleep therapy in his own practice involved putting patients to sleep for several weeks with large doses of barbiturates and tranquilizers in order to "rest the brain," giving it a chance to recover from trauma. Patients who were treated with DST often also were given electroconvulsive therapy (ECT) during this "sleep" period, a procedure that some psychiatrists thought had the effect of wiping the brain clean.[41]

A few doctors at the 312th used these battle-shocked, amytal-dosed patients for their own experiments. They tried new mixes of amytal to induce mental states mimicking schizophrenia. One physician, Anthony Sampliner, went much further. In addition to the amytal, Dr. Sampliner would drip ether onto a mask held over the patient's nose to induce astasia abasia, or the inability to stand up and walk. The patient in this state

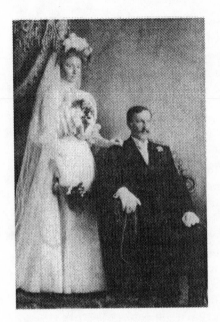

Hilda's parents.

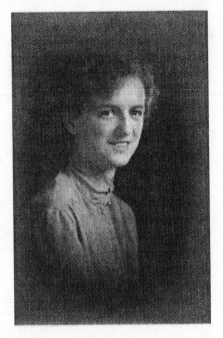

Hilda around age 18.

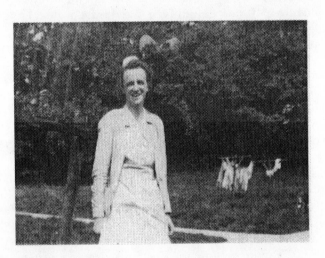

Hilda as a young nurse.

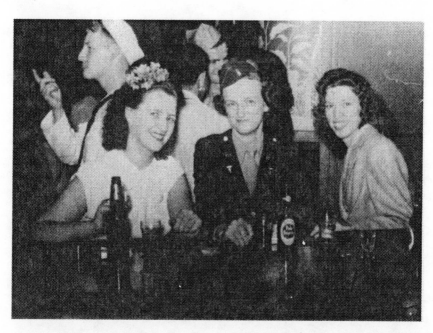

Bertha, Hilda, and Ginny Rentz at the Melody Inn in Reading, PA, 1945.

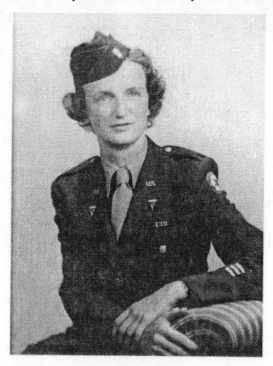

Hilda in her military uniform.

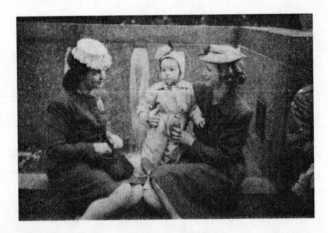

Bertha, Baby Tish, and Hilda at Radio City, in New York City, 1946.

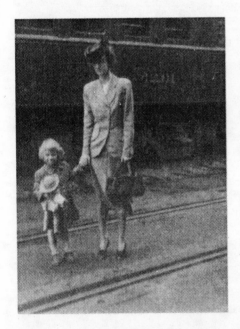

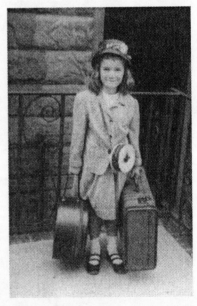

Hilda and Tish dressed for a train trip, 1948.

Tish is packed and ready to go to Cape Cod with Hilda for a vacation, 1951.

would enter a twilight zone, then begin to talk. When the ether was removed, the atasia abasia symptom would disappear but the patient would show symptoms of full-blown schizophrenia. Sampliner was fascinated by this phenomenon, and expanded these experiments as more young men arrived from the field. His practices produced "utter contempt" on the part of Peplau, and she became determined to do what she could to rescue patients from him.[42]

During the time Peplau was at the 312th Military Hospital, induced sleep involving the administration of sodium amytal remained the standard initial treatment for the battle-scarred soldiers, followed, if deemed necessary, by insulin treatment—treatments that Peplau believed to be "obscene." Through the ever-present drizzle, the trucks would arrive, and the young, limp soldiers would be carried off through the mist and unceremoniously dumped into bed where the amytal was administered and where they slept out the week. Hilda very early on let her views be known regarding this procedure. Throughout her year at the 312th, she had many discussions with both Paul Lemkau and Jay Hoffman urging modifications in the prescribed routines. She was certain that the treatments were both wrong and harmful. This conviction would continue into her later career when she actively crusaded against both lobotomy and electroconvulsive therapy as acceptable treatments in American psychiatric hospitals, believing that "talking" therapies were the ethical and effective approach. In expressing her concerns at the 312th, Hilda ultimately would be vindicated. After the war, it was Sargant, the leading advocate of deep sleep therapy, who himself sounded an alarm, describing DST as "the most problematic of all methods of physical treatment in psychiatry."[43] Today it is thoroughly discredited as a mode of treatment in such situations.

While Peplau did provide routine nursing care during the first part of the soldiers' hospital stays, when they were mostly asleep, she succeeded for a time in establishing, as patients awoke, the one-on-one bedside talk therapy that would become central to her own emerging theory of psychotherapy. Hilda had observed that patients, while in an insulin-induced sub-coma state, often exhibited signs of delirium. A patient might believe, for example, that a food cart rolling down the plank-board walkways outside the unit was a cannon and so would become increasingly agitated. To cope with these symptoms, Peplau experimented by having a corpsman sit beside a patient's bed as he awakened to try to get the patient to talk through rather than act out his frightening memories. As the patient began to calm down, he would be drenched in perspiration. Peplau would wipe his brow, encourage him to remain calm, and give him orange juice. In this way, many patients were spared the amytal and the more extreme DST treatments advocated by Drs. Sargant and Sampliner. Peplau's methods eventually would become incorporated into the standard treatment routines at the 312th.[44]

At the end of the 10 days of amytal and insulin treatment, the less severe patients had had a lot of sleep and had gained weight. They were then taken to the "training section" for further rehabilitation, which was where Hilda determined she would make a difference. She found that when they awakened from sleep therapy, the men were flaccid, disoriented, and often depressed. Many felt that because they had not withstood the rigors of battle they were failures. Those with stronger constitutions worked themselves back into shape, but others remained depressed, not caring whether they made it or not.

Observing the range of individual responses, Peplau began to work through group therapy and individualized care and treatment in an effort to help restore a soldier's sense of self-worth and dignity. She sought and was given permission to move patients out of the huts and tents as they woke and take them to the kitchen, where it was warm and where they could talk. Soon, groups of groggy patients were sitting around a kitchen table talking. Hilda was aware that she was not a sophisticated interviewer or a trained psychotherapist, but she knew both intuitively and from experience that talking was important. She'd make eggnog and toast and just keep the men talking. The topics were wide ranging—the weather, the war, home, sports, religion. If one or another seemed particularly agitated or showed an interest in continuing the conversation after the group dispersed, she would take him on long walks, talking, talking, talking.

After the massive invasion of Normandy by U.S. troops in June 1944, the workload at the 312th dramatically increased, and the psychotherapy group discussions Hilda had introduced and about which she felt such a sense of accomplishment, had to be dropped. Admissions were limited to combat cases from the continent. The initial observation period was reduced to a matter of hours, and patients were routinely treated with sodium pentothal and occasionally with ether. The emphasis became physical rehabilitation and the maintenance of "firm military discipline." At this time, according to an army hospital report, the fact that a soldier admitted to the hospital would be returned to duty "was taken for granted." Upon completion of the hospital treatment, the soldier was to be transferred to a training battalion where he would be reintroduced to long drills, retraining on antitank guns, and a requirement that he pass through a "qualification course" on the rifle range. The report acknowledges that, "There may still be some who are unable to become reaccustomed to the sound of rifle fire. They are given further treatment, until they regain their composure and the training is complete." The writer of the report justifies the accelerated remilitarization of combat-shocked troops with the sardonic observation that, "The comfortable hospitable attention and distance from a combat zone removes the one incentive needed in the treatment of nervous patients—the desire to return to the job."[45]

As a result of her Bennington internships at Chestnut Lodge in Maryland and her close attention to Henry Stack Sullivan's lectures while there, Peplau's own ideas about psychotherapeutic treatment were based on Sullivanian principles. From her interaction with the men on the wards, and her disapproving observations of the treatment they received, she began to formulate and then to implement her approach to psychotherapy. Sullivan's basic premise was that personality was formed largely through interaction with other personalities, and thus was in essence the product of "interpersonal relations." The core of anxiety, according to Sullivan, was an effort to avoid that which makes one uncomfortable, or anxious. Peplau worked with the soldiers to identify that which was factual and to accept reality, including the reality that to experience anxiety in the face of the brutal act of killing in war was a rational response. This was not accepted military dogma. Nonetheless, through her discussion groups Peplau had tried to get this message across to the men she met and with whom she worked during her tour at the 312th Military Hospital. This anxiety, which she called "combat neurosis"—and which the military identified in a more provisional way as "combat exhaustion"—was the semantic forerunner of what is known today as post-traumatic stress syndrome. During all this time, Hilda kept prodigious notes on her patients, recorded her thoughts on treatment, kept notes on lectures, summarized group discussions, made outlines, and made detailed notes of her reading. At the end of the war, she brought all this material back with her, and it provided the foundation of what later would become her first major publication, *Interpersonal Relations in Nursing*, published in 1952.

A SPECIAL FRIENDSHIP

Just as Hilda's intellectual life at the 312th was intense, so was her social life. She was popular not only because she was attractive and the ratio of women to men was 1 to 10, but also because her seriousness, together with her ability to have a good time, were valued by men whose very lives were at risk. In January 1944, Hilda complained to Bertha that "dates are a problem here. They are too plentiful." She also assured her sister that she had plenty of money, as her dates were paying for everything, and if anything was needed at home, she would pay for it. She reported that "the pubs are a great institution in England" and made dating easy. She was careful to assure Bertha, however, that the dating was not serious, but "just good times." Relationships were fast and intense, the guys came and went. You "love them, but with your heart whole, because it's a matter of days before you'll be separated."[46] She did admit, however, to meeting one new "true friend," a meeting that ultimately would change the course of her life. On January 16, 1944, less than a month after arriving at the 312th, she wrote to Bertha that:

> On my visit to London I met another wonderful guy—Deep South stuff—we did up the town and again parted for opposite ends of this war. So, I'm the original sad sack. "There's something about a soldier." So Army life is not dull from the social standpoint, but remember me—it's from the professional life that I hope to make my mark.[47]

On February 8, 1944, she reported to Bertha that she was again seeing this "*wonderful* guy . . . a southern . . . medic, very nice, though married . . . I spent Sunday afternoon wandering through the local village and nearby woodlands with [him]. That's one way to make sure you see the scenery." By February 15, she reported that "Mac the medic has gone and I'm resting." A month later the new friend, whom she continued to identify only as "Mac," had returned, for on March 12, she wrote, "This part of the country is very beautiful. Today is particularly lovely and I'm itching to be out walking with that 6 ft. 3 in. [friend] I've been seeing a lot of." She then mentioned that "he leaves on the 18th . . . and there is still work to be done on his combat jitters."[48]

Unbeknownst to Hilda, as her friendship with Mac was developing, there had been a tragedy in Reading. Her mother, Ottylie, had died unexpectedly of a heart attack on February 25, 1944. Bertha had cabled the news through the Red Cross, but Peplau's superior, the Chief Nurse, had neglected to find Peplau to give her the cable. She remembered eventually, but by that time Hilda had learned of the death in a letter from Bertha.[49] When that letter, dated February 25, arrived on March 14, the news it conveyed was totally unexpected and came as a great shock. Bertha had written:

> Dearest Hildegard,
>
> Today has been a hard sad day. There always seems to come a time when one must do something that is harder to do than anything else has ever been—that time is now. I suppose you have received the cable I sent through the Red Cross and know that mother passed away today at noon. Very sudden . . . heart attack yesterday . . . called father at work . . . got the doctor . . . resting very comfortably this morning. Another one at noon . . . With great weariness and a smile she went to her eternal rest.
>
> It's desperately sad around here today, Hildegard, and I have never longed for anyone as much as I long for you right now. I feel so very lost—and with two motherless orphans on my hands too—one as bad as the other [a reference to their adopted brother, Johnny, and to their

father, Gustav] . . . I kissed her a tender farewell for each of you. But her last words were "take care of my Johnny." And our big Boy Scout is after all a little boy and missing his mother very, *very* much. So help me, Hilda—I miss her too.[50]

In an interview in October 1994 Bertha recalled that,

Mother may have been sick, but who knew? She had a heart attack. She had taken to bed, which was unheard of. She was very sick all night, but she insisted that I go to work . . . It was the fausnachts that did her in. It was Fausnachts Day—feasting on fattening donuts—the Pennsylvania Dutch equivalent of Mardi Gras. Fausnachts were my mother's specialty—big fluffy dough, fried in deep lard, then shake them in bags of nutmeg. Gorging on these was the way to begin fasting for Lent. I'm sure that's what did my mother in. She was only about sixty-two years old.[51]

Although Hilda felt her mother had been emotionally remote during her childhood, her devastation at the time of Ottylie's sudden death was total. She felt very alone and vulnerable. Not inclined to lean on others, she found herself turning to Mac for comfort and support. On March 18 she wrote her sister that thanks to Mac she was dealing constructively with mourning for their mother, that Mac had rescued her from the defensiveness and excuses of those responsible for the mislaid cable, and that she had been given an 8-day leave. She wrote,

At the moment I am in Winchester [where Mac was stationed]. Three days here and then my friend—who got a four day leave—and I will go to Bournemouth . . . Last night the post where Mac is stationed had its first dance. It was a gala affair with steak for dinner and Irish whiskey and good music . . . I let myself enjoy most of it . . . We are staying in the vicarage with warmed sheets and pajamas, breakfast on a tray, fresh toast, and marmalade, seeing the countryside . . . having a great recuperation . . . Tomorrow we go to Bournemouth . . . Bless Mac, he called the Red Cross and managed to get rooms for us. They're scarce you know, and you sign a lot of papers to stay anywhere.[52]

The countryside near Bournemouth to which Mac took Hilda was indeed beautiful and soothing. A myriad shades of green, from the patchwork quilts of the cultivated land to the golden hues of the open fields, rolled toward the muted Channel sea. The road dipped through the dales where forests protected spotless villages and then climbed up again to the open land where the sea breezes blew to refresh the senses. Here the sheep wandered free and unfenced, unfettered by the ancient dry stone walls that marked property boundaries created by their two-legged fellows in the valleys below. Human tragedies seemed far away—whether they were war raging across the Channel or the grief on Church Street in Reading, Pennsylvania. Here the villages faded into the glory of the countryside and the glistening gentle sea. Earth and air met at the water. Here Hilda could let go of her rage and sorrow.

That Mac was stationed in England during this time was a blessing for Hilda. The week's leave and the trip to the southern English seashore, allowing for long talks, hours of comforting, and time to enjoy the sea and the sun, were amazingly therapeutic. Over the next month, Hilda wrote often to Bertha, telling of Mac's steady attention and successful efforts to secure days of leave and the use of a command car for long drives into the countryside, walks along the seashore, and trips to the "sunny south." There were visits to London, strolls along the city streets, and more talk. "Mac had made me walk, talk, and eat. You can't imagine me in that predicament, I know. But this was a blow to me. I never expected it. I have healed in Mac's very protective care." Still, she cautioned that "this is not a romance—make no mistake about that—but he is a very special guy."[53] Later still, she again referred to him as "a southern gentleman . . . and while up here he was a sad sack . . . after three campaigns. What I did for him then, he does for me [now], and it was his second dose of therapy to be able to do something for me."[54] On April 2, she told Bertha that her off-duty hours continued to be spent "touring, wining, and dining" with Mac. She had recovered enough of her spunk to strongly advise her sister to get help at home and to use the money accumulating in her bank account to make improvements and changes at 1232 Church Street. She concluded with the notation that "Mac continues in his protective role. At times like these it helps to have someone who cares."

From her letters we know that this was a special relationship, a special friendship at a time when Hilda was emotionally shattered, in a war zone, away from her family, and thus highly vulnerable in every way. The letters reveal how fortunate she felt to have the friendship of one so protective, so careful, and so giving. Yet Hilda remained extremely circumspect when it came to revealing, even to Bertha, any personal facts related to Mac's identity or his life as it existed before, or would exist after, that tumultuous year. Decades later Hilda clearly treasured memories of this time and this relationship, but continued to maintain the public silence with regard to Mac that she had kept since the spring of 1944.

It is now known that her friend and companion was a physician, whose MD was from the University of Pennsylvania. While Hilda in her letters to Bertha describes Mac as a "medic," he was in fact a surgeon when he was drafted into the army and sent with other American physicians to the 312th for the crash course in psychiatry. It was known at the 312th that Mac and Hilda became friends, but the fact was not necessarily notable, as such pairings were common during the war. At the conclusion of his training, Mac was appointed division psychiatrist for the Ninth Infantry Division and stationed in Winchester on England's southern coast. As a military psychiatrist, he was sent to the front to treat soldiers suffering from combat neurosis. It is evident from Hilda's letters that Mac himself suffered from the stress of earlier combat experiences (as is indicated in her references his to "jitters" and the "therapy" she offered him).

In the final months before her death in 1999, Hilda Peplau talked more about this very special man. Mac was probably the first man in Hilda's life who was her intellectual equal. The boys and men she dated in Pennsylvania were kind, decent, and fun-loving fellows, but not interested in ideas. With Mac, Hilda could talk about psychiatry, medicine, philosophy, and so on—as well as have fun. The contrast between his intellectual interests and those of her earlier boyfriends was striking to her. He was disdainful of people who were stupid or intellectually lazy, as was she.[55]

Given his rank as an officer and the fact that he was stationed at Winchester, Mac was able to visit the 312th with some regularity. He came immediately when Hilda notified him of her mother's death, and, similarly, made the trip when she was so ill with flu that she had to be hospitalized. Hilda was also able to visit Mac at Winchester, traveling there by train, where they continued their custom of taking long walks. Often they would sit by the river and talk. If it was very cold, they would go to Winchester Cathedral, where they would sit in a pew to talk, or visit with the rector who became a friend. At other times in Winchester, they would go to the top of the Old Bailey (the courthouse and jail) to continue their long and wide-ranging conversations. With the help of the Red Cross, which made travel arrangements for soldiers, they were able to book separate rooms in "bed and breakfasts" when they traveled together, and frequently they took small gifts of candy or canned fruit to the families that ran these establishments.[56]

Love was an issue that Hilda did not easily or willingly discuss, but it is safe to say that she loved the southern doctor in an unguarded, but nonetheless careful, way. She would later describe the relationship as a "love match" and a meeting of "soul mates." She observed that Mac was "very smart and observant. He was quick witted and humorous. He was very kind and tender." He was certainly very solicitous of her. Moreover, he was there in Hilda's time of emotional need, providing the care and nurturing she needed. She valued his company, the quality of his mind, and his thoughtfulness of her. The war letters between them show a profound personal respect, together with the appreciation of knowing one another under such stressful conditions. The question of a future, the question of "commitment," was simply not asked, nor even suggested on either side. The fact that he was married was the impediment barring any consideration on her part that they might share a future. Both seemed to have had a healthy sense of reality, an acceptance of time and place in the moment, and a deep appreciation for the essence of the other. There was no pressure on either side—simply a sharing of thoughts through extraordinary experiences, a moment in time. April 1944 was for Hilda a time of healing and renewal. It was probably the first time in her life that she felt truly loved by someone not a part of her immediate family.

In her work and her commitment to expanding her own knowledge of her field she felt a renewed enthusiasm. On April 14 she reported to Bertha, "I do what I can do. Rules are rules and my personal opinions might upset the censor." She seemed to have learned from her unhappy experience at Deshon Military Hospital in Pennsylvania. Mac's presence in her life seems to have softened her temperament somewhat, for she commented,

> My soldierly behavior remains exemplary, but below the surface my opinions remain the same. I am teaching on a ward these days and having a wonderful time with some of the enlisted men—those who want to learn and care enough. These nurses are a rigid lot and prefer to be defensive and prove that they need not learn new things . . . You get less rebellious as time goes by—you find a friend who sees what you see and you quietly raise an eyebrow instead of your temper. It's so good for the facial muscles too![57]

In addition to the many references to Mac, Hilda also often mentioned a major in the paratroopers who dropped in for long chats in front of the officers' club fireplace. "Sure is a nice fellow." If things had turned out differently, the tall, "nice," and unmarried paratrooper might have replaced Mac as her steady companion and escort, but he was quickly sent back to the front. In May, she continued to tell of going to London to meet Mac, and of the unending struggle to secure food, a drink, a room, a seat on the train, and other ordinary necessities and niceties.

About this time, toward the end of May and into early June 1944, Hildegard began to ask Bertha to send boxes of candy, particularly Fanny Farmer chocolates, and assured her that "I'm in the pink, though I find myself getting a lot of sleep these days." She saw a lot of Mac during the month of May, mentioning on May 11 that she had a 24-hour leave to go to London to see him, and later remarked that "the beauty of the city surpassed itself." She told Bertha on May 13 that she had seen Mac for his birthday and asked that a picture of her be sent for him, as well as a gift of two books for his birthday. On May 17 she reported, "Mac appears here today for a few days, and so I expect that this week will not be dull," and on May 22 that she had "just got back from a twenty-four-hour leave. Saw Mac." On May 26, she wrote that, "Mac and I were taking in the sunshine, walking through the [Winchester College] grounds, talking and talking," and then, on May 31, she asked again for a photograph, stating, "I never thought Mac would turn sentimental and want one, but there is just nothing to do about it but get it." This would be a request she repeated in every single letter every single day for the next month! She was impatient, allowing no time for the transatlantic mail.

By the end of May widespread anticipation of an Allied push into German-occupied France heightened as each day passed, and personal mobility become a problem. Hilda and Mac were both pushing the limits in their efforts to gain precious leave days and to acquire transportation by any means. Hilda had agreed to meet Mac in Winchester over the first weekend in June but suffered some apprehension over the trip. Military police were much in evidence, and as she traveled south she observed massive troop movements headed, it could be assumed, toward the coast. In fact, the tension was so great that Hilda phoned Mac, saying perhaps it would be best if she did not come at this time.

> Mac said if I didn't come, he'd be disturbed. So, I took a deep breath, got on the next train, and my fingers practically grew together I kept them crossed so tightly . . . They say there are only two kinds of soldiers—the caught and the uncaught . . . Your sister has not yet been recognized . . . For once I wished I were an ostrich. I acted like one.[58]

The trip down and back was indeed an adventure. Mac had received his promotion to major and, Hilda wrote, "there was much celebrating to be done . . . We did it." She added, however, "I saw much and was apprehensive to get 'home.'" Hilda left Mac on June 4, a Sunday evening. Forty-eight hours later, on June 6, the Allied amphibious assault on the beaches of Normandy was launched: D-day had arrived.

By June 12, Hilda was despondent, reporting that "Mac is on the beaches of France . . . Sherman was right, war is hell!" Mac was not part of the D day invasion but crossed the Channel on "D plus four," four days after D day, to set up field clinics. Hilda reported that, "The D-day was a great shock for me . . . It dawned on a Tuesday, after I'd been down to see Mac and returned on Sunday evening." She later wrote, "The colonel was in the celebrating party Friday and says I deserve a medal for courage. That's not what it was! It was sheer devotion to Mac, who's already been through Italy, North Africa and Sicily . . . When I left Mac on Sunday, it was good-bye."[59]

For all practical purposes, this was the end of the happy hours of walking along the seashore and through the lovely old town of Winchester with its famed Winchester Cathedral. Mac was again in a combat zone, and Hildegard had returned to the serious work of caring for the wounded and traumatized.

EFFORTS INTENSIFIED

As the military offensive and casualties mounted on the front, so did the challenge of the work at the 312th Hospital. Hilda wrote faithfully and prolifically to soldiers now in battle, and daily to Mac. As she reported to Bertha, both the 82nd and 101st Airborne "are in," and in each she had friends among the doctors, the product of long bull sessions on subjects relevant to mental health and life on the front lines of war, and she wrote often to these friends as well. "All are 30-day wonders—converted from obstetricians, mostly," she commented.[60] As the archival files attest, Hilda was a thoughtful, engaged, and faithful correspondent, writing literally dozens of letters every week to "her guys." The letters written to her from the front, although careful and censored, nonetheless make clear the value of her correspondence to the men at war.[61]

While she was duly impressed with the "great umbrella" formed to protect the D day invasion, Hilda cautioned, "Let me not hear of any rejoicing. So much of it is ugly!!!" She admitted to frustration at being limited to behind-the-scenes work, but nonetheless felt that "I've done a lot—here and there a GI Joe needs the kind of thinking I dish out—and they appreciated all those near-sighted medics I brow-beat into daring to humanize themselves despite the army."[62]

Although she was working very hard, and there were rewards in the appreciation expressed by those she had touched, a bit of resentment was also evident: "They let me teach here until the home team learned a little. Then they pinned silver on *them* and stuck me off in a corner."[63] Soon her letters home began to reflect frustration at the lack of promotion. Although she was confident she was doing excellent work, the obvious acknowledgment was not made. She was not alone, however, for no promotions were processed at the 312th during the latter part of 1944 and into 1945. The annual report for 1944 noted that the obstacles had been both technical and administrative, and for the "most part, unnecessary." Unimportant changes in circulars, the return of incorrectly prepared papers, and changes in jurisdiction accounted for most of the denials.[64] In May 1945, when Hilda did receive her promotion to the rank of first lieutenant, the 312th commander, Colonel Loeser, noted in her file that "she has carried out her assigned tasks in a superior manner with vigor and enthusiasm."[65]

Peplau's work was being noticed, and the feedback was good. "Now I hear occasional praise, and at the moment the colonel is perusing my scrapbook of articles on war psychology." With Mac gone, however, her repressed sarcasm was returning to the surface. "I say I got my B.A. at Bennington, but my B.S. here—and I don't mean science!"[66] Although the army and its regulations were frustrating and the protection of incompetence maddening, she was confident that she was learning and that she was making a contribution, at least in individual cases. At the end of June, 1944, she was at the top of her form, feeling well, sleeping well, and experiencing some sense of accomplishment from her work with the "30-day wonders"—despite the void left by Mac's departure and the acknowledgment of the reality of her mother's death. She did note that Mac's surgical days might be over, as he still had bouts of battlefield "tremors," but added hopefully that "he has the potential to be a good psychiatrist."[67]

At this time, the frequency of Hilda's twice-weekly letters to Bertha began to drop off notably. In the only letter to Bertha in July, written toward the middle of the month, she reported being busier than usual, especially with her efforts to keep up the correspondence with the "psychiatrists at war." She wrote that she was now in charge of a "rather important ward" and pleased with her work. She was now finally permitted to do things in her own way, and wrote,

> In an informal way, I have a school in my office. I learn about war and I hold up the mirror so the boys face themselves for a change. It is not a picnic, nor a milk run, and anyone who says it was is due to lose the front set of teeth, at least . . . Perhaps I haven't mentioned this before because I fully expect to be removed and replaced by some 1st Lt. who can barely read and write . . . Mac keeps kicking me to be a "good soldier," and by now I'm willing to sing in the choir in order to retain this job. I have all combat cases, and there's no doctor, although several drop in all day to see their own patients and watch me work.[68]

After that July letter, there is not another until August 17, nearly a month later. This letter is long and the tone intense, but the subject matter is professional.

> I've been exceptionally busy—holding down an exceptionally large and important ward . . . No doctor holds office hours. I'm in charge. The turnover must be rapid and the speed depends on my organizational ability and upon how quickly I can size up a guy's trouble. They good naturedly call me slave driven—and that I am![69]

She reported that she routinely worked 10 to 12 hours a day, while the other nurses worked 8. One day she was transferred from her ward to full-time teaching, "but three nurses couldn't manage to cover what I did in a day. It bemused me! So back I came—and that's probably my job for the duration." She attests that the job is "fascinating," and clearly found a kind of fulfillment in the tension of the job and comfort in the fact of being needed.

In this same letter Hilda went on to relate that she'd taken a trip to Scotland and indicated that the trip had given her time to reflect on the nature of her work and contributions. Indeed, it seemed that in this period, when her correspondence was slim, Hilda was consolidating her experience and giving deeper thought to the meaning of what she had learned and where she would take her growing understanding of her wartime experience. A soldier traumatized by battle and sent back from the front, she wrote,

Can wallow in grief, terror, awe of whatever it was to him—or view it in light of a changing order of reference . . . It's incredible that a nation can mobilize ten million men, send them off to fight for several years, then demobilize them and expect them to pick up their lives as though nothing has happened. It's like the flip of the coin—you're picked or not picked, you fight or stay behind the lines.

These boys need sympathy—lots of it—they've seen so much. But that sympathy must be of a *rational* order . . . There are two cultures now. Mine and yours . . . But I and every soldier here have been exposed to a rare experience—the privilege of seeing what real stress does to people and to their relationship with others. It is an experience which can add or detract from their personal growth—and the army can control most of the things we do but it cannot touch our ability to integrate one more new, even painful, experience and to make it add up constructively—for us and for society as a whole . . . For the boys the horror of war will be like the normal period of grief (as was the horror of mother's death to the people on the block)—anything that lasts longer is self-pity or even a new way of enhancing one's status without continuing constructive contributions.[70]

From this letter, one gets the impression that Peplau was preaching to herself, that she is projecting the reality of her own life plans onto the total war experience, while trying too to put Mac's experience of the war into perspective. She sees that her work is important, and she is determined to take advantage of all the experiences she has had, including the experience of tenderness and love, and fit them into a life of "continuing constructive contributions."

There are no other letters in August. On September 6 she wrote Bertha that she "had an uneventful 35th birthday." Again, this letter is lacking in personal information, focused instead on thoughts about her work. She observed that

Some of the boys think I'm wonderful when I point out this stuff—I am always helping them to save face in a rational way (when they have temper tantrums, for example) and boosting their self-esteem along the lines of the total picture. All of us have integrity of a sort—what happens to it under battle conditions is a man's business but if he's socially responsible he'll maintain it in a constructive way. He'll grow with the time.[71]

The only other letter written in September and preserved in the archives was written on September 25, when Peplau wrote a short V-mail note, mentioning the classes she now instructed. On October 3 she reported that she was continuing to work on the same ward, anxiously following the news from France (an obvious reference to Mac's whereabouts), and noted disparagingly that it was still raining. On October 7 she wrote again, mentioning that she had a day off in which to catch up on her letter writing—"i.e. the weather, the rain, the cough and the wheeze." She also mentioned, "that bank account is a grave concern to me now as the chance of this unit getting home becomes a possibility." She also talked about the continuing training of "medics" in emergency methods of psychological treatment and mentioned that all of her hutmates had gone to London for a visit but that she had not accompanied them.[72]

In fact, early in July Hilda's loneliness and abrupt termination of companionable times and shared moments with Mac took on new significance. It began to dawn on her that her ability to sleep well, in spite of worries about Bertha's coping with the situation in Reading and her concern for Mac and her other friends on the front lines in Europe, had a cause. She began to acknowledge that something she had not expected, and for which she was not prepared, had probably happened. She could no longer ignore the changes in her body. She was becoming certain—she was pregnant.

ENDNOTES

1. Letter from Hildegard Peplau to Mary Garrett, May 25, 1943, Bennington Personal File.
2. The town of Butler was known not so much known for its hospital as it was as the birthplace of the U.S. Army Jeep. In the summer of 1940, the army was quietly trying to rearm its forces in anticipation of being drawn into the war in Europe, including finding a successor to the unwieldy two-ton trucks that had been used in the First World War. When the call went out for the creation of a lighter, more mobile field vehicle, it was the Bantam Car Company with factories in Butler that responded with the prototype for the all-purpose four-wheel drive jeep. See "Built First in Butler," *Pennsylvania* (April, 1993): 18. Bantam, however, had not patented its prototype, and the government feared the little car company could not mass produce its vehicle quickly enough when war came. Thus, once the United States entered the war, Ford and Willys-Overland were given the contract to produce the Bantam prototype. Butler, however, retained the credit for the production of the first Jeep, as the blue-collar town returned to steel production for the duration of the war. The Deshon General Hospital was converted to the Deshon Military Hospital for the duration of the war.
3. Interview, Hildegard Peplau, February 10, 1992.
4. Letters from Hildegard to Bertha Peplau, Box 3, Files #60–73, Schlesinger Library collection.
5. Letter from Hildegard Peplau to Bertha Peplau, September 10, 1943, Box 3, #64.

6. Ibid, September 12 and September 14, 1943.

7. Ibid, September 15, 1943.

8. Ibid, September 17, 1943.

9. Ibid, October 2, 1943.

10. Interviews, Hildegard Peplau, February 10, 1992, and Dr. Robert Kemble, March 23, 1993, in Sarasota, Florida.

11. Letter from Hildegard Peplau to Bertha Peplau, October 2, 1943, op cit.

12. Ibid, October 5, 1943.

13. Ibid, October 12, 1943.

14. Letter from Walter Peplau to Hilda Peplau, September 14, 1943, Box 3, #66.

15. See correspondence between Hildea, Bertha, and Walter Peplau in Box 3, #65–66.

16. Letter from Hilda Peplau to Bertha Peplau, October 16, 1943.

17. Ibid, October 22, 1943.

18. Ibid, November 1, 1943.

19. Interviews, Hildegard Peplau, February 10, 1992, and Dr. Robert Kemble, March 23, 1993.

20. Diary notations and notes from Bill Borman were found in Box 3, #72.

21. Interview, Hildegard Peplau, February 10, 1992.

22. Ibid, and letter to Bertha Peplau, December 2, 1943, Box 3, #66.

23. Interview, Hildegard Peplau, February 10, 1992.

24. Diary notes in Box 3, #72.

25. Annual Report, 1944, 312th Station Hospital, U.S. Army Archives, Washington, D.C.

26. Interview, Hildegard Peplau, February 10, 1992.

27. Ibid.

28. Details taken from V-notes written by Hildegard Peplau to Bertha Peplau between January and April, 1944 found in Box 10, #300.

29. Letter from Anna Barry to Hildegard Peplau, December 14, 1943, in Box 10, File #300.

30. Annual Report, 312th Station Hospital, 1944, U.S. Army Archives, Washington, D.C.

31. The Director of the "School in Neuropsychiatry" was Major Howard D. Fabing. While at the 312th, Peplau argued "endlessly" with Fabing about "endlessly giving electric shock treatments to young soldiers for just about anything." Years later, after the war, Dr. Fabing sought her out at an APA meeting in Cincinnati, and insisted that she be at his hospital at 7:00 the next morning. At 7:00 the next morning she was at the hospital, in a room, with a patient where he proudly unveiled a new machine, one to just "tickle" rather than shock the brain. He wanted her to see that she had inspired him to modify the shock treatment. As she commented, "it was a great improvement, but I still didn't approve." Interview, Hildegard Peplau, February 11, 1992.

32. Letter from Hildegard Peplau to Bertha Peplau, May 23, 1944.

33. Letters from Hildegard Peplau to Bertha Peplau in Box 3, #69.

34. A collection of Peplau's notes from her wartime reading in neuropsychotherapy, and her lecture notes, group discussion notes, and protocols may be found in Box 10 in the Schlesinger Library collection. She was a thorough and prolific note keeper. This collection alone is worth a PhD dissertation into the treatment of mental illness during the war in active war zones.

35. Combat Exhaustion: From the School of Military Neuropsychiatry" (312th Station Hospital, APO 513, U.S. Army, 1945), 2, found in the Army National Archives, Carlisle Barracks, Carlisle, Pennsylvania.

36. Ibid, 12.

37. Interview, Hildegard Peplau, February 10, 1992.
38. "Combat Exhaustion," 13.
39. Materials found in army files of the 312th Station Hospital, marked "secret," but reclassified under the Freedom of Information Act, National Army Archives, Carlisle Barracks, Carlisle, Pennsylvania.
40. Ibid, 14–15.
41. Melanie McFadan, "The Endless Sleep," *The Sunday Independent* (Edinburgh, Scotland, June 28, 1992): 8.
42. Interview, Hildegard Peplau, February 11, 1992.
43. McFadan, "The Endless Sleep."
44. Interview, Hildegard Peplau, February 10, 1992. See also extensive notes kept by Peplau in Box 10 in the Schlesinger Library collection.
45. Historical Report, Hq. 312th Station Hospital, April 1 to September 30, 1944, 3.
46. Letter from Hildegard Peplau to Bertha Peplau, January 5, 1944.
47. Ibid, January 16, 1944.
48. Ibid, March 12, 1944.
49. Interview, Hildegard Peplau, February 11, 1992.
50. Letter from Bertha Peplau to Hilda Peplau, February 25, 1944, Box 3, #66.
51. Interview, Bertha Reppert, Mechanicsburg, Pennsylvania, October 30, 1994.
52. Letter from Hilda Peplau to Bertha Peplau, March 18, 1944, Box 3, #67.
53. Ibid, April 23, 1944.
54. Ibid.
55. Notes from Anne Peplau to Barbara Callaway, February 12, 1999.
56. Ibid.
57. Letter from Hilda Peplau to Bertha Peplau, April 14, 1944.
58. Ibid, June 12, 1944.
59. Ibid, June 17, 1944.
60. Ibid.
61. Even then Peplau had a sense that life's events have an importance of their own; thus she saved letters received from the front during the war, as well as asking Bertha to save all the letters written home. The entire collection is in the Schlesinger Library and contains a wealth of information about the day-to-day life at or near the front in Europe toward the end of World War II. It is clear the men were seeing a lot of battle, and that the nurse who took them seriously during their stays at the 312th played an important role in helping them to keep their composure.
62. Letter from Hilda Peplau to Bertha Peplau, June 19, 1944.
63. Ibid, June 20, 1944.
64. 312th Military Hospital, Annual Report, 1944, 25, National Army Archives, Carlisle, Pennsylvania.
65. Found in Personnel File #291111, unclassified under the Freedom of Information Act, and sent to Hildegard Peplau at her request.
66. Letter from Hilda Peplau to Bertha Peplau, June 24, 1944.
67. Ibid, July 1, 1944.
68. Ibid, July 18, 1944.
69. Ibid, August 17, 1944.
70. Ibid.
71. Ibid, September 6, 1944.
72. Ibid, October 3, 1944.

Transitions 5

I have settled the score with my conscience long ago . . . and consequently am almost nil on being self-conscious. It is certainly La Grande deception, and when the day of reckoning here occurs . . . I shall still have some of this backbone left.

—Hildegard Peplau
December 18, 1944

Hilda's realization in July of 1944 that she was pregnant—and the period of intense introspection that followed that realization—explains the sudden absence of the usual frequent and often breezy letters sent to her sister Bertha from the 312th Military Hospital in England. She had been writing at least twice weekly, but after mid-July weeks went by with no letters at all. When Hilda did write, the letters tended to be short V-mail notes, brief and relatively impersonal. Obviously, the intensely personal situation in which she found herself now consumed her mental and emotional energy.

It seems clear that early in her work at the 312th, if not sooner, Hildegard Peplau had confronted and made her peace with a prevailing dilemma for talented, ambitious young women of her generation: A woman might pursue a career, or she might marry—seldom both. Although she had always thought marriage was a difficult challenge under the best of circumstances, she apparently briefly reconsidered that assumption early in her army career. During the war she met many men with whom she seemed to have much in common, not just the experience of the war, but fascination with the mental work that it brought. The long conversations before the officers' club fireplace at the 312th, and the socializing during off-duty hours had caused her briefly to imagine that a marriage quite different from that of her parents just might be possible. There were several officers in her orbit, single and eligible, who held out possibilities she may have considered. Her mother's death, the relationship with Mac, and subsequent developments put an end to any such fantasies. Once Hilda determined that she would become a single mother, she never again seriously considered the possibility of marriage. In point of fact, Hilda was uncommonly dedicated to pursuit of a meaningful career in nursing, and by the end of the war she clearly believed that her opportunities for the greater service—and the greatest potential influence on her chosen field—lay in earning an advanced degree. There is no doubt that her wartime experience, and her struggles with the nursing and medical hierarchies at the 312th Military Hospital, reinforced her commitment to acquire the academic credentials she would need.

In 1944, while the war was still raging, a remarkable law was passed by Congress to reward the millions of Americans serving in the war effort. This was the Servicemen's Readjustment Act of 1944, known more simply as the G.I. Bill. Hilda was excited. The financial means for further study would be at hand when she returned home. In essence, the G.I. Bill guaranteed that the U.S. government, recognizing the sacrifices made by the men and women who served in the war, would subsidize a college or graduate or professional school education, or provide assistance and preference in finding a job for every veteran when peace came. Peplau knew immediately that she would take advantage of this legislation. She would, she concluded, become one of only a few nurses at that time to earn an advanced degree. Hilda had confided as much to Bertha in January of 1944, shortly after her assignment to the 312th Military Hospital:

> I like the job and am glad to be here . . . This is a station hospital and I can tell you little about it, but it all adds up to what will be some of the footnotes in my thesis—and to some of the ideas expressed in an earlier paper which I've written which *will* be the master's thesis eventually.[1]

FACING REALITIES

In July Hilda faced a frightening situation. At this time there were long gaps in word from or about Mac, who was then serving in a heavy combat zone. In fact rumors had reached her that he had been killed in action. This Hilda refused to believe. It could not be true. She remained firm in her belief that Mac was alive. She did not make the obvious connection— that because of the life growing within her, she felt both his presence and his absence much more poignantly than ever. Her faith was well placed. In late July, without confessing her earlier dread over his safety, she reported to Bertha that, "Mac is now doing well, bribing French children to teach him the language."[2]

A week later, she reported on a big party she attended with her good friend, Colonel Carl Lindstrom. This apparently was a last fling before

the reality of her situation set in for her. She wrote that, "perhaps by reason of my celebrated guest, all the brass was there and a few British
physicians of import." Hilda wrote that the party went far into the night,
and that she had taken the next day off, writing that she and Carl break-
fasted together before he finally "jeeped away." She mentioned that Carl
is "full of badges and things—among them the purple heart—his glider
did a crash landing." She told Bertha that she thinks he'll be back,
because "in this field you throw in your lot when you find someone who
speaks the same idiom in the language of psychiatry." She concluded,
however, by noting that she had "almost given up smoking and drinking
though you wouldn't think so if you'd seen me Saturday night."[3]

Returning to the 312th after the July trip to Scotland, Hilda had
embarked on a period of concentrated work and careful physical monitoring. The afternoon chats in the officers' club ceased. Now she would
spend long hours recording her observations, writing to her friends at the
front, and thinking through the decisions she must make as her pregnancy proceeded. To help ease the loneliness and out of practical considerations, she confided her situation to two of her hut-mates, Tish and Anne,
who immediately became most solicitous, as well as thoughtful and considerate. The dietician for the 312th Hospital also shared their hut and
she providentially provided Hilda with oranges and apples, milk, meat,
and other healthy food, including an occasional toasted tuna fish sandwich (a real treat, since no tuna fish was to be found in the commissary).[4]

Bertha must have sensed that something was wrong, because on
September 8 Hilda wrote her to provide an explanation of the apparent
renewed concern over the family finances:

> The reason I'm inquiring about the funds is obvious. The war will fold
> and we *may* get home if we're not sent to the Pacific, or end up staying
> here as an army of occupation. If we get home . . . I'll want some money
> to get around on until I find a job which suits my fancy. Otherwise, I'd
> say use it all. But that's why I've cut out all requests. However, Johnny
> can tell you what he needs and you can get it for him. I know he won't
> take undue advantage of that.[5]

She added this somewhat cryptic afterthought: "Nothing new here *yet*."
In a letter of October 7 she reiterated that "nothing else is new." By
October, however, Hilda realized that she would need to confide in somebody at home in order to carry through with the plans she was now making. She had thought through her options and taken full responsibility for
her decisions, deciding to become a single parent and to continue her
career. Thus, the most fundamental decision had been made. She had
decided to keep her child and would not consider adoption—the overwhelmingly more common solution sought by unwed mothers at that
time—however, she would need help. Bertha was the logical choice.

Hilda, at last, wrote candidly to apprise her sister of the situation and to explore the possibility of Bertha's assistance. Then she waited with some unease for Bertha's reaction. Finally, the response came. It was all Hilda had hoped for. Bertha's letter is not in the archives, but Hilda's response to it is. On October 22, 1944, she wrote with obvious relief to Bertha: "Your letter arrived today, and from the maturity of understanding in it I guess I can quit thinking of you as my baby sister. To say that I was glad to hear from you is to understate the facts quite considerably—there is need for sharing in times like this."[6] Bertha's letter provided the encouragement her sister needed to begin to think concretely and to constructively plan a future. Hilda wrote,

> I am well, only browned off about the necessity for placing a new problem in your lap . . . The two rooms upstairs [at the Church Street home in Reading] could be put into some kind of living shape. By arrangement and by putting things to use, those rooms could be ready *when and if* the war is over . . . Anyway, that's my idea—what do you think?
>
> I am quite well. I have an enormous appetite, which is killing me to control—but I do it—and hope to be here for the duration so as not to upset [anyone] at home. In line with your job perhaps you can find someone who would like to earn money [for child care] for a year—or perhaps you have some idea to offer. Again, I say, this is not your problem—you can drop the whole subject if you like—I only wanted you to know and to receive your suggestions.[7]

At this time Hilda calculated that she was 5 months pregnant and assured her sister that the "signs" were not yet visible and that she was being very diet conscious and taking "vitamins galore to make up for bulk." She also assured Bertha that she was in the best shape she had ever been in physically. Hilda's dual concern about nutrition and her close attention to weight gain became a recurring theme in subsequent letters Obviously she had put herself on a healthy but restricted diet in order to conceal her condition as long as possible. In her letter of October 7 she mentioned that she was eating well and had gained no weight, a fact she had also noted as early as September. In a note dated October 8, she again remarked, "I am well—healthier than usual—and still 132 pounds since August 1, and working."[8] It was clear that Hilda was prepared to take care of herself and the child to come.

In letters from this time to Bertha, Hilda noted, somewhat ironically, that "it seems that my talents are now recognized as valuable." She was busier than ever in her work. Nonetheless, by mid-November she wrote that she intended to request night duty, for "with careful planning and management, I believe I can keep up the deception past Christmas and I hope for a short period into January." Her plan was to delay making arrangements for the birth until it was too late for the army to send her home, and that thereby "considerable face-saving would be effected." She would stay in the army until after the baby was born—sometime in late February or early March, she calculated—and then return to the United States.

Her first impulse had been to think of her childhood home as a safe refuge, but she soon saw this as unrealistic. Both her father, Gustav, and her foster brother, Johnny, still lived at home. In the end she would inform neither of them about her situation. Hilda remembered well the circumstances of Johnny Forster's "adoption" into the Peplau family. When her mother, Ottylie, had agreed to take Johnny—the out-of-wedlock child of the daughter of a friend—in to raise, Gustav was incensed. He wanted to have no part of an illegitimate child. It was weeks before Gustav would speak to Ottylie.[9] As for the arrangements to be made in her case, by late November Hilda had decided not to return to Reading after the war at all, but to go to New York straightaway to begin work on her graduate degree. On November 22, she wrote,

> I would rather think in terms of foster care—boarding out—in Reading with you to supervise until I can take over . . . someone to take this job, which could be put forth as the problem of a close friend of yours or better—*mine*. It's a colossal problem, Bertha, but I think not unsolvable—especially if you will help. For the moment, if you would think along such lines, not making plans, but feeling out possibilities for which money will be the gain for the person who takes on the responsibility . . . Early next year I can let you know how things go and perhaps definite arrangements can be deferred until I call you [when] I am [settled] in New York—end of March. It will be simple enough, then, I believe, to put the possible wheels in motion.
>
> Here, two of my hutmates know and they promise to tell me when the fingers of scorn can be pointed. Luckily, that is not yet and by December 15 I should be on night duty for a month . . . December 15 through Christmas and New Year's, the time of the year will divert attention elsewhere. At this sitting, it does not seem difficult.[10]

In a letter written the next day, Hilda told Bertha that she had informed Mac and that he would do "what he can" financially. Clearly she did not want this to be a major issue for him. As she informed Bertha, this "will smooth out more easily later, but for now I don't want it to present an additional anxiety to him." She also assured Bertha that Anne and Tish "are not moralistic, which helps and they help cover up with the other three in the hut and have been exceedingly kind and considerate kids." Other than Anne, Tish, Mac, and Bertha, it seems Hilda informed no one at this time of the monumental change about to take place in her life.[11] She cautioned Bertha not to discuss this with anyone in Reading, including her best friends, Natalie and Betty, now both married. From here on out, she would be writing newsy letters home about her work, letters to be shared with her father and friends. More private letters for Bertha's eyes only would be sent to Bertha at the pediatrician's office in Reading where she worked.[12] Hilda's desire to protect Mac's privacy and to spare him additional anxiety, can be seen in the exchange of letters between the two in 1944 and during the immediate pre- and post-birth months. In these letters, Hilda comes across as more protective of him than of herself. She conveys little of her feelings, other than to reassure him that she is making plans and arrangements, and other than wanting him to be aware of the facts, will not require anything of him. Mac responded with a mixture of relief and guilt.[13]

THE GRAND DECEPTION

As for herself, Hilda assured her sister that sharing the "problem" with her and knowing that she would help had eased her mind. Nonetheless, she was acutely aware of the social stigma attached to unwed motherhood in the 1940s and 1950s and of the shame such circumstances brought down upon an entire family. When Hilda was growing up in Reading, gossip was a major pastime in the neighborhood. Real or suspected pregnancies were a favorite topic. She knew well that girls who "got into trouble" either married, no matter what the consequences, or were sent away to a place where an "illegitimate" or "bastard" child could be born in secrecy and given up for adoption. Similarly, as a nurse, she was aware that to raise a child born to her out of wedlock could be tantamount to professional suicide, and would most certainly be so at the highly politicized academic levels to which she aspired. She faced these facts squarely in a November letter to Bertha:

> On the personal side, there isn't much I can say. I want this and I don't . . . Naturally, I want social approval which will not now be forthcoming. Naturally, my professional future can be lost in a minute. Nursing is a very narrow-minded profession. With deception in name and your help in management and my taking over later as an adoptive parent, I believe I can have my problem and solve it too . . . I won't come back to Reading. That is final. If you can keep your eyes and ears open for an ideal family—where a foster-care plan can be supervised by you—that would be helpful . . . As far as money goes, there is enough around, and more available . . . It isn't inconceivable that you could do this for a friend, and people would believe that. And when I come home from the war for good, I can then deal with the problem unaided.[14]

She again assured her sister that she was "fit," and reported that in June she had weighed 126 pounds and at the end of November weighed only

134 pounds. Her height, her strict diet, plenty of exercise, and the cover of bulky winter clothing, as she had hoped, made the weight gain concealable. In fact in late October Hilda recounted that she had been assigned to stand retreat and that, "Yesterday I played volleyball for an hour and was not a bit stiff today, so I must be in pretty good shape."[15]

November brought not only the ever-present rain, cold, and mud, but again the very distressing news that Mac may have been killed in action. "I don't believe it and won't until I too have letters returned marked deceased," she wrote Bertha. She was aware that Mac was in Aachen, on the German border with Belgium, and that the casualties had been high in that area. Although she had not heard from him, she consoled herself with the knowledge that mail was slow when a war zone is active, and vowed she would not accept such devastating news from the informal network. Nonetheless, Hilda began making inquiries from every angle she could think of. For the first time she began to sound truly discouraged and emotionally exhausted:

> What worse could happen to me? I seem to have had a phenomenal career of ill luck in the army. You can imagine how I feel. As though again the bottom has dropped out of the world . . . I am marooned here. Mother has died. Perhaps Mac . . . This situation gives the advantage of pondering out what has happened to produce the deteriorated sad sacks we see.[16]

Typically, she attempted to deal with her own feelings of helplessness and despondency by analyzing the similar feelings she saw in the soldiers returning from the front, defeated and demoralized by the wages of war. She believed that perhaps her own "down" feelings gave her insights into the psychological states of the young men around her, and thus she wrote Bertha her observations of the division between two "separate and unlinked worlds," the world of war and senseless killing and the world of civil society and its values. In the same letter, she speculated, "the soldier maintains his hold on his civilian destiny first through conversation with his buddy, and secondly through mail from home . . . Once the buddy is killed, much, and frequently all, is lost. And the will to go on disintegrates."[17] She continued to reflect on the condition of the physically debilitated soldiers who came into her wards; but because the roots were psychological, she noted, their effort to get well "is nil."

Still she had no word of Mac, and for the next several weeks her letters home were bleak one- or two-liners to the effect that, "I am well, still no news from the front." Then new mail from the front arrived, including word from Mac. While reinforced in her hope that he was indeed alive, she wrote Bertha that she was checking the postmark dates and waiting for a letter postmarked after November 8 before she could rest assured, that being the day she was told he had gone down. On December 2 she reported to Bertha that she had "had a few more letters from the front lately, but still waiting for one dated November 8 or later to say all is well."

Other than Hilda's fears for Mac, however, she seemed again to be rising to all challenges. She reported to Bertha that as Christmas approached she weighed 138 pounds, just 12 pounds more than she weighed in June, "when I weighed last unknowingly."[18] A new, although undated, letter from Mac further revived her spirits. She assured her sister that she was feeling better than she had ever felt: "good color, excellent posture, and no insomnia." She indicated that she would undergo a physical examination in early January and that her condition would then be known—at least by her physician.

> I have settled the score with my conscience long ago and will take whatever happens to be my fate—and consequently am almost nil on being self-conscious. It is certainly La Grande deception and when the day of reckoning here occurs, now set for January 1 in my mind, I shall still have some of this backbone left.[19]

She speculated, "the end of February will bring the more immediate problem [the birth] to hand—between the 20th and the 4th of March." She hoped that when she did reveal her condition to her superiors and decisions had to be made, that they would agree to let her continue working at the 312th until childbirth was imminent. She did not know what would happen then, but planned to investigate her options after facing the "time of truth" that would come with the physical examination in January. In the meantime, there was work to be done.

> People continue to tell me how well I look, how increasingly beautiful I am becoming—I look like Mother—and how much more energetic I seem. As Tish says, I could go on to February and just no one would suspect or believe this . . . maybe so . . . I am more than able to continue on the job daily without fear . . . except for the one problem—what to do then—I am certainly OK. Be assured![20]

On November 25, 1944, she had reported, "my training program for patients is now going unusually well . . . I am feeling pretty proud of myself."[21] In other short V-mail notes, she repeatedly informed her family that she was well. It was clear that her spirits remained high in spite of the unrelenting rain and the daily arrival of new psychological tragedies from the war zone. Obviously, the challenge of work and success in it gave her deep satisfaction and a sense of fulfillment and self-worth that would sustain her in the years to come.

On Christmas day, December 25, 1944, she wrote a particularly cheerful letter to Bertha, who had sent the news that she had met and decided to marry Byron Reppert, who was in the Marine Corps. Byron was then in a military hospital recovering from a combat wound, but would be returning to Reading in a few months. He and Bertha planned to marry in May. Hilda was very happy for them and full of sisterly advice concerning where to live and what to do about furniture. Mostly, though, she was pleased that Bertha's future was now settled. The occasion of her sister's forthcoming wedding clearly led Hildegard to reflect on the value of family, and in spite of herself, she began to dream a bit about the future—a future with a career and her brothers as surrogate fathers to her child.

> I should prefer living somewhere rural—near city transportation—with fireplaces and farmland. I believe Walter would join us, Harold too—and pooling our resources we could do rather well . . . Circumstances permitting, I shall probably work in Philadelphia [or] New York . . . If all else fails, Johnny can always come with me, especially during his college years.[22]

Thinking ahead, Hilda suggested to Bertha that she persuade their father to draw up a will, and should he do that and leave the house to Bertha (or to all of them), Hilda suggested they pay off the very unconventional mortgage. Then, were her father to die, the house could be used to mortgage a country house near Reading where all the Peplaus could live together. Obviously, she was giving a lot of thought to the practical details of her future, and thinking very much that she wanted her own family around her if at all possible.

Hilda's second Christmas at the 312th Hospital was a festive one. Her secret was still a secret, and her hut-mates decided to make the holiday memorable. They found a suitable tree and made decorations out of used insulin vials. They roasted chestnuts over the coal stove, sang carols, and toasted one another. By this time, Hilda had gained only 12 pounds, and other than those "in the know," no one else had a clue.[23]

Early in January 1945 Hilda received a letter from Mac, written on November 24, 1944, describing his general state of mind after a long siege of front-line battle. His plane had indeed been shot down, and he'd seen a great deal of death and suffering. The letter was a great relief to her, but also caused renewed fears for his mental health. Too many campaigns and too many close calls too near the front lines had taken their toll. Mac was again suffering from a bad case of "nerves." He described his state of mind in emotional terms that caused her great concern and again called forth her therapist instincts. Mac wrote that he had

> Apparently dedicated myself and my thoughts and efforts to self pity and accusation, steeped in the broth of alcohol, barbiturates, and general mental self analysis . . . My thoughts and appearances are mirrored in unreal and grotesque images . . . something has happened to my

competitive urge . . . have tried to cover up in as many ways as possible
. . . exception of occasional outburst of real antagonism, I have done so.
. . I want peace, security, and an ever-present crutch to assist my punc-
tured ego . . . I guess I am tired of mud and rain, snow and sleet, innumerable inconveniences, buzzer bombs, and artillery and death—the
whole so-called military machine . . . Hostility seems to have completely overshadowed anxiety.

The next day he wrote a bit more directly about his concern over Hilda's
decisions.

Your future upsets me for I realize the inevitable must arise and I cannot clearly in my own mind plan a course of action for you. So many
factors come into play and so many people's futures are at stake.
Maybe you have a solution—I haven't—only an intense admiration for
your courage and [an] unclear conception of alternatives.[24]

He wrote again on November 27, apologizing for his letter of
November 24, and again expressing his uneasiness at not being able to be
more helpful, but acknowledging that the major decisions were hers. He
regretted that "censorship makes things so difficult to put in words," but
he did assure her, "financially I should be a position to help considerably,
and morally I am with you." He informed her that he was being returned
to England, to the 189th General Hospital, and was pleased about that,
believing that the change of scene would get him out of the "doldrums."
He signed off with "good night and good luck, Peppy. I wish I had your
courage." In another short letter dated the same day, he informed her,

Lots of mail today, several from you and one from your sister Bertha,
which pretty well sums up one end of the problem . . . I want to be of all
possible help . . . My concern over your welfare must seem infinitesimal
when you view the days ahead . . . You have a lot to offer the world . . .
Please let me know your thoughts and ideas.[25]

And she does. She wrote daily letters to Mac in December, sharing her
thoughts, decisions, and her reasoning—all the time reassuring him that
it was her problem and not his. She wrote to him of her work, and she
tried to boost his morale while stimulating him to think analytically
about his own emotional problems. She wanted to share with him her
"thoughts and ideas," but at the same time she made it crystal clear that,
because he was married, there would to be no future involvement on his
part with the child.

Hilda Peplau was not one to waste time daydreaming about unrealistic scenarios. The immediate problems to be dealt with were too acute for
such indulgences. She was determined to keep her child, have a career,
and not waste one precious moment in self-pity. This self-reliant attitude

was communicated to Mac, with the unintended result, perhaps, of inten-sifying his own sense of self-doubt.[26] His several letters in December, however, were considerably more cheerful, indicating that the transfer to the 189th General Hospital had gone well and with only elliptical allu-sions to the impending birth.

BEGINNINGS AND ENDINGS

Hilda had written Bertha about her plan to submit to a physical examina-tion early in January in what she believed would be in the seventh month of her pregnancy, after which "the facts would be known" and definitive plans for the immediate future would be made. At that point, she wrote, she would inform "those who needed to be informed" and make the nec-essary arrangements.[27] The January 2 examination did not go as planned. Hilda was astonished to learn that she was not, in fact, in the seventh month of her pregnancy but was somewhere between the eighth and ninth month! Her physician ordered her off duty immediately, and arrange-ments for her to be moved by military truck transport to the 10th Station Military Hospital in Manchester—a military hospital designated for deliveries—were hastily made. The suddenness of the discovery of the imminence of birth upset Hilda's own plans, but saved her the awkward-ness of having her pregnancy become general knowledge. She had liter-ally worked up until the day she left the 312th, her condition undetected. With the war winding down in Europe, and so many men and nurses being sent home either for reassignment or discharge, there was nothing unusual about her sudden disappearance. Because medical personnel and patients alike were in constant flux, Hilda's transition out of the 312th was much easier than she had imagined possible.

At the Manchester Station Hospital she was deemed well and healthy, and allowed to help where needed right up to the last day of her preg-nancy. On January 30, 1945, Hildegard Peplau gave birth to a baby girl. She named the child Letitia Anne Peplau, after her hut-mates Letitia Towson and Anne Anton. The birth itself seemed in retrospect exceeding-ly easy, for she was in excellent physical condition. Hilda, however, did do battle with the attending obstetrician, who wanted to do an episioto-my. Hilda objected to the procedure, and prevailed, in part because of the support of the obstetrical nurse.[28] Hilda's decision to raise her daughter rather than give her up for adoption had been a straightforward one. She never considered any other alternative and had permitted no discussion of that option once she arrived at the Manchester Station Hospital. She had given birth because she had become pregnant, and because, in her own totally rational way, she loved the father of the child, a man who could never be her husband. It was as simple and as complicated as that.

She knew that the responsibility for Letitia Anne Peplau would be hers, and hers alone. Hilda never again had a serious romance, nor imagined any alternative to single motherhood.

News of the arrival of the baby—whom Hilda called Tish or sometimes "Tisha"—was slow to reach Mac. Letters between Mac and Hilda missed and crossed one another and were sent from hospital to hospital and from theater to theater. On February 10, 1945, Mac wrote that he had received her letter of January 5, 1945, and that he was relieved to know that her move from the 312th to the 10th Station hospital in Manchester had been so easily facilitated. He clearly was not entirely comfortable with her decision to keep the child, however:

> I hope your plan for the future is the wise one and I dare not put in my two cents worth. Your judgment is and has been good and you know far better than I what you want. I want you to get through this as easily as possible, and safely, and to be as contented as you can be later on . . . Your work at the 312th was so good and appreciated and constructive and I hope it will be so that you can continue in it later.[29]

He would be surprised to learn soon after this letter was written that in fact Hilda was already a mother. The chaos at the end of the war was making it impossible for the two to get in direct touch with each other. Mac mentioned he had tried to call her, but hadn't been able to catch her before she left the 312th. On February 12 he wrote to inform her that he had a further psychological crisis and that he was to be hospitalized before being sent home. He was dismayed by this turn of events, sliding back into self-doubt: "I guess the little confidence I had in myself and the faith you placed in me wasn't so justified after all."[30]

On February 15 he wrote that her letter announcing "the arrival of Letitia Anne or Tish" had been unexpected. He said that he had been diagnosed at the 124th General Hospital as suffering from "anxiety and emotional instability." He added, "What a slap after two and a half years." The extremes of living and dying had gotten to him. The next letter from Mac, also written on February 15, 1945, was from the 124th Hospital. Hildegard had jotted a phone number, presumably his, on the envelope. In this letter he told her that he had talked the physicians out of the insulin and amytal treatment, and in fact was helping out on the wards while he waited for a hospital ship back to the states.

Hilda's response, written on February 25 (the first anniversary of her mother's death), was a long, thoughtful letter full of encouragement, reassurance, and concern for his emotional state. It was a therapeutic letter, meant to encourage and help. It reveals a mature woman able to give out of a deep concern, empathy, and love. There is not a note of self-pity, self-doubt, or insecurity in this beautiful letter. Alone with her child,

thankful for her health, her strength, and proud of her "grand deception," she wrote Mac that "we all have our limitations—even you." She
then assured him,

> I have a healthy respect for your quick brain and your alert observa-
> tions . . . great admiration for your ability to endure and work during
> those hundreds of days you've spent under fire. But, even I do not look
> up to you as superman—and sometimes one reaches the point where
> one has simply seen enough . . .[31]
>
> Another thing, Mac, don't worry about Tish and me. She is strong
> and I am stubborn, and together we will manage well . . . There is so
> much of you in Tish—in her appearance, her baby behavior: she
> intrigues me and gives me a job for the rest of my years.[32]

Apparently this long and thoughtful letter never reached Mac. It was
returned, marked "hospitalized." Hilda, however, did reach Mac by telephone in this period, and the two met one last time in March. Hilda took
the train to Bournemouth for the day. Mac met the train and they went to
a restaurant to talk. He brought a bracelet that he had purchased for the
baby. The conversation was rational and caring. They discussed their
postwar plans openly and in detail, and determined that it would be best
not to keep up contact in the future. Shortly after the March meeting, Mac
left for the States.[33] It is clear from the written sources, interviews, and
the record of the rest of her life, that Hilda herself resolutely cut off all
connection to, correspondence, or communication with Mac, who presumably returned to his family after the war and disappeared completely
from her life. The last letter from Mac had been forwarded all over
England and finally reached Church Street in Reading and was sent on
from there to Hilda. It is a fairly dispirited letter and reveals, as Hilda
would have known, that Mac never received her long letter of February
25 for in it he complains, "I still have no mail . . . except two ancient letters written early in February."[34] Several times in his letters during
Hilda's pregnancy, Mac had given assurance that he would help financially. Hilda, however, never requested such help. She insisted the break
be complete, and definitively cut off all contact.[35]

Hilda, with other wartime mothers, sailed from England on April 8
bound for Charleston, South Carolina, and Stark Memorial General
Hospital, arriving some time after the middle of the month. She befriended several women on the ship, but unlike Hilda, they had opted to put
their babies up for adoption. Hilda could not imagine the emotional pain
they had chosen to put themselves through, although she understood all
too well the shame attached to unwed motherhood. As had been agreed,
Bertha traveled to Charleston by train at the end of April, and stayed for
a day before taking Tish back to Reading where boarding arrangements
had been made with a neighbor, Mrs. Agnes Von Nieda. The separation

was harder for Hilda than even her worst imaginings. On May 5, she wrote Bertha, "I miss my Tisha terribly and am eager for news to appease my loneliness. I knew she was a real joy, but until now I didn't realize how well she filled my day."[36] Hilda remained certain that she had made the right choice in sending Tish to Reading, but she admitted that the separation from her child was extremely difficult for her to bear.

> It would be better for me to have her with me, but I don't think it would be better for Tisha . . . The important thing is that she is well-taken care of, well-loved, and thriving on it . . . She's a wonderful child, the only real jewel I've ever had . . . She was literally born with her eyes open and from the beginning had a special alertness . . . It's better if I take her after I get out . . . You will be the bridge when she gets reacquainted with me. I have no qualms about that now. You see, she's mine![37]

This had to have been an emotionally draining time, as Hilda was separated from the child with whom she had clearly bonded and whom she adored. She wrote affectionately of the first months of Tish's life, recalling in a letter to Bertha that she believed her bright, eager baby daughter had spoken her first word—albeit one of her own devising—at the age of 3 months. Tish's word, as transcribed by Hilda, was "achcook."[38]

> Funny how she thought that one up! She first said it one 5:00 a.m. aboard ship. Then three 5:00 a.m. mornings in a row. Then every time she looked pleased. It was always as though it had real meaning for her. Take good care of my golden girl for me, and keep her supplied with whatever it takes for her to keep up her enthusiastic exploration of the world.[39]

Beyond her yearning to be reunited with Tish, Hilda's thoughts while in Charleston were consumed with securing her own discharge from the army at the earliest possible date and with strategies to assure Tish's future legal and social status while allowing Hilda to raise her as an "adoptive parent." The first plan explored by the two sisters was that Bertha, who would be marrying Byron Reppert the end of May, would officially adopt the baby and Hilda would then assume the responsibility for her care. The story would be that the child had been born to a close army friend of Hilda's and that Hilda wanted to adopt her. It was to be said that because single women were not able to adopt while serving in the army, Bertha had stepped in to facilitate things until Hilda again had civilian status. Their letters in these days are filled with details of the efforts to arrange for the formal adoption. There were affidavits about support to be signed, notaries to be arranged, complications because Hildegard had managed not to name the father on the birth certificate and, ever protective of Mac, was refusing to do so now. She was working with a lawyer and dealing with the endless vicissitudes of the military bureaucracy. On May 15, Hilda despaired of the saga of army red tape. "Everything is subject to change without notice," she complained.

The lack of action, the idle time on her hands in Charleston, and the time away from her child were taking their toll, and the loneliness of her days comes through clearly in her letters. She sent her ration books to Mrs. Von Nieda, the woman caring for Tish for Tish's use, but was more adamant than ever in cautioning Bertha that

> The circumstances of Tish's background need not be told except to her. I remember that too many people knew Johnny's tale, and so let's spare Tish that . . . I haven't told Betty, Nat and so forth because I feel strongly that the privacy of Mrs. Von Nieda's home must be respected.[40]

On May 5 Hilda wrote that she feared she would miss Bertha's wedding: "I probably won't get a leave since I had one [in March] to see Mac." She was also unsure of the details of the progress of discharge papers. On May 10, she wrote "Still no news of what next . . . I hope VE day means they'll release some of us—including me."[41] Bertha was in the midst of planning for her wedding to Byron, which would take place in the Holy Spirit Lutheran Church in Reading on May 19. Still she took time to visit Tish every day at Mrs. Von Nieda's—including the day of the wedding—and to write a daily short note of reassurance to Hilda. On the wedding day, Hilda also wrote Bertha expressing her regret that instead of being in Reading, she was trapped in Charleston while the "winding and unwinding of red tape goes on and on—I continue to wonder how the army ever gets going at all . . . But this is your day and I hope that everything that happens today happens as an omen of wonderful dreams come true."[42] (For Bertha, the dreams did indeed come true. In 1995 Bertha and Byron Reppert celebrated their 50th anniversary, issuing a picture newsletter chronicling "fifty very full years of happiness.")[43]

Hilda had decided early in the summer that she could no longer put off informing her brother Walter of her true situation. She and Walter had always been close, and they communicated faithfully during the war. Their letters establish that brother and sister were open and confiding and in fact grew closer through the war. The exchange of mail continued unabated in the spring of 1945, but Hilda did not share with Walter the intimate drama of those months. She was reluctant to give him news that would cause him concern. After the birth of the baby, and especially after her return to the States, silence on this subject was becoming more and more awkward. Walter had noticed the change in their communication. The catalyst to take Walter into her confidence came in Walter's letter of May 25, 1945:

News that you were in the land of the free was surprising ... I still can't
figure out why you were in such a hurry all the time ... whatever it is
that brought you home, I hope it isn't serious ... a little news wouldn't
hurt ... it would keep me from thinking, at least ... Get yourself well
in a hurry ... you are going to be invited to a wedding.[44]

With some trepidation Hilda finally wrote Walter about Tish and waited
anxiously for his response. Again, she need not have worried. On June
10, 1945, Walter wrote from Germany:

I am so glad you wrote as you did and wish I could be of more help
than I am. Tisha is a very fortunate child and I am all for her—and
more than anxious to see her ... wish we could have a long, long talk,
HEP, there is so much to be said ... I am building up a fine assortment
of fine liquors for that long talk ... The best news is that you are on
your feet and everything is being taken care of as it should be.[45]

Walter, however, would be frustrated in his desire to get home, to see his
sister and her daughter, and to marry his prewar sweetheart. His letters
of July and August 1945 are a catalog of frustration as he was moved
around from front to front, first to Germany, then to France. As he
expressed it to Hilda in August, "my work is classified as 'essential' and
I am anything but essential—any PFC could do twice as much."[46] Most
important to Hilda, Walter had been "informed" of her situation and was
supportive. Her brother's endorsement of her plans did much to give her
reassurance that her decisions were sound.

Although Hilda was not required to work, she had taken a part-time
job on a paraplegic ward at Stark General Hospital to fill the time. Early
in June, she wrote that most of the soldiers had been released and that the
hospital in Charleston was virtually empty. For the first time in her life,
she found herself with idle time on her hands. Days were spent reading,
sitting on the beach tanning, plotting for the future, and expressing frustration at the slowness of things, until finally—"my idle brain is turned to
writing a book." She began to write about her wartime observations
about the treatment of mental illness.[47] She was still trying to arrange for
a legal adoption through the army, but was beginning to think that perhaps she should just forget it, secure her discharge, and get to New York
to make preparations to enter graduate school—in short, get her life organized so that she could reclaim Tish and then deal with the adoption
legalities as a civilian.

On June 8 she requested a discharge to be arranged as soon as possible. The affidavits concerning the details of the adoption by Bertha and
Byron had been returned for yet another "technicality." Hilda decided
that she had "had enough of this fooling around."[48] A woman of her
word, she moved quickly. On June 16, she wrote Bertha that her orders

had been put through and that she would receive an honorable discharge from the U.S. Army as of July 30, 1945. In the meantime, she had accumulated vacation leave and thus could actually leave Charleston as soon as she could pack her bags. She intended to go to New York first, find a job and a place to stay, and begin the process of enrolling in the master's degree program at Columbia University's Teachers College. Col. Jay Hoffman, the commanding officer of the 312th Hospital at the end of the war, wrote a strong letter of recommendation for Hilda, stating that her "superior qualities of judgment, tact and good common sense . . . made her one of the most valuable members of our staff."[49] When housing in New York and a source of income were in place, Hilda would return to Reading for her precious Tish.

At the time of her discharge Hilda weighed 126 pounds, just 2 pounds more than the 124 pounds she carried when she entered the army. At 5 foot 10 inches, she was a striking woman—tall, slender, and blond; but these were not her concerns as she made preparations for her move to New York. Her mind was on her daughter. She had promised Tish, on the day of her birth, that she would be loved, well cared for, and that she would see the world. Hilda vowed that her daughter would have a better life for having seen the world on her mother's wing as it were. She would keep that promise. Tish would be well loved, and she would indeed see the world. Hilda had found a sense of peace and purpose, knowing that her life ahead was the life she had chosen, not one to which she had merely consented.

ENDNOTES

1. Letter from Hilda Peplau to Bertha Peplau, January 24, 1944, Box 3, #65.
2. Ibid, July 22, 1944.
3. Ibid.
4. Interview, Hildegard Peplau, March 11, 1992, in Sherman Oaks.
5. Ibid, September 8, 1944.
6. Ibid, October 22, 1944.
7. Ibid.
8. Letters in Box 3, #72–80.
9. Although Gustav would live for 6 more years, Bertha believes he did not ever know that the child who would soon come into Hilda and Bertha's lives was in fact his biological granddaughter. Interview, Bertha Reppert, October 30, 1994.
10. Letter from Hilda Peplau to Bertha Peplau, November 22, 1944.
11. Interview, Hildegard Peplau, March 28, 1992, in Sherman Oaks.
12. Summary of letters from Hilda Peplau to Bertha Peplau in Box 3, #70–83.
13. Not all material relevant to this discussion is yet available. A sealed envelope deposited in the archives is not to be opened until the year 2025. There are, however, many letters in various files that are open to research, and from them one can glean the nature of the relationship between the two, and the great caution being taken on both sides, each to protect the other. Great kindness and deep feeling is

evident, as is the determination to do the right thing, each anxious not to burden the other. Neither passions nor regrets are expressed.

14. Hilda Peplau to Bertha Peplau, November 13, 1944, Box 3, #74.
15. Ibid, October 22, 1944.
16. Ibid, November 18, 1944.
17. Ibid, November 16, 1944.
18. Ibid, December 19, 1944.
19. Ibid.
20. Ibid.
21. Ibid, November 25, 1944.
22. Ibid, December 25, 1944.
23. Interview, Hildegard Peplau, February 11, 1992.
24. Letters from "Mac" to Hilda Peplau, November 24 and 25, 1944, Box 4, #149.
25. Ibid, November 27, 1944.
26. In addition to the sealed packet of material not to be opened until 2025, there is a file of letters between Peplau and Mac written in December 1944 marked "not open for research until 2025." The letters of November 24 and 27, 1944 were not in the "closed" file, and hence I have quoted from them. Letters "not open for research" were not opened in order to respect the wishes of Hildegard Peplau.
27. Letters from Hilda Peplau to Bertha Peplau, November 25 and December 19, 1944, in Box 3, #81.
28. Notes from Anne Peplau to Barbara Callaway, February 12, 1999.
29. Letter from Mac to Hilda Peplau, February 10, 1945, in Box 4, File #149, Schlesinger Library collection.
30. Ibid, February 12, 1945.
31. Letter from Hilda Peplau to Mac, February 25, 1945, Box 4, #149, Schlesinger Library collection.
32. Ibid.
33. Notes from Anne Peplau to Barbara Callaway, February 12, 1999.
34. Letter from Mac to Hilda Peplau, June 10, 1945, Box 4, #149.
35. Letter from Hilda and Anne Peplau to Barbara Callaway, February 5, 1999.
36. Letter from Hilda Peplau to Bertha Peplau, May 5, 1945, Box 3, #78.
37. Ibid, May 13, 1945.
38. Ibid, May 2, 1945.
39. Ibid, May 15, 1945.
40. Ibid, May 10, 1945.
41. Ibid.
42. Ibid, May 19, 1945.
43. "Bertha and Byron Reppert's Pot o' Gold News: 1945–1995," family newsletter "published" by the Repperts for their four daughters, their families, and the many cousins, nieces, various in-laws, and grandchildren.
44. Letter from Walter Peplau to Hilda Peplau, May 22, 1945, Box 2, #57.
45. Ibid, June 10, 1945.
46. Ibid, August 7, 1945.
47. This manuscript, begun on the beach in Charleston, South Carolina, would indeed become a book, *Interpersonal Relationships in Nursing*. Published in 1952, it is today a classic of modern nursing.
48. Letter from Hilda Peplau to Bertha Reppert, June 8, 1945, Box 3, #80.
49. Letter from Jay L. Hoffman, Lt.. Colonel, M.C., Commanding, July 15, 1945, Box 10, #300.

Graduate Studies and Motherhood Too

6

I would lay down my life to protect her. I tried to always think of the long-term consequences of what I was doing . . . I was very much aware of feeling rejected as a child and of the consequences of that . . . I read to her constantly and always talked to her—she had a great vocabulary.

—Hildegard Peplau
April 15, 1992

In April and May of 1945, Hildegard Peplau felt mired in the uncertainties of an army bureaucracy that she believed moved excruciatingly slowly. She was anxious to move into her new life as a mother to her child and a return to the academic world. Although Hilda felt herself to be languishing in Charleston, the fact is that massive demobilization and reintegration of millions of men and women into a postwar world already was well underway. The constant relocations—the global movements of men and equipment—made those who had been caught up in the dislocations of wartime yearn for that which would again be permanent and important in life. Under the impetus of demobilization and important new legislation being fashioned for a postwar world, life-altering choices often were made rather quickly. This proved to be true for Hilda, although she did not appreciate at the time the speed with which her own transition from army nurse to graduate student was occurring.

Hilda had left England in early April of 1945, and she left Charleston at the end of June, ready to begin civilian life in New York City. In less than 3 months—her impatience with the military notwithstanding—a lot had happened: Hilda had made the decisions to proceed with her sister's adoption of her daughter, to hasten her own discharge from the army, to go to graduate school utilizing the G.I. Bill, and to move to New York. Arrangements had been made for the care of her child, her sister had married, and her brother Walter, too, was planning a wedding.

When Hilda arrived in New York, she began inquiries about admission in September to the nursing education program at Columbia's Teachers College (TC). She stayed temporarily with her army hut-mate Anne Anton and contacted Grace Warman, her former supervisor at Mount Sinai Hospital, who promised to arrange part-time work for her while she looked for a permanent job. Because she would need a steady income to supplement her G.I. Bill stipend, she scoured the want ads, and found a notice of a job for which she seemed a natural—assistant nurse at Finch Junior College. She applied for it.

While waiting to hear from Finch, Hilda went home to Reading, where she had a joyful reunion with Tish, but was made uneasy by the stratagems required to conceal from her father and friends her actual relationship with the baby girl in Agnes Von Nieda's care. In late July she was offered the position at Finch College. A letter from Finch president Jessica G. Cosgrove stated that the appointment would provide room, board, laundry, and "$20.00 a month in cash" in exchange for 28 hours a week on duty. The offer included 3 weeks vacation at Christmas, 10 days in the spring, and summers off, during which times she could keep her room, but there would be no meals.[1] Faced with the financial realities, Hilda reluctantly concluded on this trip that the best plan for the moment was to accept the Finch position, leave Tish in Reading with Mrs. Von Nieda, who clearly adored the child, and return to New York alone. She recognized that in Agnes Von Nieda's care and with Bertha's daily visits, Tish did seem to be thriving.

Another plan, however, was taking shape. Bertha's new husband, Byron Reppert, would also use the GI Bill, in his case to complete secondary school and enter college. The Repperts decided that Byron would seek admission to the Rhodes Preparatory School in New York, and that he and Bertha and Tish would join Hilda there as soon as possible. The three adults would share an apartment and expenses, Bertha would provide child care, and Hilda and Byron would go to school. While she regretted further, even if temporary, separation from Tish, Hilda agreed that this plan made the most sense. After 3 weeks in Reading, she returned to Charleston where she was officially discharged on July 30, 1945, with the rank of first lieutenant. Letitia Anne was then 6 months old, to the day. Returning to New York in August, Hilda worked part-time at Mount Sinai and stayed at the hospital's home for nurses until September when she assumed her position at Finch Junior College and moved into the staff residence at 61 E. 77th Street. Peplau herself described the period at Finch as "a nice interlude."[2] Finch was a private junior college/finishing school for upper-class young women in Manhattan. Hilda was the live-in nurse, but students were seldom in need of medical attention. She worked with another nurse and there was a physician on call. Unlike her nursing position at Bennington, where she had been excited about the work itself and eager to learn all there was to gain from the experience, Finch was indeed just an "interlude" for Hilda.

EARNING A MASTER'S DEGREE

Hilda had been excited about becoming a full-time student for the first time since her early high school years in Reading. However, the reality of her graduate experience at Teachers College would not meet her expectations. When she presented herself for admission in mid-summer she was interviewed by Virginia Henderson, one of the great ladies of nursing. Miss Henderson doubted that Bennington College, where Hilda had earned her BA, was sufficiently established to meet Columbia's admission standards. "Are you sure?" asked Hilda. "If so, I'll go over to the Veterans Administration and inform them," a reference to the large number of service men and women then enrolling at Columbia under the G.I. Bill—and unknowingly prescient of the fact that General Dwight David Eisenhower, supreme commander of the Allied Expeditionary Force, would later become president of Columbia University. Henderson backed down and Peplau was admitted, but there never would be much warmth between the two women.[3]

While Henderson questioned whether Peplau had the academic background required for graduate level work, the opposite proved to be the case. Hilda began work on her master's degree with great anticipation, but almost immediately was disappointed by the low level of instruction offered. She soon realized that Nursing Education lacked the respect accorded Columbia University's academic programs. The reasons may be found in the history of Nursing Education at Teachers College.

The origin of the program was a 1894 request from the New York Society of Superintendents—a body with oversight over hospital nurse-training programs—that Columbia offer a course in hospital economics at TC, to be staffed and paid for by the society. From this beginning, the leadership at Teachers College saw a market and began offering courses in basic science, household economics, and elementary biology to a limited number of nurses. In 1907 Adelaide Nutting, from the Johns Hopkins University Hospital, was appointed a professor of "domestic economy" and charged with running the program for nurses. Nutting thus became the first American nurse to be appointed to a university position.[4] She changed the name of the program from Hospital Economics to Nursing and Health. It was not until 1912, however, that Nursing and Health required a high school diploma for admission. In 1923 the program was renamed the Division of Nursing Education. Its mission was to prepare nurses to teach in, or administer, hospital nurse-training programs.

Nutting was succeeded in 1925 by Isabel Maitland Stewart, whose emphasis continued to be on curriculum development in order to reform the educational experience nurses received in hospital-based schools. Nutting and Stewart lacked the academic credentials expected of administrators at Columbia University, as did R. Louise McManus, who would succeed Stewart as director in 1948. The lack of a traditionally credentialed faculty and the absence in nursing of any kind of scholarly tradition meant that, while tolerated and even appreciated, the nursing faculty ranked low in terms of the respect and status generally accorded faculty at research universities. Hilda was not oblivious to any of this.

Moreover, Hilda was one among a group of former army nurses who entered TC on the GI Bill in the immediate postwar period. A review of the college catalogue for these years reveals an instructional faculty credentialed only at the MA level, and of rather limited experience, when compared to that of the army nurses, who were more aware of a rapidly changing health care environment.[5] The faculty was not ready for these older, more experienced students. Hilda herself had spent many a night tending the young men brought to the 312th Field Hospital suffering psychotic breaks from the stress of battle, death, and destruction around them. She had ordered books and read articles seeking to understand their trauma. She was intellectually curious and single-minded by nature. She was determined that she could make a contribution to psychological understanding through her chosen profession, nursing. She was driven. Given these circumstances, it is not surprising that the TC master's degree program in Nursing Education did not in itself meet her expectations and did not offer her either the opportunities or the exciting intellectual adventure she had expected.

Hilda was busy, but not fulfilled. Over this fall of 1945 a nearly overwhelming sadness engulfed her. Until plans were complete for Bertha, Byron, and Tish to join her, Hilda was a solitary figure, going to classes, studying in her little room at Finch, exploring the city—all quite alone. She did form a friendship with Helen Manock, a classmate who, like Hilda, was a little older than the majority of TC students. They often went to the great Riverside Church together to hear Harry Emerson Fosdick preach and stayed for the luncheon seminar after the service, but Hilda did not confide any of her personal concerns to Helen.

Her work as school nurse at Finch was not challenging, and the absence of intimacy with anyone near, especially Tish, took a toll. Hilda hungered for every word about her daughter. "Your accounts of Tish are wonderful—do keep them up," she wrote to Bertha. "She is a bright child—we mustn't stamp that out."[6] It was Mrs. Von Nieda who assured her that this would not happen. At 8 and 9 months old, Tish was already "talking up a blue streak" and walking impatiently around her playpen, seeking a way out. Mrs. Von Nieda was obviously very fond of Tish, referring to her as "our little darling."[7] Hilda returned to Reading toward the end of her first term to spend a warm Christmas with Bertha and Byron, keeping a low profile as she visited her daughter in her foster home. Byron had been accepted at Rhodes, but wouldn't begin until the fall of 1946, meaning a wait of perhaps another 9 months before the Repperts and Tish would join Hilda. It was a sad and lonely woman who returned to New York in January for the start of a second semester without her family. The world seemed dark and grey indeed.

At the end of this first term at TC Hilda confronted the inadequacies of the Nursing Education curriculum. She petitioned the dean and was granted permission to supplement the program by taking courses in the Social Psychology Department at Teachers College. Later she took a course from Karen Horney at the New School, attended lectures at the William Alanson White Institute of Psychiatry and Psychoanalysis, and attended classes in psychology at Cooper Union. In addition to assuming extra coursework at Columbia and attending lectures across the city, she also was intent on completing the manuscript she had begun in Charleston, building upon her experiences and reading during the war and her reflections and thinking about mental illness and the role of nursing in its care and treatment. Thanks to her own efforts, Hilda was becoming fully engaged in what would become a far more rewarding academic program.

A FAMILY REUNITED

Good news arrived at the end of the that grim January: Bertha announced that she and Byron had decided to join Hilda in New York as soon as feasible, rather than wait for the summer.[8] In the spring of 1946, as the time approached for Bertha to take the baby to New York, Mrs. Von Nieda expressed her appreciation for Tish and her reluctance to let her go:

> Yes, we will miss our little prankster as she is so full of tricks and fun . . . She keeps quiet with a smile on her face, then YELLS and gives a little jump as if she were trying to scare us and then she will laugh right out loud . . . I will be proud to hand over a happy, healthy, contented baby and hope she continues to be that way throughout her whole life . . . She is so good.[9]

Hilda was on the alert for word of a roomy but affordable apartment—not an easy task in the postwar period—and in February she found the perfect place. It was a sunny and spacious seven-room apartment at 109 West 106th Street. Because it was on the fifth floor and there was no elevator, the rent was reasonable—under $100 a month. The apartment was owned by a Mrs. Daly, who lived on the first floor, and whose sons, all policemen, lived on the second, third, and fourth floors, promising the residents of the fifth floor great security. It was a wonderful apartment with a living room, three bedrooms, a dining room, and a small study.[10] Byron and Bertha worked out plans to arrive in March, bringing Tish with them. Unbeknownst to Hilda, Bertha was then pregnant and the Repperts were happy to get to New York ahead of schedule and get settled in the new apartment. This would give Byron time to start his studies at Rhodes before the entering class arrived, as well as earn a little extra money tending bar—a skill at which the gregarious Byron excelled. The Repperts and Tish joined Hilda in the new apartment on March 20, 1946. Hilda was at last reunited with her daughter.

While Byron worked and Hilda went to school, Bertha took care of Tish. To furnish the apartment, they frequented local secondhand stores where they found a giant oak table and six chairs. The table was a wonderful place for meals and became a place for Tish to draw. Bertha painted the chairs and decorated them with stenciled Pennsylvania Dutch designs. (Getting the table up four flights of stairs was a major undertaking, and when they moved from the apartment they simply left the oak table in its place in the dining room.) Bertha, a self-taught botanist and herbalist, filled the rooms and window sills with pots of wonderful smelling herbs and the table with flowers.[11] The lonely days were over for Hilda. A hectic academic and professional life and intense experience of mothering was about to begin. At the end of the semester, her second at TC, Hilda resigned from both Finch and the part-time work she had continued at Mount Sinai so that she could devote all her time to her studies, and to Tish. Byron also started school that summer. Life was suddenly good again—full of love, interests, study, and family life. On January 30, 1947, on Letitia Anne's second birthday, Bertha gave birth to the Repperts' first daughter, Carolynn Elizabeth.

In 1947 the term "quality time" was not yet in vogue, but this is indeed what Hilda gave Tish in every possible way. She was acutely aware of every step in her daughter's development, and was determined as a parent "to do it right." She read books on child psychology and took an interest in everything Tish did—but she was also a single mother earning a graduate degree as well as a living, and intent on having a meaningful professional career. As both a mother and a student, Hilda was intense. She read Tish to sleep every night by 8:00, and then got out her Royal manual typewriter and worked until 2:00 to 3:00 in the morning on the manuscript for her book.[12] Hilda seemed not to require much sleep. She was constitutionally strong and energetic, and her physical stamina— dating back to her time at Pottstown—had been an enormous asset to her. In time she began working evenings and weekends at Women's Hospital (now St. Luke's Presbyterian) at 114th and Amsterdam to earn extra

money. This was to keep Tish well supplied with imaginative toys. Nearly
every day Hilda went into the Creative Playthings store on Columbus
Avenue, one of the first to carry educational toys and activities materials,
asking "what's new, what's new?" Her daughter was infinitely curious
and Hilda wanted her to have every latest stimulation. Tish eventually
became a tester for new toys, so great was Hilda's enthusiasm. Although
only in her second year of life, Tish was already set in her ways. Like her
mother, she was exceedingly neat and organized. As soon as she could
walk, she wouldn't go to bed until she had put her things—toys, clothes,
crayons—away in their designated places. Recalling this period, Hilda
said, "I would lay down my life to protect her. I tried to always think of the
long-term consequences of what I was doing . . . I was very much aware of
feeling rejected as a child and of the consequences of that . . . I read to her
constantly and always talked to her—she had a great vocabulary."[13]

The 1946–1947 period was a fulfilling and happy year. While Byron
and Hilda worked and went to school, Bertha made a home and took
care of Carolynn and Tish. Bertha's cat "Faff" completed the family. The
apartment was roomy, warm, and bustling with activity. Tish had discovered artwork and spent happy hours at the little easel Hilda had found
for her. Little Tish was a frequent visitor to the TC campus, where she
delighted in feeding stale bread to the pigeons and squirrels on campus.
Although she was not yet 3 years old, Hilda took her to the zoo and to
see her first play, "Alice in Wonderland." It was a time of new beginnings
for all, but life continues and this lovely time was but another interlude.
Byron, Bertha, and Carolynn left during the summer of 1947 to move to
Sampson, Pennsylvania, where Byron would go to junior college before
transferring to Lehigh to finish his college degree. Left alone with a
seven-room apartment and a 2½-year-old child, suddenly bereft of the
child care and homemaking provided by her sister, Peplau began to experience the true challenges of single motherhood. There were economic
strains, time pressures, and the real or imagined stigma of being a woman
alone with a child.

WORKING MOTHER

Hilda's first year as a graduate student had been for the most part a lonely
time as she did double the coursework assumed by other students, and
waited to be reunited with her daughter. The second year was a far hap-
pier, though no less hectic, time. Work, home life, and her writing did not
deter Peplau from her objective, however, which was to join the slim
ranks at that time of hospital-trained nurses who would earn university
graduate degrees. Peplau completed her master's program in Nursing
Education in June 1947, in time for the Repperts to see her receive her

degree. Fewer than 200 of the country's 500,000 nurses held an advanced degree of any sort at that time. Even more rare, Hilda had chosen psychiatric nursing as her specialty. In this, she was in a truly select group, for only four other nurses held a master's degree with a clinical focus in psychiatric nursing. Ninety-nine percent of nursing education remained anchored to the nation's hospital system.

With her MA degree in hand, Hilda hoped and expected to find a position in nursing education, but was surprised to find that doors did not open for her. Her Bennington BA made her academic credentials suspect to less-educated nursing supervisors, and her Teachers College MA seemed, for a time, only to make her prospects worse. Her frustration at the low level of graduate courses in nursing education and her initiative in constructing a more challenging program for herself had not gone unnoticed, and did not help. She had worked hard, and was surprised, taken aback, and somewhat despairing when her advisor, Elizabeth Burgess, called her in at the conclusion of her MA work. "She said it was a shame I was in psych because I was bright," Hilda recalled. "She said that because my background was wrong, I could not teach, but only work in a mental hospital."[14] The fact that Hilda held a BA degree from Bennington College rather than a baccalaureate in nursing, Miss Burgess explained, would disqualify her from teaching in a collegiate school of nursing. Further, university-based nursing programs at that time required instructors to have had several years of staff duty including 2 years as a head nurse, as well as a baccalaureate degree in nursing.[15] While Hilda indeed had extensive staff duty nursing experience at Bellevue and Mount Sinai, as well as in the army hospitals during the war, her experience in the Bennington College health service was not considered equivalent to a "head nurse" position in a hospital, according to Burgess. Nor did her Bennington BA in psychology give her any credibility with this literal-minded nursing faculty member. Hence, for all practical purposes, her Teachers College MA with its focus in psychiatric nursing was simply superfluous.

While deeply disappointed, practical financial considerations precluded brooding or biding her time. Peplau had some correspondence with Karl Menninger about a position at the Menninger Clinic, but largely because there were several doctors and nurses at Menninger's who had been in the 312th Field Hospital during the war, she thought it would be a terrible idea. She had put the 312th and all its associations behind her and felt strongly that it was important to keep it that way. In her contact with physicians she had known at the 312th, the discussions were always professional. They knew nothing of her personal life now, and she did not want former colleagues from the 312th speculating about Tish.

Thus, when the Repperts left for Pennsylvania, Hilda took a full-time position at Bellevue Hospital, working the 11 p.m. to 7 a.m. shift so that she could take care of Tish during the day. For a few hours each morning, she sent the child to nursery school so that she herself could sleep. She paid for baby-sitting through the night. At Bellevue, she worked the night shift on the "Women's Disturbed Service" with two other nurses. The night supervisor was no problem. She would march in, see that all was in order, and then march out, not to be seen again that night. Hilda soon took over and shortly thereafter all was organized. One nurse did the scut work, preparing the medications, serving supper, briefing the interns, and answering the phone. Another passed out the medications and kept her eye on the 30 patients. Peplau spent her time with highly disturbed patients or patients who arrived during the night and were admitted by whatever intern was on duty. Hilda got the other two nurses to agree not to give the newly admitted patients any drugs prescribed by the interns until after she had talked with them, walked with them, and tried to calm them. The interns often were thought to have misdiagnosed when patients admitted during the night were found to be calm enough to be released in the morning.[16]

The cost of the night baby-sitters for Tish, together with the costs of maintaining the apartment and Tish's nursery school, however, were proving to be too much of a financial strain. A colleague she'd known at TC, Reddy Kehoe, lived in Riverdale, up the Hudson from Manhattan. One weekend, she invited Tish and Hilda to visit her and her family. While visiting, Hilda mentioned the strain of keeping the big apartment without her sister and brother-in-law sharing expenses. Reddy immediately suggested Hilda consider moving out of Manhattan to Riverdale. The couple across the hall had a spare bedroom they wanted to rent out, and the Kehoes had three children. Reddy could watch over Tish and provide playmates at the same time. So in October 1947 mother and daughter moved into the spare bedroom of the apartment across the hall from the Kehoes. The commute into Manhattan meant even less time with Tish, and, other than when they were in the small bedroom together, they were seldom alone. Hilda, used to her privacy, felt claustrophobic in the new arrangements.

Although Peplau enjoyed the work at Bellevue and found it challenging, she knew this was not a good situation for her. She still hoped to teach, and felt strongly she would be good at it. Furthermore, Bellevue in 1947 was not the Bellevue she knew in the 1930s. It was on its way to becoming the hellhole later described in the book and film *The Snake Pit*, which portrayed shockingly inhumane conditions in mental hospitals. Of more importance to Hilda, time with Tish was increasingly limited. After the move to Riverdale, Hilda worked the 3–11 evening shift and did not arrive home until after midnight when Tish was already asleep. Tish clearly was not happy in the mornings, and Hilda wasn't there at night to put her to bed and hear about her day. Life was becoming more frustrating than challenging. In fact, it seemed suddenly to have become unmanageable.

At Christmas 1947, Hilda took Tish to visit her Uncle Walter, who was now stationed in Asheville, North Carolina. Being with her brother and his wife, Anne, brought home to Hilda just how lonely and stressed her life in New York had become. At Walter's urging, she agreed to move to North Carolina. There was a private psychiatric hospital in Asheville and housing available next door to Walter and Anne. The day after New Year's 1948 Hilda made the short trip from Walter's house to Highland Hospital, seeking an interview for a position there. She was interviewed by Dr. Basil T. Bennett. Because she needed a job, and because she did not want to appear threatening to anyone, Hilda told Dr. Bennett only that she had graduated from a hospital diploma school and had recently been discharged from the army.[17] Dr. Bennett was impressed and hired her on the spot. First, though, she would return to New York with Tish to collect their few belongings.

Back in New York, Hilda informed the Kehoes that she would be leaving, gave notice on her room, and went to Penn Station to buy two one-way tickets to Asheville. That night, January 9, it snowed 4 feet! Nonetheless, Hilda was determined to go. Little Tish held tightly to her mother's hand and carried her own small suitcase as they slipped and slid down the hill to the subway station. Hilda somehow managed to carry her larger suitcase as well as her typewriter. At Penn Station, they were nearly the only passengers taking the overnight train to Asheville.

HIGHLAND HOSPITAL

The Asheville period would prove to be both an idyllic time and a time of enormous stress. Living near Walter was a godsend. Anne, a skilled seamstress, made little dresses for Tish, the first truly frilly clothes she'd had, clothes it turned out Tish loved. Walter often barbecued in the backyard, and there were many weekend trips and cookouts on the overlooks of the nearby Craggy Mountains. Tish flourished, and Hilda felt blessed having such a dear brother who provided so much comfort and security.

In more ways than one Walter was a father for Tish. During this period, Hilda decided to reopen the adoption issue. The scheme for Bertha to become the adoptive mother before Hilda left the army had not worked out. Now Walter offered to adopt Tish. This proved an excellent solution for Hilda who knew that Tish needed a birth certificate for school enrollment and other purposes. To protect her own career interests, however, Hilda did not want to use the military birth certificate issued with Hilda's name as the natural mother. Thus, while in Asheville, she consulted a lawyer, Walter McGuire, and reopened the adoption proceedings, this time successfully. On July 5, 1949, the adoption was complete and Walter became Tish's father for legal purposes. The fee was $56.20.[18]

Letitia Anne Peplau was issued a small birth record card in North Carolina, which gave no detailed information and which was used when she entered school, got a driver's license, and applied for a passport in the 1960s.

While Hilda's new home life was secure and nurturing, Highland Hospital was another story. Highland was just a few miles away from the Peplau home, on the north side of town. The hospital had been founded by Dr. Robert S. Carroll in 1936 as an experimental psychiatric facility and had been taken over by Duke University in 1945. Surrounded by the Blue Ridge, Smoky, and Balsam mountains, Asheville was blessed by a year-round temperate climate, which was favorable to Carroll's somewhat unorthodox treatment programs. Carroll believed that mental illness could be controlled by diet and rigorous exercise, including a 5-mile daily hike. By climbing up and down the hills surrounding the facility, Carroll believed patients learned perseverance in the face of the monotonous reality of everyday life.[19] The daily calisthenics, hikes, games of volleyball, nightly square dances, and physical work around the hospital (the patients grew their own vegetables), assured that patients were physically tired and generally slept well. The diet included plenty of natural foods. No alcohol or tobacco were permitted and there were no mirrors on the walls. Dr. Carroll's methods were considered so innovative that he lost his medical license, but he had been retained as director with much of his program intact when Highland was taken over by Duke.

The hospital housed 65 patients at a time. Patients lived in several low-slung buildings at the foot of a hill, and Dr. Carroll lived at the top of the hill in a large home, complete with a library and ballroom. Patients who did well were invited to dinner there, where the more attractive female patients got to dance with the doctor. Highland was unique in that many of the staff were hired from among the patients considered cured by their stay in the hospital. When Hilda was there, both the director of nursing and the business manager were former patients. In practice, such staff were often attractive women escaping unhappy marriages or romances. The presence of a coterie of devoted admirers made for a persistent undercurrent of heightened tension.[20] It certainly made for an unique staff. These former patients were sympathetic and empathetic with the current patients (having been there once themselves), as well as extremely loyal to Carroll.

Peplau began work on one of the wards, and worked along quite happily for about two weeks. She hit it off immediately with the physician for that ward, Dr. Irving Pine. Then the summons came: Please come back in to see Dr. Bennett (who had interviewed her initially). She couldn't imagine what she'd done wrong. She had made an effort to make no suggestions, to change nothing. She had worked well with Dr. Pine, and already some of the patients seemed to be making progress. "Well now," Dr. Bennett said, "Irv Pine tells me you know a lot, that you're pretty smart. So tell me now, what's your *real* background?" The game was up. Peplau confessed, and told him more about her experience and academic training. Far from being annoyed, Dr. Bennett was quite excited. He had been searching for someone to open a postgraduate hospital training program at Highland Hospital and had already recruited the first class of six students. They were due to arrive the very next week. Bennett's search for a director had not been successful, however, and no program had been developed. Dr. Bennett had not quite realized how few nurses there were with advanced degrees and had overestimated his ability to recruit one of them to Asheville. Now, though, it appeared his prayers had been answered: Here was Hilda Peplau! She was relieved of her ward duties and given 1 week to design a postgraduate program. She welcomed the challenge.

Almost immediately she ran into trouble. While Drs. Bennett and Pine were delighted with the true background of the new nurse, the director of nursing, Mrs. Sykes, most certainly was not. The two clashed soon after Peplau assumed her new responsibilities. Sykes wanted to place the arriving nurse-students on night duty. Peplau said no way. Only one of the six was even remotely qualified to work unsupervised in a psychiatric hospital; and Peplau was not about to supervise and teach all day, and be on call all night. After much argument, and with great reservation, Peplau finally let the one semi-qualified student be assigned to night duty, while the other five were assigned day duty. The student on night duty was to keep very detailed notes of everything she did, and Peplau would go over them with her the very first thing each morning, just before the day shift began.

The night supervisor, who had herself been a patient not so long before, was most unhappy with all this. She wanted six student nurses, not one. And she wanted those nurses to do as she said, no questions asked. The fact that the one student nurse who was assigned night duty was taking notes of her observations must have been very unsettling, probably calling forth any paranoid inclinations the supervisor might have had. There was tension. One day in early March Peplau found the night supervisor sitting outside the office of the director of nursing, rocking furiously. In Hilda's opinion, appearing clearly psychotic.[21] Hilda went to her own office and phoned Mrs. Sykes, who did not seem concerned. Hilda, however, felt great anxiety, so great that she literally could not think straight. She went for coffee and ran into Dr. Pine. He asked if she felt all right, and she told him she was feeling "strange." At his urging, she went home to get some rest. In retrospect, Peplau believes she was suppressing knowledge of impending disaster. She remembers that consciously she had experienced alarming anxiety but could not identify the cause. That night—March 10, 1948—Highland Hospital burned to the ground.

At home, Hilda slept through the fire, the excitement, and the sirens screaming throughout the night. She awoke the next morning, saying, "I must get to the hospital." When she arrived she found the hospital surrounded by fire engines, police cars, and Red Cross ambulances. Peplau's initial reaction was one of pure anger: All of this was happening without her! She hurried up the hill to Dr. Carroll's house and went directly to the library where patients were gathered. Dr. Pine arrived and told Hilda what was known about the fire. It was already clear that this was arson. Peplau now realized the source of her anxiety of the day before. She was now sure she knew what had happened, but she couldn't even speak of it. She felt as though she'd been rendered mute.

There were several suspects. Eventually the night supervisor was arrested and taken to Winston-Salem, where, under sodium pentothal, she confessed. The night of the fire, she had given a double sedation to the patients she did not like, and for good measure, had locked them in their rooms. She had told the student nurse, the one Hilda had reluctantly assigned to night duty, to stay in the office doing charts that night— that she herself would see to the patients. The student dutifully recorded all of this in her journal, but feeling uneasy, she decided to check up on things. She is the one who discovered the fire, and when she tried to call for help found to her great horror that the phone line had been cut. She had to go to another building to phone in the alarm. She was even more horrified to discover that about half the patients were trapped in locked rooms. Staff and firemen struggled to free them, but were hampered by heavy chains on the outside windows and the rapid incineration of the wooden external fire escapes. In all, nine patients died, including Zelda Fitzgerald, who was then a patient at Highland Hospital.[22] Peplau herself was so traumatized by this experience that she was never been able to recall the name of the student nurse who lived through such horror. For years, this nurse would reintroduce herself at professional meetings, but each time Peplau would be so overcome with feelings of guilt she would in consequence suppress her name.[23]

After the fire, Dr. Bennett raised the possibility that Hilda might stay on as director of nursing at Highland Hospital, but soon thereafter Bennett himself left Highland, which was sold by Duke University to Dr. Charmen Carroll, the adopted daughter of the founder. Charmen Carroll offered Peplau the directorship of the hospital and a partnership in the business—an opportunity that Hilda declined. The fire had been traumatic, and former patients still comprised a large portion of the staff. As tempting as it was to stay in this lovely city where her brother and his family lived, and to have the freedom to design a psychiatric nursing service as she thought it should be, she could not suppress the intuition that for her this would be a mistake. Peplau realized that she really wanted to teach and do research. She made the decision to leave, but in later years she would often wonder what her life would have been like had she stayed in Asheville at Highland Hospital and designed a nursing service and nursing education program to reflect her own principles. Although she would have a challenging and fulfilling career, she would often rethink the decision to leave Asheville.[24] It had not been an easy choice, but in her heart Hilda knew she belonged in an academic setting.

RETURN TO TEACHERS COLLEGE

While Peplau had been both dismayed and disappointed when her TC adviser told her that her background did not qualify her to teach at the college level, she soon learned that others did not share that view. In January, shortly after she settled in Asheville, Katharine Tucker, the dean of nursing at the University of Pennsylvania, inquired whether Hilda would be interested in developing an advanced program in psychiatric nursing there, assuming Penn received a grant under the aegis of the new National Mental Health Act of 1946.[25] In April, Martha Smith, the dean of the Boston University School of Nursing, wrote to express surprise that Hilda was in Asheville: "I didn't know you were at Highland Hospital. You should be in a university . . . Please contact me if you might be available."[26]

Shortly after the fire Peplau attended a conference at Duke University. Her old friend, Dr. Maurice Greenhill, whom she had known in the 312th Hospital, was there, as was Dr. Helen Nahm, one of the few nurses in the country with a doctorate, who was then working at the new National Institute of Mental Health. Dr. Greenhill and Dr. Nahm both urged her to return to a teaching environment where, they asserted, she was sorely needed.[27] Teachers College also tracked her down at Highland Hospital. On July 19, 1948, R. Louise McManus, who had assumed the position of director of the TC Nursing Education program the previous fall, wrote to ask Hilda to call immediately if she would be interested in returning to TC as an instructor.[28] Hilda made the call. The next day McManus wired to inform her that Miss Ruth Gilbert would be in Richmond the following week and could interview her there. Hilda wired that she would be there, and then rode the bus all night to keep the date. In early August Hilda received another letter from McManus offering her the position of instructor of psychiatric nursing at a salary of $3,300, plus tuition remission for two courses toward her doctorate.[29] Peplau wrote back immediately accepting the offer, stating, "I trust that you will find my abilities equal to the challenges the position presents: I can assure you of my interest in doing my best."[30] She gave 1 month's notice to Highland Hospital and took the long train ride back up to New York to look for an apartment and to enroll Tish at the Midtown Children's Center, one of the nation's first and most progressive centers for early childhood education. There Tish was introduced as the niece she was raising, the adopted child of her brother.

One of the attractions of the position at Teachers College was that it allowed Hilda to study for a doctoral degree as well as teach. Hilda decided she very much wanted this degree. Surely no academic institution would question her Bennington BA if she held both an MA and a doctorate in nursing education. In spite of her misgivings about the quality and nature of nursing education at Teachers College, the TC nursing program was the largest in the country and one of only a handful that offered nurses the opportunity to earn advanced degrees. The program enjoyed a national reputation and had at least one endowed chair, the Professorship in Nursing Education funded by the Helen Hartley Foundation, and a steady input of grant money from Mary Todd Rockefeller personally as well as from the Rockefeller and Kellogg foundations, which assured that nursing education at TC was well funded.[31] Hilda was excited by the potential for a career in academe where she could combine her intellectual, practice, and research interests, and for this reason the opportunity at TC, which was then considered the most prestigious nursing education program in the country, seemed very promising. She would again lay claim to the G.I. Bill, and that, together with her teaching stipend and tuition waivers, would make it possible for her to pursue a doctoral degree while providing adequate child care for Tish.

Search for a Home

Even with the income provided by her instructorship, Hilda found that housing for herself and Tish would become a greater problem than she could ever have anticipated. Their return to New York marked the beginning again of both the best of times and the worst of times for mother and daughter. On the one hand Hilda in this period would enjoy the delights of exploring both the educational and recreational opportunities of the city with her bright and companionable daughter, while on the other hand she and Tish would endure a truly horrifying series of housing misadventures.

At the time of her appointment to the TC instructorship, she placed an ad in a New York newspaper for a room and board arrangement for herself and Tish and was contacted by a couple who had an apartment on West End Avenue at 86th Street. Hilda knew that between teaching, attending classes, working on the manuscript for her book, and doing part-time work for extra money, she would not have time to shop and cook. In early September 1948 mother and daughter took the train back to New

York, carrying one large suitcase, the ever-present old Royal typewriter, and two coats. They splurged on a taxi to the apartment at 495 West End Avenue, where they met their new "family."

Hilda had misgivings from the beginning, but felt they could remain until other arrangements could be made. She and 3-year-old Tish shared a large room and bath. Under the room and board arrangement breakfast for both would be provided and Tish would be given dinner each evening. Hilda left at 7:00 every morning, and Tish was taken to her preschool bus at 8:00 a.m. Hilda would return after dinner and take Tish to their room to talk about her day and read her stories, making shadow figures with her hands on the walls to illustrate. After Tish went to sleep, Hilda either studied or worked on her manuscript until midnight.

At Christmas, Hilda and Tish had a happy family reunion with Bertha, Byron and Carolynn Reppert at their home in Bethlehem, Pennsylvania, together with Hilda and Bertha's brother Harold and their father, Gustav. Walter's adoption of Tish was not yet complete but it was in process. If Gustav had any idea about Tish's true parentage, he did not acknowledge this. Bertha believes he did not know. This would be the family's last Christmas with Gustav, who died of a stroke in September of 1949.

One evening in February, Hilda arrived home at the apartment on West End Avenue to witness a most distressing scene. Tish was a very particular child. Everything had to be just right. She was sitting at the dinner table stubbornly refusing to eat some fried carrots. Smart, but not devious, Tish finally stood up and dumped her carrots on top of the garbage, at which point the landlady hauled off and slapped the child hard across the face. Hilda had never struck Tish, and was truly appalled. Hilda took Tish to their room and comforted her, assuring her that they would leave. "Promise?" asked the little girl. Hilda promised. They got up early the next morning and again packed all they owned, into two suitcases this time, took Tish's favorite doll and the old typewriter, put on their coats, and walked out. The landlady tried to stop them, assuring Hilda this would not happen again. "If you did this once, you'll do it again. We're leaving now," Hilda told her.[32] She later discovered this couple had lost custody of their two daughters after beating them nearly to death. Back to the train they went, this time to go out to Byron and Bertha's home in Bethlehem, where Byron was a student at Lehigh University. Once again Tish stayed with the Repperts, while Hilda returned to New York to find another place to live.

It wasn't easy, but she did find a one-bedroom fourth-floor walk-up apartment at 322 West 88th Street for $150 a month—exactly half her monthly income. A student in one of Peplau's classes passed along to them a cot, four chairs, and a table which did double duty as a dining room table and desk. Money was so tight they were lucky if there were cans of soup or spaghetti at the end of the month.[33] Child care on 88th

Street at first appeared to be easily solved. Another single woman lived on the first floor and had a daughter, Britony, who was Tish's age. The mother offered to collect Tish from her school and the two girls would play together until Hilda got home around 6:00 in the evening. Hilda was somewhat concerned when Britony would become quite distraught when it was time for Tish to leave, but assumed that the behavior wasn't entirely abnormal. After all, Tish seemed to be the child's only friend. Just as Hilda was counting her blessings, however, the police arrived. It was then that Hilda learned that the mother was a prostitute who drugged Britony at night while she either went out or brought home "dates," when more drugs would be used. The child sensed something was wrong in her home, and dreaded being there alone with her mother. Soon, both were gone. The next tenant in the first-floor apartment was a nurse who had served in the Pacific during World War II, and who immediately volunteered to help with baby-sitting. After an outing with Tish and this new friend, Hilda discovered that her typewriter was missing. It had vanished from the apartment—in which there was little else to steal. The next day, when visiting in the nurse's apartment, Hilda had an uncanny feeling that her typewriter was in a chest in the living room. Hilda casually lifted the lid. There was her typewriter. When the nurse opened her coat closet, Hilda noticed a row of clothes with tags still on them. The new neighbor and volunteer baby-sitter was a kleptomaniac.

Peplau was learning the hard way the vicissitudes of being a single mother in New York City. She was fortunate, though, in having a bright and highly adaptable child. Tish was thriving at the Midtown Children's Center, which was run by Ethel Abrams, a cousin of the famous composer Leonard Bernstein. Tish's precocious intellect and self-possessed ways were immediately noted. One day a child fell on the playground and starting screaming hysterically. Tish immediately and instinctively gathered the other children together, shepherded them into a corner and got them playing a game while the teachers dealt with the emergency. Tish's individualism was also apparent At Midtown the girls were encouraged to wear slacks so that they could play vigorously. Unfortunately for Hilda, Tish adamantly refused to wear anything but skirts and the pretty dresses made for her by her Aunt Anne in Asheville. In an era before synthetic fabrics, when cotton dresses had to be ironed, this domestic chore became quite a burden for Hilda.

Tish had playmates at school and invited classmates to her fifth birthday party, which was held at the 88th Street apartment on February 4, 1950. Finding appropriate playmates outside of school, however, remained a challenge. After the setbacks with little Britony and the kleptomaniac baby-sitter, Hilda thought a solution had been found. At the Children's Center, Tish had met a bright young girl whose father manufactured children's clothing. Tish loved to dress up and had a flair for putting together exotic outfits. The parents had sent a box of clothing seconds in Tish's size to the Peplaus, and Tish was in seventh heaven. Whenever Hilda was held up at TC, Tish was invited to the apartment of her new friend to play until Hilda could come for her. One day when Hilda asked, "And what did you do today?" Tish replied that they had played a game called "nudity." "And how did that go?" asked a shaken Hilda. Tish then explained that when her playmate's father came home from work, he undressed and the girls climbed on his bare back, beating him as he galloped around the apartment! Needless to say, Tish never returned to that apartment to play. From experiences such as these, Hilda learned to be ever vigilant where her child was concerned.

Better times lay ahead. Soon after this distressing incident, Kay Nelson, a fellow faculty member at Teachers College, stopped Peplau in the hall and mentioned that she was going away for a year and had a nice apartment on 110th between Broadway and Columbus, just a few blocks from the Cathedral of St. John the Divine and within easy walking distance of TC. If Hilda would like it, Kay would be happy to sublet it. The rent was $5 a month less than what Hilda was paying on 88th Street, the neighborhood was pleasant, and the building well maintained. So Tish and Hilda moved up to 504 West 110th Street. Kay Nelson did not return at the end of the year, and the Peplaus remained happily settled in this apartment for more than 3 years. Here, Hilda was fortunate, for finally she met a wonderful neighbor with a child Tish's age. Tish and Mary Alameda soon became very close friends. Mrs. Alameda was home all day and loved to have the well-behaved Tish playing with Mary. As often as not, the children would play at the Peplau apartment, which was amply furnished with childproof furniture and where Tish's creative imagination was allowed full rein. Life in the Peplau apartment was, indeed, very child-centered. Tish would turn a card table into a "house" by covering it with a sheet. Chairs for the playhouse were made from fat New York City phone books covered with washcloths. A towel suspended by safety pins created "rooms." Sometimes an even larger playhouse was made by suspending one end of an old curtain from the bedroom windows and tying the other end to the bedposts. When Tish later acquired a record player and a collection of 45 rpm records, she would construct a "city" in the hallway of the apartment using dominoes and blocks as walls and records as the floors for skyscrapers and other inventions.

Hilda, in turn, was able to make a real home at last in this apartment. In the early 1930s she had purchased a handsome set of cherry wood bedroom furniture from a friend in Pottstown, which included a double bed, two bureaus, and a framed mirror. This set had been in storage for many years, but was retrieved when Hilda and Tish moved to the 110th Street apartment. The cherry wood pieces remain to this day in the family, as do the graceful child's rocker and a doll cradle made by Hilda's father and which completed the bedroom furnishings at 504 W. 110th Street. The combination living room and dining room was more eclectically furnished and over time became quite crowded. Hilda had an antique love seat and an antique cherry drop leaf table with four chairs. There was also a sofa and two upholstered chairs, and a number of bookcases crammed with books and files. In 1952 space was made for a prized purchase, a baby grand piano, purchased with the advance Hilda received when her book was accepted for publication. Tish, too, had her own furniture, notably a child's play table and chairs and, later, a crudely constructed coffee table made by Tish in a carpentry class and prominently featured by Hilda among the more sturdy pieces of living room furniture.

MOTHER AND DAUGHTER

While the years of Hilda's tenure as an instructor at Teachers College would prove to be tumultuous for her professionally, this period—from the fall of 1948 through 1952—was a happy time for mother and daughter as Tish grew older and the two discovered the delights of the city together. Sundays were made special when they walked to the bakery at the corner of Broadway and 110th to purchase sweet cinnamon buns for breakfast. A very special occasion warranted a trip to Schraft's where they would sit in a green leather booth and Tish would be treated to a chocolate ice-cream sundae, served in a silver sundae dish with butterscotch sauce and chopped walnuts. Money was always tight, but in 1950 Hilda enrolled Tish in a once-a-week program at a creative dance school—at a cost of $25, which for Hilda was a major investment. That summer Hilda had agreed to teach summer school at TC to earn a few extra dollars to provide these advantages for her daughter. The problem was, she herself had no summer dresses suitable for work. At the end of May, Hilda took the subway down to the bargain stores on 14th Street in lower Manhattan where she bought five dresses for $3 each. For the next 6 weeks she wore one of those five dresses each day of the week. She was afraid to wash them for fear that they would fall apart. At the end of the 6 weeks, she simply threw them away. They had served their purpose, and she had saved the money she might have had to spend on a better wardrobe.

Hilda's frequent outings with Tish included more summer trips to the children's petting zoos at the Central Park and Bronx zoos and to the Statue of Liberty in the New York Harbor. At Thanksgiving there was the famous Macy's Parade. At Christmas they went to see the lighted tree at Rockefeller Center, to watch the skaters on the tiny rink there, and to wonder at the magnificent holiday window displays at New York's elegant department stores. They went to free concerts, to museums, and to an occasional play, including *Peter Pan* starring Mary Martin. There was also a trip to the *Howdy Doody* television show where Tish had her picture taken with Howdy, Clarabelle, and Buffalo Bob. Coney Island was also a favorite destination.

Franny Burgess Martucci, a friend who had been a student with Hilda at TC, was in 1951 a private-duty nurse. Her patient was George C. Tilyou, who in 1897 had opened a 15-acre amusement park, called "Steeple Chase—The Funny Place" on Coney Island.[34] It was the Disneyland of his day. Tilyou lived in a grand Brooklyn home, and almost every day in the spring and summer Franny would take him to sit in the sun and watch the Steeple Chase parachute ride. Tish and Hilda got into the routine of taking the BMT subway to Brooklyn where Hilda would sit with the garrulous Mr. Tilyou while Franny took Tish off for a few hours roaming the park. At the end of the day Tilyou would take them all to dinner at his favorite Italian restaurant.[35] Eventually Tilyou gave Hilda a lifetime pass to Steeple Chase and a pass for all the rides for Tish. For months to follow there were weekend trips to Coney Island.

That summer and fall, nearly every Saturday, they got on the BMT subway and joined the platoons in summer shirts and shorts heading out to the beach at the end of the line. With Tish in shorts and Hilda in skirts, they carried one little bag with their sandals and towels. Their companions on the subway carried bags of groceries, cases of beer, buckets of ice, folding chairs, sand pails and shovels—all bound for the beach. There Tish mastered the art of weaving through the crowds, avoiding the blankets of strangers, finding a path to the boardwalk, Steeple Chase, or to the ocean. Coney Island in the 1950s was a vivid melding of sights, sounds, and smells. The symbol of the park was a huge grinning face, a slightly menacing joker. A mechanical race course ran around the edges of the park, with carved wooden horses carrying human riders moving into the dells and over water and above hedges, while music played on a blurred sound system. The rides and runways were teeming on the weekends with thousands of people, eating corn on the cob, cotton candy, ice-cream cones. Tish loved every minute of it, and so did Hilda.

As fall moved into winter, Tish and Hilda often went out to New Jersey where Byron and Bertha were now living in the small town of Green Brook. In contrast to the crowds and wild laughter of the summertime Coney Island line, they sedately rode the train under the Hudson River and out into the quiet New Jersey countryside. They both looked forward to these trips to the Repperts' warm home where green plants grew in every nook and corner and the walls were adorned with Bertha's drying herbs and Byron's growing collection of jugs. Bertha created beautiful centerpieces and arrangements from materials in her garden, inspiring Hilda and Tish to create an arrangement of their own from a graceful, silvery branch they found when visiting the Repperts. That branch, hung on the wall at the 110th Street apartment, was decorated with a string of lights at Christmastime and with colored eggs at Easter. Later, when Tish and Hilda themselves moved to New Jersey, the holiday branch went with them as a memento of their New York home.[36]

Hilda felt it was important to expose Tish to religion, since her own upbringing had been religious. Not having a particular allegiance to the Lutheran church of her youth, Hilda selected a Methodist Church at 86th and Amsterdam. There Tish earned several bars on her "perfect attendance" pin. When Hilda picked Tish up from her Sunday School class, she would listen intently as the child explained what she'd learned. Hilda's interest did not go unnoticed, and in 1951 the pastor asked if she would teach a class for adolescent boys. Hilda knew nothing about adolescent boys but was intrigued by the challenge. She accepted, and each Sunday she would discuss the assigned lesson for 5 minutes, then ask the boys to open their Bibles and point to a passage at random. The class would then discuss the meaning of these randomly chosen passages and their relevance to the boys' everyday lives. At first the boys were sullen, then skeptical, then they began to get really interested. Soon, Hilda's class was lively and excited. This too did not escape notice. Parents were concerned by her unconventional approach to the Bible and perhaps also to the freewheeling discussions that ensued in Hilda's class. The matter was brought to Hilda's attention by the pastor who clearly hoped she would adopt a more customary teaching style. "I don't have time for this," she replied. "So fine, let one of those complaining parents teach"[37]— and with her characteristic low tolerance for nonsense, she walked out. Such a forthright abruptness and straightforward reaction may be understandable, but it was bound to cause problems in the years ahead.

An Uncommon Teacher

It is difficult to imagine how Hildegard Peplau could have made time for the many weekend excursions and enhanced learning experiences she personally provided Tish in these years—much less take on a Bible study class. She was in every respect an uncommon teacher, and the path she set for herself in the period from 1948 through 1952 was continually accelerating. Within a very short period of time Peplau forced an innovative instructional program on a conservative and unimaginative Division of Nursing Education. Her director, R. Louise McManus, was at first very supportive, then resistant, and eventually hostile, but Peplau had to be tolerated. Her classes were popular, and, of more importance to McManus, Peplau had begun to bring funding from the National Institute of Mental Health to TC, funding that not only sustained her programs but also enhanced the reputation of the TC Division of Nursing Education. Moreover, although she was only an instructor, and in the process of earning her doctorate at that, by 1950 Peplau was quite active professionally and was beginning to develop a national reputation as a leader in psychiatric nursing. Her ideas about nursing education were groundbreaking, and her view that nurses could participate in the treatment of mental patients was absolutely radical. It is not surprising that her career as a teacher at TC would prove to be a rocky one.

ENDNOTES

1. Letter from Mrs. Jessica Cosgrove to Hildegard E. Peplau, July 23, 1945, Box 9, #306.
2. Interview, Hildegard Peplau, March 30, 1992, in Sherman Oaks.
3. Virginia Henderson passed away early in 1996. In 1989, the International Council for Nursing established nursing's most distinguished prize, the Christiane Reimann Prize. The first prize was given in 1992 and there were two nominees, Hildegard Peplau and Virginia Henderson. The first prize went to Virginia Henderson. Five years later in 1997, the second Christiane Reimann Prize was awarded to Hildegard E. Peplau.
4. See Barbara Anne Pedersen, *The McManus Years: Advances in the Division of Nursing Education, Teacher's College, Columbia University* (PhD Dissertation, Columbia University, Ann Arbor: University Microfilms, 1992), pp. 24-26.
5. *Bulletin, Teacher's College, Columbia University,* 1947–1949, Box 14, Schlesinger Library collection.
6. Letter from Hilda Peplau to Bertha Reppert, October 10, 1945, Box 5, #178.
7. Letters from Agnes Von Nieda to Hilda Peplau, January–March, 1946, Box 5, #178.
8. Interview, Bertha Reppert, October 30, 1994, in Mechanicsburg, Pennsylvania.
9. Letter from Agnes Von Nieda to Hilda Peplau, March, 4, 1946, Box 5, #178.
10. Interview, Hildegard Peplau, February 11, 1992.
11. In 1968 Bertha established Rosemary House in Mechanicsburg, Pennsylvania, a very successful "flavors and fragrances" shop and internationally known mail-order business related to herbs. By 1993 she had written 10 books and been awarded many awards, honors, and prizes for her work as a herbalist, author, lecturer, and entrepreneur. It has been said that, "Bertha is to herbs what Hilda is to psychiatric nursing."
12. Interview, Hildegard Peplau, March 2, 1992.
13. Ibid, April 15, 1992.
14. Ibid, March 2, 1992.
15. Interview, Grayce Sills, June 1995, in Washington, D.C.
16. Interview, Hildegard Peplau, February 6, 1992, and letter to the author, August 25, 1998.
17. Ibid, January 25, 1992.
18. See correspondence with Walter McGuire in Box 2, #52.
19. Nancy Milford, *Zelda* (New York: Avon Books, 1970), 369.
20. Interview, Hildegard Peplau, March 2, 1992.
21. Ibid.
22. Materials on the fire at Highland Hospital are in Box 15, #488–493.
23. From newspaper clippings and notes on the fire written by Hilda Peplau, Box 8, Schlesinger Library.
24. Interview, Hildegard Peplau, January 25, 1992.

25. Letter from Katharine Tucker to Hilda Peplau, January 2, 1948, Box 10, #306.
26. Letter from Martha Smith to Hilda Peplau, April 5 and May 4, 1948, Box 10, #306.
27. Interview, Hildegard Peplau, January 25, 1992.
28. Letter from (Mrs.) R. Louise McManus to Hilda Peplau, July 19, 1948, Box 9, #306.
29. Letter from R. L. McManus to Hilda E. Peplau, August 2, 1948, Box 9, #306.
30. Letter from Hilda E. Peplau to R. Louise McManus, August 5, 1948, Box 9, #307.
31. Interview, Arthur Levine, New Brunswick, New Jersey, February 16, 1994.
32. Interview, Hildegard Peplau, January 25, 1992.
33. Ibid, April 15, 1992.
34. Pete Hamill, "Coney Island," *New York 26*, (June–July, 1993): 57.
35. Interview, Fran Martucci, April 15, 1992, in Santa Monica, California.
36. Interview, Hildegard Peplau, April 15, 1992.
37. Ibid, March 30, 1992.

Teachers College: Beginning a Career

7

I believed that interpersonal techniques could be devised and utilized in teaching . . . I believed that these techniques, rather than modifications of medical-surgical technical learning, are the crux of nursing education . . . their idea was brush your teeth, brush your mind!
—*Hildegard Peplau*
February 2, 1992

Peplau was approaching the age of 40 when she returned to Teachers College (TC) in 1948 as an instructor. She had been disappointed in her days as a master's degree student at TC, and she was excited by the challenge of giving her own students a very different experience. In particular, she was convinced that Sullivan's theories of interpersonal relations could be applied to teaching as well as to psychotherapy.[1] In essence, the core of interpersonal relations theory is that mental health is established by harmonious interaction between conscious and unconscious mental processes and drives on the one hand, and adaptation to the requirements of the outer world and to relationships with other people on the other.[2] Peplau believed that students' experience in the classroom itself could and should be used to promote learning, and further that such learning would be more effective than traditional or didactic forms of instruction.[3] She was not naive nor unrealistic about the tension between traditional nursing education, where students learned largely by rote, and the expectations of a college education where students should be taught to think independently, to question, and to extend knowledge rather than to simply absorb existing knowledge. She hoped that in a great university, her ideas about using interpersonal relations theory as a new tool of instruction in nursing education would be welcomed.

Peplau's goal at Teachers College was nothing less than to make a substantive contribution to nursing education. Her overall ambition was to teach in such a way as to enable nurses to become independent thinkers

167

who could solve problems on their own, work autonomously, and thereby contribute to the advancement of human welfare as well as to the advancement of their own profession. In order to do this, she had concluded that lectures weren't enough. In learning to think for themselves, students must observe and record their own behavior in the classroom and get detailed and specific feedback, first from their peers, then from their instructor, in order to understand the impact of their own words, actions, and reactions on each other and their learning. Finally, in their coursework nurses needed to learn and be able to apply the concepts and theories of a wide array of thinkers, not just learn the standard procedures of patient care. Nurses needed to see themselves and the particular ways in which they talked to each other and to patients as part of a therapeutic process.[4]

The factor Hilda failed to consider in all this was the resistance she would meet at Teachers College. On the surface, it seemed that R. Louise McManus, the new director of the Division of Nursing Education, and Hildegard Peplau had much in common. McManus was an innovator and a solicitous mentor to her staff. In fact, a majority had studied with her. She had supervised their dissertations as a faculty member and as director continued to mentor them through their academic careers[5]—as in fact Peplau would for staff in later years.

Louise McManus was no newcomer to Teachers College. After receiving her nursing diploma from Massachusetts General Hospital in 1920, McManus earned her BSc from TC in 1925 and her MA in 1927. She had joined the staff in 1925, the year that Isabel Maitland Stewart became director of the Nursing Education program. In 1940 McManus became chairman of a joint committee of the National League for Nursing, the Association of Collegiate Schools of Nursing, and Teachers College, established in 1938 to develop state board tests for RN licensure. She also worked on a major curriculum study funded by the Rockefeller Foundation, and through these positions had gained recognition as a leader in the field of nursing education.[6]

The nursing program was the largest program in Teachers College, which, in turn, was the largest unit in Columbia University. Moreover, the TC Division of Nursing Education was then considered the country's leading graduate program in nursing. Hilda's own education in the field of psychiatry, however, had gone far beyond anything that the TC nursing program had to offer. She had taken courses with Erich Fromm and Joseph Chassell at Bennington, and attended classes taught by Harry Stack Sullivan and Frieda Fromm Reichman at Chestnut Lodge. During the war she had worked side by side with physicians who by 1948 were assuming or held positions of leadership in American psychiatry. For several years Hilda had been thinking seriously about what nurses could do in the field of psychotherapy and how they could do it. She was excited by the intellectual challenge of developing courses that excited students intellectually as well as prepared them for therapeutic work with the mentally ill. She looked forward to making major curricular contributions in mental health nursing and to graduate education in nursing.

As director of the Division of Nursing Education, McManus's goals were to establish a firm financial base for the division through grants and endowments and to "advance a professional ideology for nursing."[7] McManus emphasized that the graduate nurse should "spend her time in professional activities supervising others rather than in actual nursing."[8] She believed there should be a clear separation between preparation for service and preparation for education. The emphasis at TC was to be on "professional nursing," and thus the curriculum was to focus on supervision, administration of schools of nursing, and teaching.[9] Nothing could be more diametrically opposite to Hildegard Peplau's evolving vision for the future of nursing built around clinical specialization and graduate education based on research in patient care.

AN INNOVATIVE TEACHER

Peplau's reputation as a gifted and innovative teacher took root almost immediately. In her first semester at TC as an instructor she was asked to teach the introductory course, "Mental Hygiene and Nursing." Because "their idea of mental hygiene was brush your teeth, brush your brain," that is, learn the routines and don't think, Hilda requested that the course title be changed to "Interpersonal Relations in Nursing."[10] Since there were no materials she thought appropriate for an introductory graduate course in nursing, Hilda created the course outline as she went along. Instead of lecturing students on how to establish and maintain order on a typical hospital ward, Peplau emphasized making a positive contribution to patient care and recovery. As she would later state it,

> The emphasis in psychiatric nursing is *not* on managerial activities. Historically, these have been aspects of custodial care with restraint, protection, cleanliness and order the dominant themes . . . these are *not* professional activities . . . can be better performed far better and more cheaply by high school graduates . . . they are largely busywork which keeps the nurse away from direct contact with patients.[11]

She invited two psychiatrists, Dr. John Rosen and Dr. Jacob Moreno, to lecture on establishing relationships with both doctors and patients. In addition to guest lectures, she used films and psychodrama to illustrate her points. Students played the part of doctors, then patients, and then nurses. Miss Peplau's class soon became very popular. Word spread, and other instructors began to send their students to the class. Then, the instructors themselves began attending. Eventually, TC would make this course a part of its core program required of all students.

Peplau's participatory and interactive approach to teaching raised eyebrows then, but this was nothing compared to the concern about an approach added the next year when she involved her students in group therapy experiences. At that time she contracted with Dr. Joseph Geller, a New York psychiatrist, to meet in group sessions with her students to "try out the possibilities in bringing the skills of a group therapist to bear on the teaching of psychiatric nursing."[12] The purpose was for the students to learn to use group therapy techniques in their future work, whether as teachers or as mental health practitioners. Peplau secured a stipend for this project and was able to offer Geller $10 per session per person for his efforts. Dr. John Schimel from the William Alanson White Institute later joined Geller in conducting these sessions. Group work proved to be an intense experience for many of the psychiatric nursing students and a factor that tended to set "Miss Peplau's students" apart from the general student population. This approach to teaching was indeed innovative and did not go unnoticed by Peplau's colleagues. Some were curious, some were puzzled, and some were hostile. None was oblivious to the fact that Hildegard Peplau was beginning to do very different things in her classroom.

Peplau carried the title of instructor, but with her appointment to the Teachers College faculty she had also been named director of a new program in Advanced Psychiatric Nursing. In the fall of 1948 the program existed in name only: There were no courses, no curriculum, no funding, and basically no faculty. Peplau would have to construct the program, develop the courses, find the clinical field placements, and apply for funding to support both the program and the students. In the first year she succeeded in getting National Institute of Mental Health (NIMH) funding for developing the program. Because she considered her own clinical/practicum experiences when she was an MA student to have been boring and a waste of time, Peplau decided that her students would have meaningful clinical assignments. In addition to NIMH funding for program development, she also submitted a training grant to the Public Health Service (PHS). The grant was funded, with the result that all her students would be supported by fairly generous PHS stipends during the years Peplau was at TC. Early on she determined that the students in her graduate program would focus their learning on the nurse/patient relationship itself, and not something called "processes of education," a vague catchall phrase used to describe the content of most courses in nursing education at TC.

Oblivious, or perhaps merely indifferent, to the fact that she was at odds with the philosophy of the school, Peplau plowed ahead. In contrast to merely observing others caring for patients or learning how to administer units in a mental hospital, her students would be "talking with patients." The distinction between "talking" with patients and "caring for" patients is critical. Nurses at that time "cared" for patients only in the physical sense—bathing, giving medications, and taking temperatures. Peplau's concept of what nurses could and should do on the wards of psychiatric hospitals was a far different thing.[13]

BROOKLYN STATE HOSPITAL

In order for her students to study a nurse-patient relationship, Peplau needed patients with whom students could work without interference. Such a situation was not easy to find. Hilda canvassed the New York City hospitals, seeking such a placement for her students, to no avail. Finally, the nursing director at Brooklyn State Hospital, Florence Unwin, agreed to help. Mrs. Unwin was a diploma nurse, but she was convinced that nursing could indeed do a great deal to improve patient care in public mental hospitals if given the opportunity. Florence Unwin wanted to help, but she had first to clear the project with the hospital's director, Dr. Clarence Bellinger.

Coincidentally, Bellinger was a childhood friend of Harry Stack Sullivan. In fact, each had been the other's only childhood friend.[14] Hilda had not forgotten the impact of Sullivan's seminars at Chestnut Lodge and since that time had read most of Sullivan's writings. She considered him to be her greatest intellectual influence. Bellinger and Sullivan both had lonely childhoods, and both had gone to medical school and taken residencies in psychiatry. In the 1920s both had become interested in research. But, while Sullivan moved to higher levels of theoretical sophistication, Bellinger sought appointments in state hospitals where he could conduct statistical studies of various sorts. Bellinger had become the superintendent of the Brooklyn State Hospital in 1935. As adults, the two psychiatrists had not remained friends.[15] Fortunately for Peplau, she did not know of the childhood connection and never spoke of Sullivan to Bellinger.

Dr. Bellinger was willing to meet with the new nursing instructor, but was skeptical about her ideas. When Hilda met him, he talked and talked about how difficult his job was, but expressed no curiosity as to why Miss Peplau might want her students to talk with patients. She listened quietly and attentively, and when he wound down, she remarked; "This is precisely why I want students to talk to patients—so we can better understand how difficult your job is." Bellinger was flattered and agreed to let Peplau's students work in his hospital, but gave the nurses access only to the most "hopeless" patients in the back wards—patients who had been given multiple electroshock treatments or lobotomies. There were no nurses on these wards, only surly attendants who did not appreciate the invasion of their territory. Many hours were spent by the students and the professor analyzing how to work effectively with patients without drawing Bellinger's attention or upsetting the attendants.[16]

It was not easy. Many of Peplau's students had been staff nurses in state mental hospitals before returning to school for graduate work, and were resistant to the notion that something could be done with patients as sick as these.[17] Their conventional understanding of mental hospitals was being challenged. Peplau replied that, contrary to their understanding, students needed to study the pathology of the ward to determine its dynamics and look for points of possible change. With Unwin's help, each student was assigned to a patient and required to spend an hour with that patient twice a week for one academic year, taking verbatim notes, no matter how disjointed or incoherent the conversation. Before the days of modern copy machines, the notes were painstakingly rendered in duplicate by means of carbon copies. Peplau went over these notes word for word and wrote voluminous suggestions on the transcripts.[18]

Gradually the patients with whom the students were talking began to improve. Someone was interested in them as individuals, and the results were evident. They took showers, dressed better, combed their hair, asked for shaves and haircuts, and became more coherent. The attendants began paying attention to the work the TC students were doing. They noticed the progress patients were making and improvement in the atmosphere on the wards. The attendants reported this to the physicians, who maintained that changes observed were only superficial, that there was no actual improvement in the mental state of their patients. The doctors complained to Bellinger who concluded that physician supervision of the students' work was required. He issued a directive that TC students must attend a weekly seminar with Dr. Nathan Beckenstein and his staff before reporting to work on the ward. This was not in Peplau's plan. She did not want physicians supervising what she and her students were doing. A diversion was devised to head off potential interference.[19]

Peplau decided to introduce a new course into the curriculum, entitled "Preparation for Field Work." This course was open only to students doing fieldwork at Brooklyn State Hospital. Peplau impressed upon her students the importance of protecting the confidentiality of the patients. Therefore, she directed, no patient data were to be shared with the doctor. Instead, Hilda and her students came up with theoretical or clinical questions to pose for Beckenstein—in effect, to seize control of the agenda, consume the hour, and divert attention from their individual case studies. Each student was assigned two questions to ask every week, and the rotation was mixed up so that the questioning would appear spontaneous. At first, the students were terrified. The idea of questioning Dr.

Beckenstein left them shaking in their shoes—but they feared the wrath of Miss Peplau more. With the proper degree of temerity and respect, they began asking the questions.[20] Beckenstein was taken aback by the depth and seriousness of the issues these student nurses raised. The plan worked for about 6 weeks before he put two and two together. He called Peplau and demanded, "What's going on here?" Thinking quickly, Hilda replied that because he could give more expert answers then she, she urged the students to take their classroom questions to him. Like Dr. Bellinger, Beckenstein was flattered, and then satisfied with her answer. Later, Dr. Beckenstein would become one of Peplau's closest friends.[21] The back ward patients at Brooklyn State were the first of many such patients that Peplau students would see over the years.[22] Out of these early nurse-patient relationship studies Peplau began to define the concepts and the processes of psychotherapy she would use in teaching her students throughout her career.[23]

A Growing Audience

Three-and-a-half-year-old Tish was happy and appreciated at the Midtown Children's Center. When mother and daughter moved to the apartment at 504 W. 110th Street that was to become their first real home together, they met the Alameda family, and their luck with neighbors changed dramatically and for the good. The Alamedas had three children: Mary, who was Tish's age, and two younger siblings, James and Celeste. Mary's mother had died, and her widowed father married his wife's sister. Mrs. Alameda was a full-time homemaker, and the father, of Italian Catholic heritage, was a strict disciplinarian.

Mrs. Alameda's presence and her interest and her pleasure in having Tish as a playmate for Mary allowed Hilda to accept invitations to lecture to associations of nurses around the city, where she literally sang for her supper. Nursing groups could rarely afford honoraria, but they did offer dinner. In these situations, Hilda was able to bring home such things as bread, rolls, and cookies—the little extras that often made the difference in days when money was always a problem. Rent for the apartment, Tish's school costs, and the contributions that Hilda had made since the day of Tish's birth to an education fund consumed virtually every penny of Hilda's modest salary. Eventually her hosts at speaking engagements began to give her paper bags full of "goodies" in lieu of a fee. By 1949 Hilda was invited to lecture outside the New York City area. Honoraria were still basically nonexistent in nursing circles. But travel, food, and lodging were provided, and key rings, handkerchiefs, or inexpensive jewelry were offered. All were trinkets Tish loved. Her wardrobe accessories grew as her mother's reputation spread. After 1950 or so, Hilda began to take Tish with her on her out-of-town trips, thus honoring her pledge that the child would "see the world." Eventually nurses across the country would look forward to the visits of Hilda and her beguiling "niece."

In many ways the academic life was also very accommodating. The schedule was flexible. Many nurses who were at TC during the years Hilda taught there comment on how involved they were with Tish and her development.[24] They were accustomed to seeing Hilda's little "niece" in the office, sitting quietly with her books, crayons, and coloring books while Hilda worked at her desk. Tish was allowed to dress as she wished, and had a lively imagination. "She used to appear in the most amazing get-ups."[25] By the time Tish was five, students often baby-sat or took the child on afternoon expeditions.[26] As one student at the time commented, ". . . psych nursing students at the time had what was in effect a clinical experience with Tish. Tisha was our clinical experience in child development!"[27]

As a result of her meetings with local nursing groups, Hilda was invited to speak at state nurses association meetings. She began to speak more widely on issues involved in the development of graduate education for nursing, the development of psychiatric nursing as a speciality at the graduate level, and issues of professional development. Peplau's visibility on the state level and then on the national scene was enhanced as word spread about the truly unique and exciting graduate program in psychiatric nursing that she was developing at TC, and she was soon invited to accept appointments to a number of national committees and advisory panels.[28] Her correspondence grew enormously, and she began to engage in her lifelong commitment to answer every letter with a substantive response to any idea ventured or mentioned, or any professional concern expressed.[29]

One of the first of her many appointments to national panels came about as a result of her wartime experience and her ongoing correspondence with physicians with whom she had worked during the war. These included Dr. Robert Felix, the first director of the National Institute of Mental Health, who named Peplau the nurse member of the National Advisory Mental Health Council.[30] This board, which was a significant adjunct to the National Mental Health Act of 1946, was constituted to advise the Public Health Service, the National Institutes of Health, and the National Institute of Mental Health on the funding and development of all mental health training grant programs.[31] This was a key position for Peplau and one that provided her access to the rapidly developing field of mental health theory and practice.

Louise McManus no doubt valued Peplau's contact with these major government funding agencies. McManus, herself, had worked long and hard to gain her own position as a power in the National League for

Nursing, which restricted itself to issues related to the evaluation and accreditation of nursing programs from a nursing perspective. Hildegard Peplau, though, was moving in much wider circles involving a much broader range of mental health issues at the national level. While the League offices were just down the street from the TC campus in Manhattan, Peplau was constantly on the train to Washington, D.C., for meetings with key federal agencies.

MASTER TEACHER

It was during the years from 1948 to 1952, while developing the program in Advanced Psychiatric Nursing at TC, that Peplau systematized her own ideas about the teaching of psychiatric nursing, about the nature of graduate programs in nursing, and about the impact nurses could make on the care of the mentally ill, particularly in the public mental hospitals. During these years she developed and introduced direct, one-to-one nurse-patient relationship studies to determine what kind of nursing interventions actually helped patients or provided them relief from their demons.

Her teaching method was at its heart Socratic. She would pick a problem—for example, patient anxiety—and examine it bit by bit and piece by piece. Students would read relevant psychiatric theory and observations on anxiety, look for signs of it in their clinical placements, record what they saw, bring their observations back to class, analyze them in the context of theory, and then devise appropriate nurse interventions to relieve it. Peplau would then encourage her students to think of what they could contribute to an understanding of patient anxiety, or whatever clinical problem was under study, thus getting many intriguing conversations under way.[32] Whether following this foray into psychiatric concepts through old territory or onto new ground, there was always much to be learned about the investigative process itself. In this way, Peplau introduced her students to the fundamentals of research methodology and the scientific method.[33]

Her innovative teaching methods continued to require time in a clinical setting as well as in a classroom. In the clinical setting, each student was required to have a regularly scheduled interview with the same psychiatric patient each week over the course of the semester. These interview data were recorded verbatim, at first handwritten, then, as technology advanced, tape-recorded, and eventually videotaped.[34] Hilda carefully reviewed and analyzed these data with each student. Theory application in class and testing in practice were the aim. Ultimately this method led the class to generate explanatory concepts relevant to clinical practice and to begin to understand the nature of theory based on empirical clinical research. It is not surprising that before long Peplau's students felt competent to engage in psychotherapeutic work on their own.

Peplau also worked to push psychiatric nursing onto solid conceptual and theoretical ground of its own. She examined an issue such as anxiety, hallucinations, or loneliness in relevant theoretical literature, whether in psychiatry or psychology, while pointing out the gaps in the data or the conceptual framework and asking what nursing could contribute. These observations and questions were then set aside for further discussion after the students gained experience, or when new knowledge could be brought to bear on a puzzling facet of the matter. In this process, students learned to juggle a variety of problems and concerns within the field, to think conceptually, and to be open to new problems, new solutions, and new conceptualization of what they were observing. Whether with her students in the classroom, or in conversation with colleagues, Peplau's lively intellectual curiosity was never at rest.[35] Whether making casual observations, or engaging in intellectual conversation, she put all her energy into making accurate observations and formulating interpretations. Her mind was never idle. While a few found this trait stimulating, many of her colleagues found Peplau's active, questioning intellect uncomfortable, if not unsettling.[36]

THE WILLIAM ALANSON WHITE INSTITUTE

Just as when studying for her MA Hilda had supplemented the program offered at TC by taking courses outside the Division of Nursing Education, so as a doctoral candidate, she continued that practice. She was intensely interested in the process of psychotherapy, and believed strongly that there was an important role for nurses to play in this developing field. As a result, she was intent also on expanding her own knowledge of the interactions that occurred in therapy and her own ability to lead students' training for a speciality in psychiatric nursing. In 1950 she applied to the Veterans Administration to use G.I. Bill benefits to earn a certificate in psychoanalysis at the William Alanson White Institute (WAW) in New York City. The VA agreed to this highly unusual request. The White Institute was an outgrowth of the Washington School of Psychiatry and was one of only two psychoanalytic institutes in the United States at that time with an academic structure. It had remained closely affiliated with the Washington School, where Frieda Fromm Reichman and Harry Stack Sullivan held sway, and reflected Sullivan's view that interpersonal relations were central to the development of personality. Not coincidentally, Erich Fromm, Hilda's Bennington College psychology professor, was also affiliated with the Washington School of Psychiatry. The White

Institute was unique for another reason: Two of the great women of American psychiatry were among its founding directors, Clara Thompson and Janet Rioch. The White Institute and the Washington School of Psychiatry were at the forefront of a radical rebellion in American psychiatry against the strict confines of classical Freudian theory that had set the boundaries of American psychiatry up to that time. The White Institute, however, unlike almost every other similar institute, never suffered a major division or alienation of a significant portion of its membership. It was a very compatible place.[37] As Peplau began writing and developing her own theoretical understanding, she became more and more Sullivanian in her focus, her teaching, and her work. It was only natural she would be attracted to the WAW.

In 1950 the WAW had a certificate program in psychoanalysis for teachers. This was the program to which Peplau applied. Her initial interview was with Dr. Harry Bone, the director of the education program. Dr. Bone described Peplau as "the type of self-made woman, a little rigid, straight, somewhat detached and sober, but very serious and a hard and thorough worker. She is likeable, sincere, and unaggressive."[38] He concluded with the observation that she is "exceptionally able and creative. I expect her to reflect favorably on the Institute."[39] On June 16, 1950, Dr. Edward S. Tauber notified Peplau that she had been admitted as a candidate for the Certificate in Applied Psychiatry for Teachers.[40]

The building that would later be renamed the Clara Thompson Building at 20 West 74th Street in New York City is a gracious brownstone just off Central Park West. It provides, in the tradition of psychanalytic institutes, large, lovely, heavily paneled, high ceilinged rooms for classes and social affairs. Although the brownstone was the center of academic pursuits and social interaction between members, the real work of the would-be member, or candidate, occurred through his or her own personal analysis. Every candidate for admission was required to undergo analysis with a member of the institute. This was not an easy or speedy process. For a woman to be accepted into such an institute in 1950 was unusual. For a nurse to be accepted was truly exceptional. Peplau was one of only two nurses during the next decade to receive the certificate in psychoanalysis.

Hilda was hoping to work with one of the "grey ladies" of the institute, Janet Rioch or Clara Thompson, but instead was assigned to a young, new member of the staff, Earl G. Witenberg. In 1950 Witenberg, who would become director of the WAW in 1962, was an analyst-in-training. As was the case with Hildegard Peplau, World War II had been a defining experience in terms of how he wanted to practice therapy. A physical chemist by training, Earl Witenberg served in the Navy as a medical officer on an attack transport where he became interested in the psychological effects of war on naval and marine personnel. After medical school, he moved into a residency at Bellevue and entered analytic training at the White Institute in 1947.[41] Hence, when Peplau began to work with him, he was several years younger than she in age and only a few years ahead of her in training and education. Dr. Witenberg said of himself, "My position is, I love all theories, but I fall in love with none of them."[42] Thus, he emphasized tolerance for ambiguity and uncertainty in psychoanalytic work. Others said of him, "He does not suffer fools gladly, but he respects courage."[43] Another associate stated, "Earl Witenberg embodies the profoundly American view, broadly labeled interpersonal psychoanalysis."[44] Although Peplau knew that Dr. Witenberg was not much more experienced than she, she trusted him absolutely.[45] He was clear in his belief that, "the relationship between two people in analysis creates a dynamic through which people can change."[46] This insight ratified both Hilda's own understanding of what nursing could contribute to recovery from either chronic or acute mental illness and the theories she was working with in the book she had begun to write when she left the army. Increasingly, Peplau would use what she learned at WAW in her own teaching and in her workshop presentations.

ROUGH WATERS

While Peplau's role in the development of psychiatric nursing as a clinical speciality at the graduate level continued to grow, she did meet resistance, even among her colleagues in other graduate programs. In the spring of 1950, as she began her work at WAW, Hilda participated in a 2-week NIMH-funded workshop at the University of Minnesota convened to explore "appropriate curricular content" in psychiatric and mental health programs at the graduate level.[47] This was an opportunity that Hilda had hoped for, one in which she believed her own groundbreaking work in her course in Advanced Psychiatric Nursing at TC would find a forum. Instead, it was one of the stormiest conferences she would ever attend and in the end proved to be an enormous disappointment to her. At the time there were only 11 graduate programs in mental health nursing in the country, and 8 of these—including the TC program directed by Peplau—had come into existence after the passage of the National Mental Health Act of 1946.[48]

During the conference, in spite of all they had in common, the directors of these programs could not agree on the basic content of graduate work in psychiatric nursing nor on what it was psychiatric nurses would be doing once they had their graduate degrees. This lack of consensus on program content and objectives caused problems for the funding agencies. The central bone of contention was whether what nurses holding graduate degrees in psychiatric nursing did in "counseling" patients could be called "psychotherapy." While all could agree that the nurse had an important role to play in counseling patients and were willing to acknowledge that Peplau's emphasis on the nurse-patient relationship was important, the majority of the program directors feared retribution from physicians should they ever even hint that their student nurses were conducting "psychotherapy." They finally agreed to use the term "psychotherapy approaches" to describe what such nurses would or could do.[49] Hilda was not happy with the final report and was disgusted by the meekness and lack of courage evidenced by her fellow directors.[50]

At this time, Peplau also began to take an active interest in the definition of nursing as a profession. In 1950 the American Nurses Association (ANA) commissioned a study of "nursing functions" and funded a research team that included the sociologist, C. Everett Hughes. As it happened, Hughes taught a course in research methods for TC nursing students during the summer of 1950. Hilda, too, taught summer school that year.[51] She engaged Hughes in conversation early in the session, and almost every day thereafter Hughes brought his lunch to Hilda's office where the two talked about nursing and the nature of a profession. Her colleagues Lydia Hall and Edith Roberts often joined them. Although Hughes introduced many of these ideas in the course of the ANA project, in the end the study merely outlined in great detail "the nature and boundaries" of nursing "work." A study of timed functions was the core of the project. This consisted of observers shadowing nurses on the job and classifying their activities on a pre-coded checklist, noting the amount of time spent on each task.[52] In Hilda's view, nothing could be more deadly to the development of a professional orientation. Then, as now, most nurses seemed to view nursing as a job rather than a profession. The issues and concerns of nursing centered around issues of wages and security, thus keeping nursing associations more in the mode of labor unions than advocates for a profession. Peplau and her colleagues often discussed this fact and strategized on ways they might help change this orientation.

While the 1950 ANA conference and Peplau's conversations with C. Everett Hughes did not in the end contribute to the professionalization of nursing, the events did capture Peplau's attention and launched her on what would become a lifelong commitment: working to elevate nursing's evaluation of itself. In 1951 she published her first scholarly article, "Toward New Concepts in Nursing and Nursing Education," in the *American Journal of Nursing*, the journal of record in the nursing profession.[53] It was a beginning.

In 1950 Peplau also became involved in a Teachers College project that had been launched in 1948, before Hilda's return to TC. It was a NIMH-funded project between Teachers College, the Norton Memorial Hospital School of Nursing in Louisville, Kentucky, and the University of Louisville School of Medicine. The goal was to evaluate the content of psychiatric nursing education in three different learning environments (TC, a hospital-based school of nursing, and a university hospital) in order to compare and evaluate the results. The project had not really gotten off the ground, and Peplau was asked to step in. Representing TC, Peplau was to work with two physicians on the project in Louisville, Dr. Spafford Ackerly and Dr. Billy Keller. Three times a year she would fly to Louisville to monitor the progress of the evaluation. Dr. Ackerly, the chief psychiatrist at Norton Memorial Hospital, was prominent in the American Psychiatric Association and was regarded as quite innovative, but he had no real interest in nursing. Dr. Keller, another well-known psychiatrist in Louisville, was chief psychiatrist at the Louisville University Hospital, and the spokesman for the two physician codirectors. For Hilda, both would become problematic.

Soon after Peplau's appointment to the project, Dr. Keller invited her to come to Louisville University Hospital to see the results of an experiment he had been conducting. He had given several patients electroshock treatments every day for a year "just to see what would happen." The patients, who in those days had no rights and few advocates, had, as would be expected, lost all trace of personality. This brought back Peplau's worst memories of her wartime experiences with amytol and insulin experimentation at the 312th Military Hospital. She found it difficult to be civil to Dr. Keller after that.[54] Nonetheless, when trouble arose on the project, Peplau would fly to Louisville. Dr. Ackerly also soon gave Peplau cause for concern. On one visit Ackerly sought her out at the hospital and said, "Come and see something new, something fantastic." At the elevator, he gallantly motioned Hildegard in, saying, "You first." Stepping into the elevator, she sank knee deep into soft, spongy foam. Her immediate reaction was one of panic and anxiety. She told Dr. Ackerly that he must warn patients before placing them in this elevator. The elevator had been especially designed for protection when transferring violent patients who often attacked either the walls of the elevator or the staff person accompanying them. Hilda was not impressed.[55]

In spite of her growing reservations about the physicians overseeing the project, Hilda took her responsibilities there very seriously, and after each visit wrote pages and pages of recommendations to all concerned—to the nursing staff, to the hospital administrators, to the medical school staff, and to the doctors. She submitted outlines for courses, outlines for experiential learning, evaluation instruments, clinical objectives, student objectives, and class objectives. When she was in Louisville she presented therapeutic workshops to illustrate what nurses could do. In the end, she presented full outlines for a course on "Psychiatry and Psychiatric Nursing" and another on "Psychiatric Nursing for Basic Nursing Students"[56]; but Peplau was not on the scene on a day-to-day basis, and no one else had her energy or her commitment to the project. Also, interestingly, Peplau had not used her own beliefs in interpersonal relations in developing these materials. As a result, no one in Louisville had a vested interest in the project, and nothing much came of it. The grant was not renewed. She appreciated getting to see something of Kentucky, including a Kentucky Derby, but Peplau regarded the project as a federally funded flop, and often told Dr. Keller and the NIMH so.

EMERGING LEADER

It was not only as a teacher that Peplau was beginning to make her mark. Late in 1951, she began to work within the National League for Nursing when she was sent as the NLN representative to a large national conference on the preparation and training of nurses working in mental hospitals. This conference was held in Peoria, Illinois, under the sponsorship of the National Association for Mental Health. Peplau clearly made an impression, as witnessed by a letter from the Paul Harris, III, the director of the conference, to Julia Miller, executive director of the NLN:

> I write to thank you for participating in the Psychiatric Aide Programs Workshop in which Miss Hildegard Peplau participated as the representative of the League . . . I am very pleased to learn that Miss Peplau was impressed with the proceedings, and that you continue to be interested in developments with this group and others concerned with the problems of providing adequate nursing service in mental hospitals . . . Her contributions to the Peoria meeting were invaluable, and we have the greatest hopes that her schedule will enable her to be with us at the Manteno [Illinois] meeting in January . . . Only by thoroughly blending the strengths of our several professions can adequate care be developed.[57]

For the next several years, Peplau conducted a voluminous correspondence with physicians working in state mental hospitals and with leaders in the National Association for Mental Health concerning what content might be appropriate for education programs for psychiatric aides.[58] She attended conferences where she conducted nursing workshops and lectured on her ideas for interactive nursing care. These workshops marked the beginning of her involvement with state mental hospitals on a national level. In May 1952 she conducted a workshop for nurses working in mental hospitals in Indianapolis, Indiana, and continued to do so in various states across the country for the rest of her career.[59] In her childhood Hilda was treated in the way that she saw nurses treating patients, and she was committed to changing this. She believed nurses could do better, and that patients deserved better. These workshops had an enormous impact on the nurses who attended them, and would eventually transform the role played by nurses in mental hospitals.[60]

Shortly after the Peoria conference, Peplau agreed to serve on the NLNE Advisory Committee on Psychiatric Nursing with a former student, Claire Mintzer Fagin. This involvement was short-lived, however. Within months she resigned from both the NLNE Advisory Committee and the National Nursing Accrediting Service, stating that there were too many disagreements and she had more important things to do. The NLNE preoccupation with wording and the lack of focus on long-range goals drove her to distraction.[61]

Peplau began to work on the international level when she was asked by the Expert Nursing Committee of the World Health Organization to write a working paper on psychiatric nursing that would set the theme of an October 1951 international conference on nursing held in Geneva.[62] In this report Hilda demonstrated just how thoroughly and seriously she would take any assignment. The paper was 333 pages long![63] She also began consulting in 1951 with the Veterans Administration. Each consultation was followed by long, dense, and very detailed reports. In August of that year she was invited by Dr. "Bud" Hall, director of the Menninger Foundation, to participate in a Menninger-sponsored workshop for psychiatric nursing aides. He was particularly hopeful that Hilda would attend because, he wrote, "You have more than anyone else to contribute to a meeting like this one."[64]

From as far back as her days at Bennington College, Peplau had attended conventions of the American Psychiatric Association (APA) whenever she could, and in 1952 she presented a paper—"Psychiatric Concepts: How Nursing Personnel Learn Them"—to the APA convention held in Atlantic City. At this conference, as at all others she was able to attend, Hilda took in as many theory panels as possible and kept copious notes.[65] In this way she kept up to date with current thinking in American psychiatry and was able to build upon ideas she gathered in these conference settings. In 1952, in addition to the meetings of the APA, she attended the annual meetings of the American Hospital Association, the Mental Hospital Association, and the joint APA/Mental Hospital Institute in Columbia, Ohio, where she again made a presentation outlining her views on the importance of psychiatric theory to nursing education and practice. She also conducted workshops for the Illinois State Nurses Association and continued to consult for the Veterans Administration, writing a lengthy report that year for the VA Hospital in Little Rock, Arkansas.[66] In these efforts, she stressed the positive contribution interactive nurse-patient relations made to patient well-being.

> The aim of nursing care of psychiatric patients is to assist the patient to struggle toward full development of his potential for productive living in the community. This aim requires nursing strategies which will aid the patient to resolve obstacles that stand in the way of full development . . . for healthy social interaction in the community.[67]

Thus, early in her career as an instructor at Teachers College, Hildegard Peplau had gained recognition as a national leader in nursing. Her reputation as an exceedingly bright, conceptual, serious, and reliable contributor to the mental health discussion at the national level was widely acknowledged.[68] In the summer of 1952 she was invited to give commencement addresses to graduates of nursing programs in Atlantic City, Little Rock, and New Haven—a sure sign of a growing national reputation.[69] It never occurred to Peplau that others might envy or resent her national and international involvements. She was on the march. With Peplau, it was always "the work, the work, the work."[70]

The year 1952 marked a major milestone for Peplau. Her groundbreaking book, *Interpersonal Relations in Nursing: Offering A Conceptual Frame of Reference for Psychodynamic Nursing*, was published by G. Putnam and Sons.[71] Most of this book was actually written during 1948–1949 in the evenings after Tish went to sleep. Initially, she had difficulty getting it published. The major publishers were uneasy publishing an academic book written solely by a nurse. Several publishers were interested in the manuscript, but would agree to publish it only if she were willing to incorporate a physician's input. This Peplau steadfastly refused to do. Putnam and Sons tried to persuade her to compromise by asking a physician to write an introduction, at least. Eventually they reached a compromise when Peplau agreed the publisher could ask a physician to review the manuscript. Publication was enthusiastically urged, and what was to become one of the all-time classics in nursing was published. Peplau did give a nod to propriety by agreeing to ask Mrs. McManus to write the foreword for the book. She almost immediately regretted even that decision, however, as days and then a month went by with no foreword being produced. Eventually, Hilda took the matter into her own hands and drafted a foreword, sending it to McManus with a note suggesting, "perhaps you might wish to say something like this." Mrs. McManus accepted the suggestion by simply signing her name to the drafted statement.[72]

Tish, too, was gaining some small celebrity of her own in this period. In 1950, to show how children could enjoy Halloween constructively, the director of the Midtown Children's Center, Ethel Abrams, arranged for her students to paint Halloween scenes on the windows of New York's Tavern on the Green restaurant in Central Park. The *New York World Telegram and Sun* ran a picture on October 30 of Tish Peplau there, "hidden by her masterpiece." The caption read "Another Smear Campaign." The *New York Herald Tribune* also covered the event and ran a photo of Tish and two classmates with a glowing pumpkin. The next spring Tish was back in the news with a photo of a Children's Center May Day celebration at Tavern on the Green.[73] Tish stayed at the Midtown Children's Center through the equivalent of the second grade, and celebrated her seventh birthday there. The following September, 1952, Hilda enrolled her in the Agnes Russell School, the Teachers College experimental one-room school where each child was given an individual program. Now mother and daughter could walk to school together, and when Tish's school day was over Hilda could fetch her and bring her back to the office, where she delighted Peplau's own students.

Although her national and international commitments were growing, Peplau did not neglect her responsibilities at TC, where she was making major contributions to a large curriculum study, directed by Mrs. McManus. The faculty at TC had several times in the past decade made an effort to distinguish between material to be taught at different levels of nursing education. They thought it important that college level material be clearly distinguishable from that offered by the hospital schools. Essentially, Peplau urged that college level education focus on the development of clinical skills and on nursing's clinical contributions to patient care.[74] Graduate work at TC, however, was focused on basic teacher education or hospital administration, not on clinical nursing care. While Peplau's work was most helpful in moving the study along, it can be imagined that it was not necessarily appreciated by colleagues who had very different ideas about what constituted nursing education.

Peplau also tried to move nursing into closer relationship with other Teachers College programs through curriculum proposals of her own. In the spring of 1952 she submitted a huge course outline with a massive bibliography to the TC curriculum committee proposing to merge courses in sociology, psychology, and nursing into an interdisciplinary course entitled "Human Interrelationships."[75] This course outline represented an enormous investment of time and thought. In what would become an increasingly obvious characteristic, however, Peplau expected the proposal to stand on its own merits and thus had not done the political spade work needed to introduce such a radical departure from the normal nursing curriculum. She had not consulted the relevant department chairs, nor had she discussed her proposal with them. She had worked long and hard on it, but in isolation from her colleagues, and submitted it directly to the college curriculum committee where it was met with more curiosity than serious consideration.[76] There were members of the committee who were intrigued with this nurse who seemed to have so many creative ideas, but no one volunteered to work with her to implement the concept. The proposal went nowhere, and—as was now becoming typical of her—Peplau could not understand why.

ANOTHER EXPERIENCE AT CHESTNUT LODGE

Soon after returning to Teachers College in 1948, Peplau reestablished her ties to Chestnut Lodge, the private psychiatric hospital in Maryland where she had done her Bennington field study in 1942 and where she first became acquainted with the work of Harry Stack Sullivan. In January 1949 she submitted a grant proposal to the Public Health Service to support students in an 18-month course designed to prepare educational directors for psychiatric hospitals. The course would include a 3-month summer clinical experience at Chestnut Lodge. The director, Dr. Dexter Bullard, whom Hilda had known from her Bennington days, was very supportive. The Chestnut Lodge segment commenced in the summer of 1949, and immediately ran into difficulty. She had consulted on her program with Dr. Bullard, but not with the director of nursing, Miss Emmy Lanning. This second Chestnut Lodge experience illustrates some of the reasons Peplau would continually have problems working within the nursing establishment in the years ahead.

Peplau believed that the education at the graduate level should include on-site clinical experience that would be described in detail by the students. They should gather data, analyze it, and formulate hypotheses leading to generalizations about this experience that could then be compared to other experiences. In other words, Peplau expected nurses in graduate programs to understand, appreciate, and contribute to research through their clinical experiences. This is the process that she had introduced, with a demonstrable measure of success, in the Brooklyn State Hospital field experience she had initiated in her first year of teaching.

The TC students who would be working at Chestnut Lodge had developed goals and objectives for their summer experience as part of their spring coursework with Peplau. The director of nursing at Chestnut Lodge had not been consulted, however, did not understand, and definitely did not approve of these goals and objectives. Chestnut Lodge had its own established routines, and Miss Lanning had her own ideas of how nursing students should be utilized during the summer session. The students almost immediately felt caught between the two sets of expectations.[77]

During the second summer, in 1950, tension at Chestnut Lodge continued to build. Before the third summer, in May 1951, a meeting was arranged to include Hildegard Peplau, Dr. Bullard, Mrs. McManus, and Miss Lanning, to resolve their differences. While McManus tried to make everyone comfortable, Peplau addressed the problem head on. Lanning was tense, angry, and flustered. Dr. Bullard sided with Peplau and expressed his support of what she was trying to do. In June Peplau wrote expressing her appreciation for his support and sent a copy to Lanning.[78] That summer, not surprisingly, the students found the tension higher than ever. They felt "trapped" between TC theory and Chestnut Lodge practice—and between loyalty to Peplau and obedience to Lanning, who was their on-site supervisor. In August Dr. Bullard wrote Peplau announcing his intention to reorganize the Chestnut Lodge Education program in such a way as to lessen the tensions.[79] Two students were invited to remain at Chestnut Lodge that September, thus extending the clinical experience from 3 to 6 months, June–December. Yet even under the new guidelines and extended time frame, tensions continued to mount.[80]

In December Peplau again visited Chestnut Lodge to try to resolve the problems and lay a better groundwork for the next summer's work. At this time, a psychiatrist on the staff tried unsuccessfully to mediate a meeting between Lanning and Peplau. Peplau's position was that an educational experience for graduate students should bring things into focus more clearly and faster than the normal clinical experience for undergraduate students. Graduate students should be expected to selectively draw conclusions and generalize from what they observed. Perhaps adding insult to injury, Peplau expressed frustration that "Miss Lanning is unwilling to describe in ways other than very general ones what her objectives are and what methods, procedures, and techniques of education are being used in the program." Lanning complained about Peplau's requirement that students write everything down. She feared that the students were practicing therapy under the guise of education and did not believe that nurses could or should offer patients anything approaching psychotherapy. She said she felt "the nurse can be therapeutic" but did not define what she meant by this. Peplau reiterated that her requirements differentiated between education and the actual practice of therapy.[81] Thus, even at Chestnut Lodge—where Harry Stack Sullivan's theories of personality as rooted in relationships were paramount—there was disagreement as to where psychiatric nursing fitted into a therapy program for patients because the director of nursing and the innovative teacher could not agree on this issue.

The physician charged with mediating the differences between Peplau and Lanning could see the situation was hopeless. He concluded the meeting by asserting that Chestnut Lodge would "design its own program and state its own objectives for the program for nurses" and would let Peplau know whether or not there would be a place in it for TC students.[82] Peplau left in frustration, sadly realizing that this experiment had failed.[83] She did not apply for renewal of the grant at the end of the year, and wrote a final note to Lanning explaining that she was "cognizant of the difficulties involved in attempting to implement at considerable distance the philosophy of the Division of Nursing Education, for which reason the project is being terminated at this time."[84] Peplau would never return to Chestnut Lodge.

In spite of the disappointment of the Chestnut Lodge experience, Peplau remained convinced that the ability to apply classroom theory to clinical situations, to gather and analyze data in the clinical setting, and then to interpret such data and generalize from it were critical to graduate education in nursing. Peplau's work in classrooms and hospitals resulted eventually in major changes in undergraduate and graduate nursing curricula, as she began to write about her teaching methods and argued for their adoption in other university-based nursing degree programs. It is remarkable that Peplau began to go down this path in 1948, in her first teaching position and while she was still only an instructor. At that time, nurses were expected to keep busy performing technical procedures and routine activities, not to actively participate in patient recovery. This split between what nurses in general did, and what psychiatric nurses increasingly were doing, persisted until Hildegard Peplau's retirement, and reflected divisions within nursing between those who lived it as an occupation and those who wanted to professionalize it. Peplau would spend her entire academic career trying to get nursing to make a cognitive shift from skilled technical labor to professional practice and intellectual self-examination. She would not succeed in this pursuit, but she never stopped trying.

ENDNOTES

1. For an excellent summary of Peplau's use of interpersonal relations theory in both teaching and in nursing practice, see Anita Werner O'Toole and Sheila Rouslin Welt, eds., *Interpersonal Theory in Nursing Practice: Selected Works of Hildegard Peplau* (New York: Springer Publishing, 1989).
2. Harry Stack Sullivan is generally acknowledged as the "founder" of interpersonal relations theory in psychiatry. Sullivan was one of the original three founders of the Washington School of Psychiatry in Washington, D.C., which in turn was closely connected to Chestnut Lodge in Maryland and to the William Alanson White Institute in New York—which itself was originally created as a branch of the Washington School. Clearly Sullivan's theories had a great impact on Hildegard Peplau. Sullivan's writings, however, are both highly technical and highly compressed. While it is easy to surmise his overall theory, it is very difficult to find a succinct quote that summarizes his definition of interpersonal relations theory. Therefore, the summarization used here is taken from the writing of Sullivan's contemporary and Hilda's mentor at Chestnut Lodge, Frieda Fromm Reichman. See Frieda Fromm Reichman, "Recent Advances in Psychoanalytic Therapy" in *A Study of Interpersonal Relations: New Contributions to Psychiatry* (New York: Grove Press, Inc., 1949), 122–130.
3. See Hildegard Peplau, "What is Experiential Teaching" in O'Toole and Welt, 139–148.
4. Hildegard Peplau, "Interpersonal Techniques: The Crux of Nursing," *American Journal of Nursing 62* (June 1962), 50–54.
5. Interview, Joyce Fitzpatrick, October 21, 1997, in Philadelphia, Pennsylvania. See also letters written to Hildegard Peplau referring to events related here and to Mrs. McManus from Terry Fernandez, Gwen Tudor, Marguerite Termini, and Kay Delaney in Box 14, #480. Forty years later, in personal interviews, these women all had nothing but praise for both Mrs. McManus and Hildegard Peplau, claiming little or no knowledge of the events described later in this chapter by Peplau.
6. Teresa Christy, *Cornerstone of Nursing Education* (New York: Teachers College Press, 1969), 28–81.

7. See Barbara Pedersen, *The MacManus Years: Advances in the Division of Nursing Education, Teachers College, Columbia University* (PhD Dissertation, Columbia University, Ann Arbor: University Microfilm, 1992), 28.

8. Christy, 210.

9. Pedersen, 64–68.

10. Interview, Hildegard Peplau, February 2, 1992.

11. Hildegard Peplau, "Interpersonal Techniques: The Crux of Nursing," 53.

12. Letter from Hildegard Peplau to Dr. Joe Geller, June 25, 1953, Box 14, #473.

13. While at TC Peplau used the word "counseling" to describe the work her students did with patients. When she went to Rutgers in 1954, however, she stressed that her students were engaged in offering "psychotherapy." In 1948, however, when she began her teaching at TC, no such words could or would be used in connection with nursing.

14. Helen Swick Perry, *Psychiatrist of America: The Life of Harry Stack Sullivan* (Cambridge: Harvard University Press, 1982), 312–313.

15. Ibid.

16. Interview, Kay Delaney, May 15, 1994, in Montrose, New York.

17. Interviews, Kay Delaney and Kay Norris, April 29, 1994, in Tucson, Arizona.

18. Several sets of these notes are in the Schlesinger archive, Box 10, #308–317. The density of the material and the meticulous attention to every detail Peplau gave to her students and the patients is most impressive.

19. Interview, Hildegard Peplau, February 2, 1992.

20. Interview, Evelyn Zimmerman, October, 1994, in Spring Valley, New Jersey.

21. Interview, Hildegard Peplau, February 2, 1992.

22. It was not until the late 1960s that she met a chairman of psychiatry, Dr. Irwin Pollack, who would give her students access to acutely rather than chronically sick patients.

23. A large collection of these early student studies may be found in Box 13, #419, 427–428, and Box 14, #449–467.

24. Interviews with Marguerite Termini, October 15, 1993, in Bethesda, Maryland; Evelyn Zimmerman, April 18, 1993, in Spring Valley, New Jersey; Claire Fagin, October 29, 1992, in St. Louis, Missouri; and Fran Martucci, April 10, 1992, in Santa Monica, California.

25. Interview, Marguerite Termini, October 15, 1993.

26. Correspondence with Terry Fernandez, May 14, 1996.

27. Interview, Evelyn Zimmerman, April 18, 1993. In a later conversation with Claire Fagin, however, she emphasized that she herself was not one of the students who thought it a good idea to be involved in Tish's development. She emphasized, therefore, that not *all* the psychiatric nursing students at TC at that time spent time with Tish or were in any way a part of Peplau's personal life.

28. Interview, Claire Fagin, October 29, 1992.

29. Her large and phenomenal correspondence is now archived at the Schlesinger Library. It provides an enormous resource for anyone seeking to explore the development of professional nursing in this country.

30. See letters of appointment and related correspondence in Box 17, #617–618.

31. See letters of appointment and related materials in Box 18, #628 and 629.

32. Interviews with Shirley Smoyak, Bruce Mericle, Sheila Welt, Fran Martucci, Marguerite Termini, Bill Reynolds, Gwen Tudor Will, Claire Fagin, Evelyn Zimmerman, Suzy Lego, Anita O'Toole, and Ann Clark, 1992–1994. Also, Box 12, Files #355–371 contain pages and pages of typewritten notes on ideas for classes, for lectures, and for conference presentations.

33. Interviews and discussions with Grayce Sills, June, 1994, in Washington, D.C.

Several sets of notes for research topics are in the Schlesinger archive, Box 10, #308–317. It is hard to convey the density of the material and the meticulous attention to every detail given to this work.

34. When tape recorders became available after 1950, Hilda received permission from the government to use grant money to purchase machines for her students. Getting Dr. Bellinger's permission to use tape recorders at Brooklyn State Hospital was another matter, however. She had many conferences with him, pleading that her students were missing a lot by trying to record by hand verbatim interviews. He finally relented by granting permission for one tape recorder to be used in the ward.

35. Interview, Martha Rogers, March 14, 1993, in Phoenix, Arizona.

36. From her first day of teaching, it was obvious that small talk, the forte of nursing conversation, was not in Peplau's repertoire. On the first day of classes, a fellow instructor, Catherine Spaulding, walked into her office and as an opening gambit, asked Hilda if she believed in God. Preoccupied and somewhat taken aback, Peplau asked her to clarify the question—did she mean God as a person, God as a father figure, or God as a cosmic concept? Spaulding was not amused. Without another word, she left the office, never to speak to Peplau again. Interview, Hildegard Peplau, March 13, 1992.

37. Interviews, Earl G. Witenberg, November 15 and January 19, 1993, at the White Institute in New York City.

38. Peplau Confidential File, William Alanson White Institute, note by Dr. Harry Bone, April 24, 1950. At Hildegard Peplau's request, all records concerning her at the WAW were open to the author. Peplau also gave her written permission to Dr. Earl G. Witenberg to help in any way he could in seeking to understand her life.

39. Peplau confidential file, WAW Institute.

40. Letter from Edward S. Tauber, MD, Acting Director of the William Alanson White Institute, to Hildegard E. Peplau, June 16, 1950, Box 10, #307.

41. Interview, Earl G. Witenberg, November 15, 1993.

42. Interview, Earl G. Witenberg, January 19, 1993.

43. Interview, Carol Mann, WAW, October 19, 1994, in New York City.

44. Interview, Ammon Issacharoff, MD, October 19, 1994, in New York City.

45. Interview, Hildegard Peplau, March 21, 1994.

46. Interview, Earl G. Witenberg, November 15, 1993.

47. See materials on this conference in Box 17, #613, and Box 18, #639.

48. Under this act funds were provided for graduate education in mental health fields, which included psychiatric nursing, social work, and psychology, in addition to psychiatry. For this reason, psychiatric nursing became the only nursing specialty to develop primarily at the graduate level.

49. *Report of a Workshop on Graduate Programs in Psychiatric Nursing*, held at the University of Minnesota, 1950, Box 18, #640.

50. Interview, Hildegard Peplau, February 2, 1992. In fact, just 3 years later Peplau resigned as the Psychiatric Nurse Consultant to the National League for Nursing, in part because of her frustration in working with this group of graduate program directors. "I feel that . . . the reports of the Program Directors suggest the general directions they wish to move . . . as the only dissenting member of the committee . . . I have a responsibility to identity these disagreements and then to retire from the Committee." Letter from Hildegard Peplau to Kay Black, February 16, 1953, Box 18, #655.

51. See Contract for Summer School, July 1, 1950–August 31, 1950, Box 10, #306.

52. Everett C. Hughes, Helen MacGill Hughes, and Irwin Deutscher, *Twenty Thousand Nurses Tell Their Story: A Report on the American Nurses Association's Studies of Nursing Functions* (Philadelphia: J. B. Lippincott, 1956).

53. Hildegard E. Peplau, "Toward New Concepts in Nursing and Nursing Education," *American Journal of Nursing* (Winter, 1951), 722–724.
54. Interview, Hildegard Peplau, February 11, 1992.
55. Ibid.
56. Box 12, #352, "The Louisville Project," including Hildegard's voluminous reports entitled *Evaluation of the Strength and Adequacy of the Learning in Similarly Designed Learning Experiences in Psychiatric Nursing in Three Different Structured Situations.*
57. Letter from Paul Harris, III to Julia Miller, November 20, 1951, Box 18, File #639.
58. This correspondence is found in the Schlesinger Library Collection, Box 18, File #341.
59. See material in Box 18, File #642. From these notes she began to develop her ideas for a new vision of the nursing profession and ways of bringing about the necessary reforms. These ideas were introduced in summer workshops conducted during the late 1950s through the 1960s across the country. The first workshops, however, were held at TC during the summers of 1950 and 1951. Voluminous materials developed for these first workshops are in the files.
60. Interviews with Grayce Sills, October 29, 1992, in St. Louis, and Liz Carter and friends, September 4, 1994, in Lake Hopatcong, New Jersey.
61. Material related to this committee is in Box 18, #630. The committee issued a report on "Desireable Functions and Qualifications of Psychiatric Nurses," which provided guidelines for the future development of graduate psychiatric nursing education. Shortly after the report was written, Claire Fagin too resigned from the committee and took a position in Washington, D.C.
62. See letter from Olive Baggallay, Chief, Nursing Section, World Health Organization to Hildegard E. Peplau, May 28, 1951, Box 17, #621.
63. Report of the Expert Nursing Committee to the World Health Organization, November, 1951, Box 17, File #621.
64. Letter from "Bud" Hall, MD to Hildegard Peplau, August 15, 1951, Box 17, File #627.
65. These notes, along with others taken at various non-nursing meetings, are in Box 18, #644.
66. These reports may be found in Box 18, #647–650.
67. Hildegard Peplau, "Psychotherapeutic Strategies," *Perspectives in Psychiatric Care 6* (1959), 264–270.
68. Interview, Martha Rogers, March 14, 1993, in Phoenix, Arizona.
69. These invitations and talks may be found in Box 18, #633.
70. Interview, Hildegard Peplau, February 11, 1992, and March 21, 1994.
71. Hildegard E. Peplau, *Interpersonal Relations in Nursing: Offering a Conceptual Frame of Reference for Psychodynamic Nursing* (New York: G. Putnam and Sons, 1952). (Reissued, London: Macmillan, 1988 and New York: Springer Publishing Company, 1994).
72. See draft of the Foreword and notes in handwriting of Hildegard Peplau, Box 17, #610.
73. News clippings sent by Hilda and Anne Peplau to Barbara Callaway, February 28, 1999.
74. Material on the curriculum study is in Box 13, #420.
75. This course proposal and related correspondence is in Box 13, #422.
76. Ibid. The committee agenda and course materials with Peplau's comments are in Box 13.
77. For details regarding these matters, see Box 12, #342.
78. Letter from Hildegard Peplau to Dr. Dexter Bullard, June 10, 1951, Box 12, #342.
79. Letter from Dr. Dexter Bullard to Hildegard E. Peplau, August 15, 1951, Box 14, #484.

80. Interview, Gwen Tudor Will, February 17, 1994.
81. "Summary on Conference at Chestnut Lodge, December 3, 1951. Dr. Adland, Miss Lanning, Miss Peplau," 3. Found in Box 14, #494. The author of these mimeographed notes is not cited.
82. Ibid, 6.
83. In her defense, Peplau had outlined for those at the meeting and for Dr. Bullard and others all she had done to help Miss Lanning reach a different level. She had gotten her an appointment as a clinical faculty member at TC; she had sent her course materials and copies of papers presented at meetings; student records were made available for her review; Peplau had invited her, and paid her travel expenses, to the Cincinnati meeting on psychiatric nursing education; and had taken her on a trip to visit the Louisville project. Peplau felt she had done everything possible so that Miss Lanning would have a chance to exchange ideas with leaders in other university programs and projects. Peplau had urged Lanning to attend the APA meetings, had invited her to participate in classes at TC, and had invited her to participate in workshops, but all invitations were declined. It is clear that Miss Lanning was simply overwhelmed with all this, and became angry and resistant to Hilda Peplau and the TC program as a consequence.
84. Letter from Hildegard E. Peplau to Emmy Lanning, June 11, 1952, Box 11, #342.

Academic Nightmare: A Career in Crisis

8

Believe me, I have never suffered as I have these last three weeks. The fatigue and anxiety and pain have been so unbearable. To me it was inconceivable that in a great and supposedly democratic institution, injustice could be served when administrative ineptness and unconscious hatred mix up with pathology . . . life in a mental hospital is simpler than such complex pathology in a work situation.

—Hildegard Peplau
February 6, 1953

It was Monday, January 5, 1953, and Hilda was returning to Teachers College quite relaxed for the beginning of a new semester. She had taken Tish with her to a conference in Miami, Florida, where Hilda presented a paper and conducted workshops. There she had met new people and had felt confident rather than anxious about new experiences.[1] This trip was the first real break Hilda had allowed herself since the birth of her daughter and her return from military service in England in 1945. The hard times, it seemed, were behind her: the initiation into single parenthood, the rigors of graduate school, the trauma of the Highland Hospital fire, and the challenges of teaching and building a hard-won reputation as an innovative nurse educator. Tish, now nearly 9 years old, had been especially delighted by the red and gold hibiscus and other flowers blooming in Miami in midwinter. Both had enjoyed the guest house provided for them and had been excited to have freshly squeezed juice from oranges Tish picked from the trees surrounding their little cottage. After the conference, they had spent time together at the beach. Hilda had a suntan—in January! On the way back to New York, they had stopped in North Carolina and had a good visit with Hilda's dear brother Walter and his wife Anne. It was a happy, wonderful time for mother and daughter. Hilda returned to Columbia rested, looking forward to the new semester, looking forward to leading her students into new territory, pleased to have a spring semester leave from teaching to finish her doctoral dissertation, pleased that her first book had been published. Life at last seemed focused and on course.

The atmosphere on Monday, her first day back at Teachers College (TC), seemed tense. A delegation of faculty members, including Hilda, were then preparing to go to an important meeting in Michigan being sponsored by the Kellogg Foundation. Hilda was surprised that R. Louise McManus, director of the Division of Nursing Education, missed the planning meeting that day and that the other delegates seemed preoccupied and distant. While Hilda noted the reticence and tenseness in the air, she did not explore it, for she was preoccupied herself. She was to play a leadership role in Michigan, and she would have to leave Tish for a week. Although she knew that her daughter was in good hands, she still fretted. Tish had been enrolled in the experimental Agnes Russell School since the previous September, where her intellect and creativity were finding full expression. It was to be the beginning of a new semester for both of them.

On Tuesday morning, January 6, 1953, everything changed. The hallway in Dodge Hall seemed eerie and quiet. It felt unexpectedly lonely. Where were Hilda's colleagues? Where were her students? Was it her imagination, or was everyone fleeing her approach? Then the summons came: "Please meet with Mrs. McManus immediately in her office."[2]

As she walked down the hall to the director's office, Peplau sensed something was definitely wrong. Everyone seemed to be avoiding eye contact, giving her only downcast looks. She had expected to attack her schedule with vigor, to get everything in order at TC, then head out to Michigan for the Kellogg nursing education conference, and after that proceed to Washington, D.C., for a meeting of the National Institute of Mental Health review board. When Mrs. McManus's secretary summoned her to this meeting, Hilda knew something was seriously amiss. Nonetheless, she went in with her chin up and tried being cheerful. There was no response, just cold silence. Then, as Peplau recalled, McManus spoke. Her first words were, "I think you are sick, you need help. If you need money, I can give it to you." Mrs. McManus continued, "There are rumors. You are psychotic. You are an alcoholic. You are a lesbian. You are immoral. You are causing us embarrassment."[3] Peplau's reaction was shock. She was dumbfounded. Then she was furious. "What rumors? What evidence? Who has said these things?" She felt paralyzed. Then she felt consumed with rage and a growing sense of fear. Nothing in these astonishing charges squared with the facts of her life. How could any such rumors possibly be taken seriously?

Ignoring Hilda's request for information about the origin of these charges, McManus issued an ultimatum: From this day forward, Peplau was to have no social interaction with students outside of the classroom.

Hilda was enraged as she realized that allegations of this nature could be made and that she was to be given no opportunity to confront her accuser or accusers. Guilt, it appeared, was a foregone conclusion. She felt the same deep anger she had felt when the unjust, and untrue, charge that she had been guilty of talking in class led her to leave high school in Reading. This was an insult to her integrity that she could not tolerate. Compounding the insult was McManus's conclusion that Peplau was "sick"—in the sense of being mentally ill—and the suggestion that Louise McManus would personally pay for therapy for *Hilda!*

Peplau immediately verbally resigned her position at Teachers College.[4] A formal, written resignation followed a week later. Thus began the most complicated and traumatic experience of her career to that time. It was a nightmare, a painful and devastating time that changed her life. Peplau never truly recovered from both the corrosive effects of these rumors and the way in which the TC administration dealt with them. She never again felt she could trust those around her, that she could relax, that she could take for granted her own reputation and knowledge of herself. It took 4 years—from the time of the confrontation with McManus in early 1953 until 1957 when she was given tenure at Rutgers—to rebuild her professional reputation and standing. The Teachers College "incident," as she would call it, was something over which she had no control and which over time she would struggle to understand.

THE FORCES AT PLAY

There were, as will be seen, a set of underlying events involving the personal circumstances of two or three students that appear to have provided the germ of the rumors. Hilda would later characterize these student grievances as a "smoke screen" for larger issues and animosities being played out at her expense. The students' problems, however, did act as a catalyst in December 1952, fueling simmering resentments that grew into the conflagration that resulted in Peplau's resignation from Teachers College.

In retrospect, it appears that a number of internal and external forces fed into the January 6th confrontation.[5] The first, and by no means the least of these, was McManus's own situation as the new director of one of the nation's most visible graduate programs in nursing education. While an able educator at TC, McManus had problems as an administrator—organizing her schedule, getting reports and information in on time, and keeping the lines of communication open to upper level administrators. In addition, she had recently succeeded the legendary Isabel Maitland Stewart as director of the Division of Nursing Education when Stewart retired in 1948, after serving more than 2 decades in the position. McManus, then, was not only relatively new in her job but had also been raised and trained in the old school of nursing education. Coming into the director-ship in the postwar period when enrollments at Columbia's Teachers College surged to unprecedented numbers, she found herself facing not only totally new administrative challenges but pressure for change with-in the field of nursing education itself. The fact was that Louise McManus was insecure in her position in late 1952 and knew that she was vulnera-ble to criticism from her superiors in the college administration.

This insecurity may have been compounded by professional jealousy, for at this time Peplau's career had begun to take off. Her book was becoming widely acclaimed, her articles were appearing in the major journals, she was serving on important national and international com-mittees, and students were coming to TC from near and far just to study with her. She was developing innovative teaching methods and new ped-agogy and had a deep interest in finding and creating new knowledge. She was an emerging leader in her profession and was increasingly seen as the mentor of her students. Peplau's teaching methods, as it will be seen, may have also caused alarm in someone concerned with maintain-ing the status quo at TC.

It is possible that there was another issue lurking in the background. On the surface, the two women had some things in common. McManus, like Peplau, was a single mother. She was a widow who had raised six stepchildren, but she kept her personal life very much separate from her professional life.[6] Peplau was just the opposite. Tish was often with Hilda in her office, and Hilda made sure both staff and students knew that she was the star of her class at the college's experimental school, and was a precocious and very independent child.[7] Tish's brightness, while a source of deep satisfaction and appreciation for Hilda, inevitably caused resent-ment in some quarters.[8] There were other personal factors in the mix. It is clear from the tone of Hilda's memos that she did not meet McManus's expectations for respect. Hilda was courteous but never deferential. It is also true, however, that with the pressured life she led and her innate impatience Hilda was not an easy, or readily accommodating, personality.

A SEARCH FOR UNDERSTANDING

Peplau made many attempts over a considerable period of time to step back, analyze, and try to understand the events and forces that led to the 1953 crisis in her career. At one level, especially in the first weeks after her fateful January 6 meeting with McManus, she struggled to put the pieces together and to deal with the powerful emotions that consumed her. While she was intellectually aware of many—but not all—facets of the situation, and while she had understood since her youth in Reading the pernicious nature of gossip and rumor, she remained incredulous that such a thing could actually happen to her. Again and again over the years Peplau would turn over these events in mind. This is a common reaction to great psychological stress. Many people in the aftermath of a traumatic experience talk, even obsessively, about the experience. By reliving the events, they may desensitize powerful emotions and achieve enough distance to gain intellectual insight. This is precisely the process by which Peplau treated battle-shocked soldiers at the 312th Field Hospital in England, encouraging them to talk about their trauma. The difference in Hilda's own situation was that there was no one in whom she could confide. Tish was too young, her sister and brother were far away, and she was prohibited from talking with colleagues and students at TC— and would not in any case have done so. Hilda's response was to undertake a personal "talk therapy" on paper, reviewing the events in writing again and again over the 1953 calendar year, and yet again as late as 1994.[9]

On January 29, 1953, she wrote a 5-page summary of all that had happened as she knew it. On January 30 she wrote a long letter, that was never sent, to McManus, examining the facts and explaining her position. The next day she took a very creative approach to "talking through" her feelings: She penned a fictional story featuring a character she called Ellen and another she called Mrs. McCormick. The story goes on, recounting detail by detail the events of January 1953.[10] The following September, Hilda wrote a 27-page letter to Dr. Maurice Greenhill, a psychiatrist she had known at the 312th Military Field Hospital during the war and who was then affiliated with the medical school at the University of Maryland. In this letter she again reviewed all the events connected with the situation as she understood them.[11] In addition she collected folders full of materials on rumors and on Communist witch-hunts in an effort to try to give the events in her life context and perspective.[12] Her own accounts provide an extensive and valuable record of the factors involved and the forces at work, as Hilda came to know them, and provide the framework for the reconstruction of events presented in this chapter.[13]

STORM CLOUDS GATHERING

The series of incidents that precipitated the January crisis seemed innocent enough in and of themselves. The first issue can be traced back to the fall of 1950, when a student named Betty was admitted to graduate work in nursing education at Teachers College. By November Hilda had become concerned about her manic behavior and discussed her concern with the TC dean of students, Dr. Beulah Von Wagonen. Subsequently Peplau recommended that Betty withdraw from school and enter private psychotherapy, which she did. In 1952, she was readmitted to the program, based on her therapist's verbal statement to Dr. Von Wagonen attesting to the student's ability to benefit from graduate work.

In October, 1952, shortly after her return to TC, Betty obtained a key to Peplau's office for the purpose of consulting books needed in her course. These books were purchased with grant monies and were kept in Peplau's office for student use. It was TC protocol that a faculty member be present to lend such books out. This protocol was broken when Betty borrowed a key from Peplau's secretary—and neglected to return it.[14] In mid-October, late on a Thursday afternoon after class, the student used the key to enter Peplau's office, ostensibly to borrow a book. She was aware that her student notebooks and notes of Peplau's observations of her were housed in an unlocked file. The temptation was overwhelming. She found her file and began reading it. What she read upset her a great deal. Distraught, she called her husband, who, reportedly, advised her to bring the file home where it could be reviewed in a calmer environment.[15] The student took the file and left a note saying that she had used the phone and left 14¢ for the call on Peplau's desk.[16] Hilda was concerned enough about the note and the 14¢ to report the matter to McManus, but she had no reason to suspect that Betty had taken a file from the file drawer, let alone removed it from the office. After reading the file at home, Betty took it to her psychiatrist. The psychiatrist felt the contents of the file were inappropriate and were disturbing to his patient. He contacted Dean of Students Von Wagonen at TC to express his concern. Because the student's father was the CEO of a major company and her husband was a surgeon, there was soon concern at the highest levels of college and university administration. The matter was communicated through Dean Von Wagonen to the TC provost, M. C. Del Manzo, and perhaps also to the office of the president of the university. Columbia University had a vested interest in accommodating the family, who were generous contributors.

Concern at the top administrative level was conveyed to McManus. This information must have caused her some alarm. She was already aware that the provost had some misgivings over administrative matters in her division. She could not have been pleased to learn that allegations involving the daughter of a prominent New York family, who had been readmitted to the Division of Nursing Education after a psychiatric leave, had been brought to the attention of the dean of students and the college provost.[17] On October 29, Dean Von Wagonen invited McManus, Peplau, and Betty to meet in her office to discuss the matter. Peplau, who believed that Betty's readmission to graduate studies should have been made contingent on a written statement rather than merely verbal assurance from the psychiatrist to begin with, suggested that he be included in the meeting. She did not prevail, and the meeting proceeded without the student's psychiatrist. Dean Von Wagonen framed the issues as Betty's use of an unauthorized key and the security of faculty offices. According to the notes of the meeting, McManus evaded these issues and instead assured the student that the nursing faculty wanted only to help her and to do what was best for her. In the end, McManus recommended that Betty withdraw from school once again, assuring her that "this might be best, because the provost was very upset." She added, "This incident has caused administrative criticism of the Nursing Division . . . it is a judg-ment of us all."[18]

In its simplest form, however, the issue continued to be security of facul-ty offices and files. This was a principal concern of Provost Del Manzo at this point in the saga. On November 20 McManus sent a memo to the faculty:

> There have been several serious incidents of students using the faculty offices and being given unauthorized keys. Dr. Del Manzo asked me some time ago to notify the staff that this practice must be stopped, and I so reported to the staff at a staff meeting on October 20 . . . If anyone knows of unauthorized keys, we will change the lock on your door.[19]

On November 24, Peplau wrote McManus repeating a request she had made twice before for a locked file in her office. She explained that as a part of their preparation as psychiatric nurse specialists, students were required to keep records of their interactions with nurses on the units where they worked, with supervisors and physicians with whom they came into contact, with patients, and with their peers. Students recorded these interactions verbatim in their notebooks and submitted the note-books weekly to Peplau. She read each one exceedingly carefully, made detailed notes for the students, and kept, for the permanent record, a sep-arate log of her own perceptions of the student and her progress in the program. She destroyed the verbatim notebooks at the end of the course. This had been explained in previous memos to McManus. In one such memo, Peplau informed McManus that this material is "potentially explosive." McManus did not respond to the request for a locked file and instead suggested that "the administration" would be concerned were it known that Peplau was generating such material in the first place.[20] Peplau replied to this in a November 24 memo, stating,

> I consider I have sufficient insight to know when a student is placing me in the role of therapist and I have consistently rejected this role—taking time, always, to aid the student to secure the kind of professional and personalized assistance that is needed. I would like the administra-tion to accept and trust my judgment on this point and to respect my intentions as an educator with regard to the kinds of records I need . . . But, I do believe such material should be in a locked file, and therefore I request for the third time that one be provided for me.[21]

The issue was kept alive, no doubt by McManus who was now focusing her efforts not on the security question but on Peplau's record keeping. On December 5, Provost Del Manzo came to a nursing division faculty meeting and addressed the original issue, informing the faculty that "attorneys for TC have advised that any confidential information regarding students must be kept under lock and key." He also noted that there were "problems with the control of the use of space."[22]

On December 14 Del Manzo sent McManus a memo directly addressing the matter of confidential records. In this memo the provost reminded her that confidential records in any TC department should be under the division director's control. It is notable that other than keeping confidential material in locked files in the director's office, no instruction was issued that would have the effect of modifying Peplau's teaching practices. Dr. Del Manzo stated,

> May I advise you that it is the practice of TC to keep all highly confidential records in the office of the director of a division or the head of a department. Under no circumstances should such records as we discussed at that meeting be available to students . . . confidential student data should not be accessible to students . . . the College has therefore followed the practice of keeping such records in the director's office . . . under lock and key.[23]

TRACING THE SOURCE

At this point in the story a more mysterious influence enters the picture in the person of a dentist who had indirect and ultimately problematic connections to Hilda Peplau. He was a personal friend of Louise McManus who had a summer cottage on Cape Cod where the dentist was her next-door neighbor.[24] Although a dentist, he had had since his service in WWII an interest in psychotherapy and had both a quasi-professional and an intimate relationship with Hilda's one-time mentor, Dr. Frieda Fromm Reichman of the Washington and William Alanson White institutes.[25] In 1950 he had received a Public Health Service grant to work with Fromm Reichman as coinvestigator exploring "Conditioning Emotions Under Hypnosis."[26] In the fall of 1950, McManus asked Peplau to find several students who would be willing to volunteer to serve as subjects in a project using hypnosis as a tool in psychoanalysis. Because Fromm Reichman was involved, Peplau assumed the project would have credibility. Four students volunteered, all of whom would later manifest psychological problems. One of these students had been Betty, who was then in her first short-lived term as a TC graduate student.[27]

Hilda met the dentist only once that she could recall. On that occasion, in the fall of 1950, she'd gone with McManus to the dentist's office in

New York City to hear him make a presentation concerning his approach to "therapy."[28] Peplau thought that he had not welcomed her presence, and she had sat in the back of the room. Hilda was appalled by what she heard, more particularly so since at her suggestion several of her students were participating in his research project. She left the meeting after asking a couple of hostile questions. Peplau then largely dismissed the matter from her mind. Three of the four students who volunteered for the project had withdrawn before the January 1953 crisis. He may have been angered by the defection of three of Peplau's students as it appears that hostility toward Peplau was communicated to Edna, the only one of Peplau's students who remained in the project. In August of 1952, Edna notified Peplau that she would not be returning to TC, and therefore would not be using her stipend that fall, but she would be continuing her work with the dentist/amateur psychotherapist.[29] During the fall of 1952 and through the winter and spring of 1953, Edna continued to write chatty, inviting, warm, and affectionate notes to Hilda Peplau. Hilda, however, was wary and cautious in her replies, especially after the events of January 1953.[30]

Hilda would not learn until decades later the extent to which the dentist's machinations behind the scenes contributed to the crisis that was brewing in the winter of 1952. It is significant that he had already written, with no result, to the campus medical officer and to the dean of students expressing concern about Peplau's use of "interpersonal relations theory" in her classroom teaching.[31]

McManus's specific reference to rumors concerning alcoholism and lesbianism appears to have emerged from reports about holiday season parties—one held during Thanksgiving week toward the end of the fall 1952 semester and the second about a month later, between Christmas and New Year's. In regard to "student parties," it should be noted that the students in Peplau's Advanced Psychiatric Nursing program were not young graduate students. Typically, Peplau's students had graduated from either hospital training schools or from undergraduate programs a decade earlier and brought with them at least 10 years of experience in various nursing settings before returning to school. As a group they stood apart from the general body of students in the Division of Nursing Education. Moreover, because her teaching methods, both in clinical settings and in the classroom, were introspective and emotionally demanding, her students tended to form intense interpersonal relationships within the program, often to the exclusion of social interactions with students in other departments. Several had relaxed relationships with Hilda and Tish as well, often baby-sitting Tish or joining mother and daughter on outings in the city.[32]

In the first week in December, McManus told Peplau that she was concerned about reports of drinking and drunkenness at the psych students'

Thanksgiving weekend party, which had been held at the home of a student's parents. Peplau assured McManus that while some of the students had gotten a little "hilarious" as a way of releasing the tensions of the semester, there had been far too little alcohol at the party for anyone to get drunk, and that in any event the student's parents had been present.[33] The source of the complaint appears to have been a male student, Tom, who did not drink and made it clear he disapproved of the presence of alcohol, no matter how little the quantity, at student parties. He apparently complained about the Thanksgiving party to Dr. Von Wagonen, the dean of students, who reported the complaint to McManus. Shortly after Christmas the students held another party, this one a dinner at the home of another student in Spring Valley, New York. The students feasted on a large turkey and all the trimmings, and "a little wine."[34] At this party, two incidents occurred that may have had a connection to the subsequent rumors. Before the Christmas break, Tom had hallucinated in class, claiming to hear the voice of God. When he tried to talk with Peplau about this at the Christmas party, she suggested he consider dropping out of school and seeking professional help. Tom would later acknowledge that he was aggrieved at what he perceived to be a rejection. In a letter to Peplau in 1957 he indicated he may have been responsible in part for the rumors, but stated that, "I meant you no harm and wish you all the best in the future."[35]

There was yet another student having problems that year who most likely figures into the unfolding events. At the Spring Valley party, this student rested her hand on Hilda's shoulder and eventually sat down and put her head in her lap, until Hilda, feeling slightly uncomfortable, gently moved away. Several days later, the student came to her office and laid her hand on Hilda's thigh, sighing. Peplau removed her hand, asking " What is this all about?" The student explained she had told the dentist/therapist of her feelings of warmth toward Peplau as a "mother figure." He, she said, suggested that she had been having homosexual fantasies about her instructor and advised her to act on these feelings to see what would happen. Not getting a response she could interpret one way or the other, she had, at his suggestion, decided to try again.[36]

THE ATTACK ESCALATES

On Monday morning, January 5, 1953, the day before she was summoned by McManus, Peplau wrote three memos to her—one advising that she would be away at the Kellogg conference and in Washington, D.C. until January 10, one giving instructions about the allocation of Edna's stipend for the spring semester, and one asking for a conference with Dr. Von Wagonen, to include Betty's psychiatrist, to discuss how to monitor Betty during the spring term. It will be remembered that Hilda in the

1952–1953 year was completing requirements for her certificate in applied psychiatry from the William Alanson White Institute (WAW). On that Monday afternoon, January 5, Mrs. McManus called Dr. Clara Thompson, the director of the institute, at her private offices in the Hotel Croydon, requesting a meeting with her and with Peplau's analyst, Dr. Earl G. Witenberg. She wanted to discuss rumors concerning Hilda Peplau at Teachers College.[37] Dr. Witenberg refused to talk with McManus without Peplau's permission, but sometime that afternoon McManus did meet with Clara Thompson, informing her that "Hildegard Peplau is creating problems at TC" and relating matters, according to the institute files, concerning "file, mattress, Letitia, homosexual rumors."[38] The notation of a "mattress" appears to have been a red herring, referring to an incident when a student set fire to a mattress on a dormitory floor where several of Peplau's students lived. The reference to "Letitia" was far more significant. After meeting with McManus, Thompson conveyed the content of the meeting to Witenberg. Dr. Witenberg saw Hilda on the afternoon of January 6.[39] In that session Hilda related that she had been called into McManus's office that morning and told that she was "sick" and in need of help, and that she was an alcoholic and a lesbian. She reviewed the charges made by McManus in detail and discussed her reaction to them.

Dr. Witenberg, however, had knowledge of yet another very serious charge—especially given the context and time. But this was a charge that Peplau would not know had been raised in the effort to discredit her. It was a matter that Witenberg, as her analyst, could not bring up in the session because she had not discussed it with him. Although Peplau was in analysis with Witenberg and trusted him implicitly, she had not revealed to him what was arguably the most important fact of her life to that date; namely, that Tish was her own biological daughter. So pervasive was the condemnation of childbirth out of wedlock that Hilda had told no one, outside of her family, that Tish was her daughter. So far as she knew, the world believed Tish was her niece. Unwed mothers were not employed by major universities in the 1950s.

What McManus had revealed to Clara Thompson the afternoon before her confrontation with Hilda was that she "knew" that Tish was Peplau's daughter, not her niece. The source of that information was the dentist/therapist who claimed to both Frieda Fromm Reichman and Louise McManus that he had been at the 312th Military Field Hospital where Hilda was stationed during the war, that he knew her companion "Mac" well, and that he knew that Peplau had been pregnant before the war ended.[40] This information was so sensitive that it could not be discussed in any public forum.[41] As it turned out, it was also information that could not be confirmed. Hilda, it will be recalled, had taken the precaution of having her brother Walter officially adopt Tish. So, legally, she was in fact raising her niece. Try as she might, McManus could not get around this point. Her mission in seeking a meeting with Hilda's analyst was to ask Witenberg to confirm beyond doubt that Hilda Peplau was an unwed mother. This was information that even he did not have, and that in any event he would not have revealed. This rumor, however, is the one that had substance and thus was most likely the one that gave Louise McManus her moral zeal in the developing crisis.[42] The dentist's motives are more obscure, but it would be understandable that he resented the fact that Peplau's students elected to leave his project and care. He may have also been angered that Peplau had judged him wanting as a therapist and a researcher when he knew she should be the most humble of women, an unwed mother who was deceiving the world about that fact. It was a situation in which Hildegard Peplau's professional career was on the line.

A CAREER ENDANGERED

Peplau's immediate reaction when informed of the presumed rumors against her had been to insist that she be allowed to confront the source of the rumors. McManus, understandably, was not interested in pursuing the sources; and, at this point, the only rumors she could substantiate were related to student parties. It was in this context that she issued her directive that Hilda was to "have no contact with students of any sort off campus."[43] Angered, Peplau had informed McManus on the spot that she would resign rather than conform to a prejudicial policy devised just for her in response to unsubstantiated rumors. Always true to her word, when she returned on January 10 from the Kellogg and Washington conferences, Peplau handed McManus her formal letter of resignation:

> I hereby tender my resignation effective June 30, 1953. On that date I will have given five years of effort in developing creative relations with students and a constructive program in psychiatric nursing. Now it seems appropriate that I move on to a new work situation . . . I appreciate the many opportunities for making a professional contribution to nursing that have been opened to me in the course of my five years of employment at Teachers College and through my relations with members of the Faculty and staff.[44]

Hilda later explained, "I was angry, but I wasn't stupid—I gave myself six months to finish the dissertation and see the students through the year."[45]

Word of Peplau's resignation, or the circumstances surrounding it, created much tension and anxiety among her students.[46] On Saturday, January 18, a group of three psychiatric nursing students called Mrs. McManus to ask if she would meet with them first thing on Monday morning. They said they had been hearing rumors "about our group" and wanted to talk

with her about their concerns.[47] McManus insisted that the students
come to her home that night. The students were there from 8–10 p.m. At
10:00, they called Peplau and asked to see her. Hilda kept notes of the
ensuing conversation and asked the students to write down what they
could remember of their conversation with McManus, much in the way
they did in class. Thus, the written record here is fairly complete.
Specifically, the students were upset about the rumor of homosexuality
and feared it reflected upon the psychiatric nursing students as a group.
It was this concern, and not Peplau's problems, that had them upset.

According to the students, McManus neither asked them about their
concerns nor was she interested in listening to them. Instead, she wanted
to be sure the students understood her side of the story about Peplau's
resignation. As recorded by the students, McManus claimed that Peplau
had been warned against attending student parties, but had insisted on
attending anyway; that her "bad" behavior at these parties had been
reported to the dean; that information about her problems had also come
through the medical office (although not identifying the source as the
dentist's letter to Dr. Von Wagonen); and that although Peplau had developed the best program in psychiatric nursing in the country, her judgment was defective.

McManus then cast the issue in an entirely new light, suggesting now
that the problem was Peplau's innovative instructional program. She
claimed that rumors related to Peplau's "unorthodox" teaching methods
were causing concern in the dean's office. When asked how rumors
should be handled, she stated that "the rumors don't bother me . . . and I
didn't get upset about them until it came from the dean's office." Mrs.
McManus talked about how difficult, high-handed, hardheaded, and
uncooperative Peplau was in not agreeing to simply cease to use such
"controversial teaching methods." She further alleged that Peplau's problems were becoming so well known that other universities were refusing
to send students to TC.[48]

After this meeting with the students McManus seemed to have second
thoughts. It appeared that the situation was escalating out of her control.
While it is true that Hilda Peplau's teaching methods had attracted attention, although not necessarily censure, at the upper administrative levels,
it was also true that Peplau was a valued member of the faculty, bringing
not only national recognition to the TC nursing education program but
also a significant input of federal funding. Peplau's vision for students in
the program in Advanced Psychiatric Nursing had from the beginning
differed from Louise McManus's concept of the proper role for Division
of Nursing Education graduates. In now asserting that "concern" on the
part of administrators at the highest levels over Peplau's "controversial"
teaching methods was the *cause* of the problem, however, McManus may
have gone too far. She must have realized this. It will be recalled that the

provost in his response to the issue surrounding the confidentiality of Hilda's notes had not suggested that Peplau modify her procedures, but rather that McManus take better precautions.

On January 23 McManus again called Peplau into her office. According to Peplau's notes written immediately after this meeting, McManus asked her to reconsider her resignation but repeated references to Hilda's "defective judgment" and to "being sick." McManus stated that she knew "the drinking was only temporary." The focus of the discussion, as it had been in their first meeting, was charges related to personal behavior, not teaching methods. Peplau again insisted that the rumors be cleared up, since they were untrue. She asked that McManus call in both students and faculty members who had been at the two parties in order to "get the facts about those parties" from them. She again pointed out that "a restricting and discriminatory policy being laid down for one individual" indicated that unsubstantiated rumors were being regarded as true.[49] McManus claimed that she had called Peplau in when she first heard the rumors. This statement made Peplau even more furious, for by then she knew that over the Christmas holiday McManus had called an emergency meeting of several faculty to inform them of the rumors. Only one of those present (Margaret Adams) had asked for evidence. Hilda had also learned that before her January 6 meeting with Hilda, McManus had discussed the rumors with Clara Thompson of the William Alanson White Institute and had wanted to meet also with Witenberg. Peplau stormed out, after calling McManus a liar and assuring her that she would "never, under any circumstances, work with a person who set up individualized policies on the basis of rumors—and thus discriminated against individuals in terms of a problem too tough to handle—that the resignation submitted was final."[50] The die was cast and now there was no turning back on either side.

It should be noted that had McManus's intention simply been to remove Hilda from her position, that could have been accomplished rather easily. Peplau was only an instructor, not a tenured member of the faculty. McManus could have simply let her contract lapse by not reappointing her for the next academic year. At this point in time, the reasons for McManus's "missteps" in regard to Peplau cannot be known, if ever they were clear.

What is known is that on January 26, 1953, McManus forwarded Peplau's resignation to Dean Harold Caswell with her own cover note:

It is with regret that I am forwarding to you herewith the resignation of Hildegard Peplau as Instructor of Psychiatric Nursing effective June 30, 1953.

I am sorry that I was unable to secure her cooperation on the plan which we agreed seemed desirable in view of the widespread and persistent unfavorable comments directed toward the psychiatric group this fall which had come to our attention from a variety of sources.

Miss Peplau has said that I have failed in my duties as an administrator in the Division in not tracking down and exposing the source of each rumor . . . I regret that she finds it impossible to accede to the administrative request made of her in the interests of the program as I see it, and to continue as a member of the instructional staff.[51]

The letter made no reference to Peplau's innovative teaching methods and alluded only to an "administrative request," presumably that Hilda have no interactions with students outside of the classroom situation.

ISOLATION

In spite of her letter to the Dean, McManus now seemed in fact to focus on Peplau's "controversial" teaching methods. Some groundwork for this new diversionary tactic existed. During the fall of 1952 Peplau had completed a draft of her doctoral dissertation, tentatively entitled "Methods of Evaluating the Instructional Process," focusing on instructor-student interactions in her courses on "Interpersonal Relations in Nursing" and "Trends in Contemporary Nursing." She had applied for and been given a leave for the spring 1953 semester to revise and complete the dissertation. A phone call from McManus on December 19, 1952, alerted Peplau that trouble might be brewing in regard to her dissertation. Hilda's note of the call reads: "Says the provost is concerned (not enthusiastic) about the Trends study—thinks it will hurt the college."[52] No indication is given of what concerns the provost may have had. It is unlikely that the provost of the college would be involved in a dissertation project, but if that were the case, it is evident that the "concern" would have been generated by McManus, who chaired Peplau's dissertation committee. According to Peplau, McManus suggested that Peplau drop the project, implying that the dissertation would never be approved.

On Monday, February 2, McManus met with Division of Nursing Education non-professional staff in the morning and with the division's part-time instructional staff in the afternoon to explain the "dangers" of Hilda Peplau's instructional methods.[53] A day later the dean himself, Dr. Harold Caswell, met with the faculty and professional staff regarding Hildegard Peplau. In that meeting, Hilda was told, Dean Caswell

Says an analyst of one of my students has written Dr. Von Wagonen about the dangers of closeness in the classroom with unstable students and about my instructional methods. Homosexuality was not mentioned, but implied . . . the issue is really on the mode of teaching, not rumors.[54]

On February 6 Hilda wrote to her sister Bertha and her brother-in-law Byron telling them about the events of January, informing them that she'd resigned, and instructing them to discuss this with no one. She then described something of her emotions and feelings:

> Believe me, I have never suffered as I have these last three weeks. The fatigue and anxiety and pain have been so unbearable. To me it was inconceivable that in a great and supposedly democratic institution, injustice could be served when administrative ineptness and unconscious hatred mix up with pathology . . . life in a mental hospital is simpler than such complex pathology in a work situation.[55]

She went on to tell her sister that college officials had decided that she was "mentally ill," and therefore should not be allowed to finish her dissertation, but that she had requested an appointment to see the dean the following week to discuss this. There is evidence of sardonic humor here when Hilda remarks on the ludicrous nature of the charges: "Of course, if I'm a homosexual, I'm a Communist too."[56]

In February Hilda's brother Walter wrote a very supportive letter, assuring her that he and his wife Anne would "take Tish at any time, have her placed in school and all that sort of stuff, so if this thought comes to your mind you can rest easily . . . goes without saying the door is open."[57] Walter also included $100 to be used to hire a typist to edit and type the final version of her dissertation, which he was sure somehow would be accepted.

Hilda's experience of the month of February is recorded in the many notes she made at this time. They describe colleagues ignoring her, turning their backs, refusing to sit with her at the lunch table, looking embarrassed when she spoke to them, and so forth. Miss Peplau had become a pariah. She had many discussions with students who came by to see her, or who continued to baby-sit Tish. While concerned for her, the students' principal worry was for their own reputations. Their hope was to be supportive of their mentor, while at the same time staying out of the line of fire and finishing their work at TC unscathed.[58] Above all else they wanted to escape any taint of the damning charge of lesbianism.

Peplau observed that once homosexuality had been hinted at, people began to edge away from her. This is not surprising given that there was a prosecutorial climate at large in America in the early 1950s that had the effect of endorsing tactics of defamation and innuendo that characterized what came to be known as McCarthyism. The main McCarthy era rumors were that the person being targeted was either a "commie" or a "queer."[59] Hilda was an unlikely candidate for the Communist label, but the lesbian charge was an easier one to level against a single woman. The stigma of lesbianism, or sexual "perversion," was often used to discredit women who chose not to marry, to follow an independent path, to be their own person marching to their own drummer. Men suspected of homosexuality were run out of the state department and discharged from the armed services. The same was true in women's professions such as teaching or nursing, and Hilda was committed to both. The accusation could and did destroy. Family, career, friends, everything could be swept away in the face of such rumors; and mere rumors were enough to bring ruin to a reputation. For this reason, no charge could have enraged and terrified Peplau more than this one, and no charge could have been more upsetting to the students in her program.[60]

THE CRISIS PLAYS OUT

At the William Alanson White Institute, a most unusual decision had been made. On February 13, Dr. Witenberg called Hilda to ask her permission to allow Dr. Harry Bone, the director of the teachers' program at the institute, to go see Dean Caswell on her behalf. Hilda readily agreed.[61] The situation was complicated because administrators at WAW knew of the personal relationship of the dentist to Frieda Fromm Reichman and to Louise McManus. More to the point, they also were aware that he had told McManus that Hilda was Tish's birth mother. Hilda did not know that McManus had gone to the WAW hoping to confirm this information. The leadership at WAW was convinced that the charges related to alcoholism and lesbianism and other alleged behaviors were entirely false. They were concerned that a very promising career in nursing was about to be destroyed.[62] The decision of the medical professionals at WAW to intervene in this situation was an extraordinary act of support for Peplau and a credit to her reputation at the institute. Dr. Bone's specific purpose in going to TC was to provide Dean Caswell with expert opinion regarding Peplau, based on the institute's own experience and knowledge of her character and her personal life as well as her professional standards. The WAW evaluation would certainly neutralize McManus's allegations and cast doubt on her motives in taking her tales to the provost. Bone, however, in his meeting with Dean Caswell would not be able to discuss the allegations about Hilda's actual relationship to the "niece" she was raising as this was information Peplau had not revealed, even to her analyst.[63]

Dr. Bone's visit did have an impact. On February 27, 1953, Dean Caswell's secretary telephoned Peplau, informing her that the dean would like to meet with her on March 2.[64] When Peplau met with Dean Caswell, he explained that he had had a visit from Dr. Bone that caused him to wonder whether he had all the facts in regard to her resignation.[65] He asked Hilda to tell her story. Unfortunately, Hilda had not prepared a succinct summary of the events nor a careful statement of her position in regard to them. Instead, she used the occasion for a cathartic release of all her anger and frustration at what she perceived to be great injustice.[66] The hour was soon up. Dean Caswell apparently made no comment at this time but assured her he would review the facts leading to her resignation and would meet with her again.

On March 23, Peplau had the promised second meeting with Dean Caswell. It was very short. He informed her that he'd reconstituted her dissertation reading committee, essentially removing McManus as committee chair and adding non-nurse faculty members to the committee. Caswell then indicated that the circumstances leading to her resignation were too complicated to untangle. Rather than try to work through the many layers of individual problems or, worse yet, get involved in the messy details himself, the dean concluded that the university would let matters stand. Peplau had resigned, that was the salient fact of the matter—but she was to proceed to complete the requirements for her doctorate. His advice to her was to keep matters simple. Hilda protested, saying that McManus was talking to people constantly but she, Hildegard Peplau, was being silenced. "You are oversimplifying for your own reasons," she declared.[67] Dean Caswell ignored her protests, repeating again that she would have a special committee for her dissertation, "so you will have every opportunity to get your doctorate."[68] In exchange for the reconstitution of her committee, the dean wanted Peplau to agree to cease her demands that all allegations and rumors be investigated. Hilda continued to protest until Dean Caswell adjourned the meeting, summarizing the official conclusions as follows:

> You and Mrs. McManus disagreed about teaching methods and you resigned, period. That's the way she sees it—it was your teaching methods. You'd better get your thesis done as fast as you can and make simple statements about why you resigned. Instructors never stay here long. You and Mrs. McManus disagreed and you resigned. Problems like this come up in colleges all the time and the best way is to get rid of it. She understands this and the less you say the better for you and the college.[69]

Hilda was outraged and despairing that she was not to be allowed to clear her name or respond in any official forum to charges she felt to be outright slander. Her image of herself as a dedicated and creative teacher, a responsible colleague, a person of great integrity, and an independent, self-sufficient woman had been assaulted by charges that she was inappropriate with students, neglectful of her responsibilities, and of questionable moral character, not to mention "sick" and in need of "help." Moreover, her image of the university as a fair and open-minded institution, a bastion of truth and learning, had been irrevocably damaged in the encounter with administrators whom she now believed valued expediency above justice. How, she had asked in her letter to Bertha, could a great and democratic institution be so unfair? Hilda had developed an idealized concept of the university and of higher education in her years at the NYU camp and at Bennington College. At Teachers College she experienced a loss of innocence and idealism.

The rest of the spring seemed to proceed on two levels. On the personal level, Peplau was devastated, not only by the accusations themselves, but even more so by the fact that with one exception (Margaret Adams), no other TC faculty member came to her defense. Among her friends in the profession at large, and there were many, the unanimous advice was simply to "move on."[70] As if with one voice they urged her to put the whole situation behind her. No one, however, offered any concrete suggestions as to just how she was to move on and where she might go to put all behind her. On another level, as the professional that she was, Hilda maintained her public composure. She acknowledged all letters, and never denigrated the advice offered. She sent very formal and proper memos to Mrs. McManus about her students, her files, her projects, her grants, and her plans.[71] She answered each and every letter from her students with proper politeness; but, the personal warmth was gone. Few seemed to notice.

Dr. Arthur Jersild was appointed to replace McManus as chairman of Hilda's dissertation committee. It was an excellent appointment. A developmental psychologist, Jersild was a professor of psychology and education who had spent decades studying the ways in which schools could foster self-awareness among both students and teachers.[72] Two members of the nursing faculty, Margaret Adams and Lavern Thompson, continued to serve as members and were joined by Dr. Stephen M. Corey of the psychology department. On March 24, Peplau had her first meeting with Arthur Jersild and found that he would be a supportive chair. Since her thesis was in effect finished, all she wanted to do was hand in the final copy. In May Peplau submitted a 300-page dissertation entitled "An Exploration of Some Process Elements Which Restrict or Facilitate Instructor-Student Interaction in a Classroom." Although Dr. Corey was critical of the weak statistical analysis, the dissertation was accepted as presented.[73] Peplau, though, had long since lost almost all interest in this dissertation, and in interviews in later years could not even recall its topic.

Hilda knew she would have to leave Teachers College, but she had been too engaged in the events unfolding around her to think seriously beyond the spring semester. She had thought she would at least have the summer, after defending her dissertation, to sort it all out and find alternative employment. That hope too was destroyed, however, when she received a short formal note from Dean Caswell on April 24, 1953, stating that "no appointment for the summer session has been made for you, since you resigned from the College effective July 1."[74]

As the academic year drew to a close, Hilda kept her counsel and, following the dean's advice, had confided in no one other than her brother and sister about her reasons for resigning. She was on leave, but continued to be active professionally. Her students continued to drop in to see Tish or just to visit. Hilda was courteous but unresponsive to the efforts to reach out to her. Her students grew increasingly alarmed by her silence. At the end of May they asked to meet with Mrs. McManus yet again. They wanted to be assured that nothing *they* had done had led to Miss Peplau's resignation. They asked why Miss Peplau would not talk with them about her reasons, and they wanted to be assured that her reasons would not reflect upon them. McManus played the good mother. She said that Miss Peplau's reasons were her own, that her resignation was neither sought nor requested, but rather "her reasons are personal and will be respected."[75] Mrs. McManus praised Peplau's work and urged the students to go forth and be good nurses, assuring them that "what you can do for yourselves and her is to live up to her high standards."[76]

Hilda had given her word under duress not to discuss the situation and she continued to keep her word, even when faced with questions from concerned friends and colleagues outside of Columbia and Teachers College. To colleagues generally she said nothing. At meetings of the national committees on which she served, however, Peplau continued to hear one way or another that rumors about her were rampant. Through the National League for Nursing, McManus had a wide network, and it is in the nature of rumors that once started, they spread. This news, and the knowledge that no one was countering the rumors it carried, increased Hilda's devastation and also made her very angry. She knew that these kinds of rumors could ruin a career. Certainly they might have destroyed a person with less personal strength and sense of integrity than Hildegard Peplau. Sleep was difficult. Her mind spun much of the night trying to think of ways to cope, of ways to understand, of ways to counter the rumors without compromising her principles.

In spite of the traumas of that spring, Peplau continued to function as a conscientious faculty member, fulfilling her responsibilities on examinations and thesis committees and making a superhuman effort not to let the academic nightmare affect her professional responsibilities to her students or interrupt her many commitments. Peplau's last official act at TC was to type a detailed, 9-page single-spaced report on the Psychiatric Nursing Program for McManus.[77]

Moving On

After submitting her dissertation in May, Peplau set about seriously looking for new employment. There was immediate interest on the academic front, but she couldn't afford to wait to work through these possibilities. She had to be sure Tish was provided for. Her own anxieties inevitably had an effect on her daughter, and she was determined to interrupt Tish's life as little as possible at this time. Peplau signed on at the Adele Posten Registry, where she had worked when she first came to New York 20 years earlier. She would once again care for private psychiatric patients. She was immediately assigned to cases, and found the one-on-one work that summer very engrossing. She appreciated the opportunity to see how her new insights into mental illness could be applied to individual patients. She informed the physician in charge of her first case that she wanted to spend at least an hour a day "talking" with the patient. "He just said, yeah, yeah, yeah, sure."[78] After all, what did a nurse know? In fact, she was working out her approach to patient therapy. Private-duty nursing employment meant, however, that she worked 20-hour days, 6 days a week. During the work week, she was expected to live in the patient's home. At night, Hilda called Tish before she went to bed. Fortunately, her good neighbor, Mrs. Alameda, was quite happy to take care of Tish along with her own daughter Mary, who was Tish's best friend. It was a happy arrangement, but Hilda missed Tish, and knew that this was not a situation that could continue for long. Tish's education was a matter of particular concern. Hilda was aware that because she was no longer affiliated with Teachers College she would not be able to enroll Tish in the TC Agnes Russell School again when fall came.

With the completion of her dissertation, her own G.I. Bill stipend had also expired. Since the stipend was paying for her analysis at the William Alanson White Institute, the analysis ended when the stipend did. By this time, she had completed the requirements for the WAW Certificate for Teachers, which was officially awarded in June 1954.[79] With so much pressure on her, and with her mind elsewhere, when she was notified that the stipends would stop, Peplau simply stopped going to see Dr. Witenberg. She didn't have time to discuss it with him.[80] He often wondered what had happened to her.[81]

Although she had no one with whom to share her thoughts now, Hilda knew she wanted to be back in an academic institution as soon as possible. She began correspondence with the Universities of North Carolina, Maryland, and Colorado.[82] Early in July, she went to the University of Maryland for an interview, where she got along exceedingly well, both with the nursing faculty and with the two psychiatrists in the medical school with whom she hoped to work and whom she had known in Europe during the war, Dr. Maurice Greenhill and Dr. Harvey Finesinger. The interviews went so well that she stayed over several days to look at real estate, and even found a house she was prepared to buy. Almost immediately after her return to New York, Hilda received a note from the dean at Maryland, Florence Gipe, saying "Welcome . . . all but the formalities have been taken care of . . . please send references."[83] On August 3, Dr. Greenhill wrote to an administrator at the University of Maryland College of Medicine informing her that "the Psychiatric Nursing position is filled—Hildegard Peplau will have that position."[84] It seemed as though all was set. Peplau was preparing to join the University of Maryland faculty as soon as she could wind up her work in New York City. All came to a crashing end when, on August 21, with no forewarning whatsoever, she received another letter from Florence Gipe:

> Your application has been reviewed by the President and Personnel Office . . . your qualifications, although high academically, would not meet the present needs of an institution such as the University of Maryland. Florence Gipe, Dean.[85]

Peplau was stunned. The academic nightmare was not yet over. On her visit to Maryland, no one had made the slightest suggestion that there would be any trouble at all. Peplau kept her cool, writing back to Florence Gipe that she would like to discuss the situation and requesting a convenient time to call. The response was a definitive telegram from Dean Gipe: "I refer you to the letter of August 21. The decision is final."[86]

Greenhill telephoned a week or so later to tell her that the Maryland Board of Nursing had vetoed her appointment. Because she thought it necessary and the professional thing to do, Hilda had listed Mrs. McManus as a reference, trusting that she in turn would also be professional and not discuss the "rumors" of the spring. Such was not the case, however. When Dean Gipe telephoned McManus, not only did she not give a good reference for Peplau, but she used her contacts at the National League for Nursing to telephone the Maryland board, threatening Maryland with loss of accreditation if it employed someone so "immoral" as Peplau.[87]

In early September, Peplau sat down and typed a 27-page single-spaced letter to Maurice Greenhill. That letter, dated September 9, 1953, provides an exhaustive review of the events at TC over the winter and spring of 1952–1953 as Peplau understood them. In the letter, she strove to record every event of relevance, but confessed that "this is not an easy problem to comprehend or solve." She expressed her frustration that she could not secure the position she sought at Maryland, even though she was one of only two psychiatric nurses in the United States holding an earned doctorate at that time. The letter is exceedingly detailed. For example, there is a long paragraph outlining eight different parties and social activities in 1952 given by other TC nursing faculty members for or with students when alcohol was served—much more alcohol than at the two psychiatric nursing parties McManus had questioned her about. (This account alone must have exhausted Greenhill.)[88]

In October, Greenhill wrote with the good news that due to strong letters of recommendation sent on her behalf to Dr. Harry Byrd, the president of the University of Maryland, was open to having the whole matter
reconsidered. Notable among those letters was one from Louis Webster
Jones, who had been president of Bennington during Hilda's senior year
there and who was then president of Rutgers, The State University of
New Jersey. By January 1954, however, the issue was dead. Dr. Byrd had
retired from Maryland without having resolved the matter, and the new
president decided he did not need to ruffle his dean of nursing by forcing
a controversial appointment onto the faculty. On January 14, 1954,
Greenhill wrote to inform Hilda that the "controversial letter of reference
which the personnel office received early in the fall" continued to cause
problems and that at best there would be no full professorship with
tenure until after a "temporary period of getting acquainted and removal
of doubt after the unfortunate Columbia rumors."[89]

Peplau herself had earlier come to terms with the fact that an appointment at Maryland would be unlikely, for she wrote a letter of inquiry to
Lulu Hassenplug, the dean of a new nursing program at the University of
California at Los Angeles. Hassenplug had arrived in Westwood in 1948
as the UCLA Medical Center was being established, and as dean of nursing was spearheading a movement to move nursing education from hospitals to college campuses. The UCLA program she was creating was the
first university-based undergraduate program for nurses on the west
coast, and Hassenplug's philosophy of graduate nursing was actually
much more compatible with Hilda's than was anyone's at TC. While TC
would continue to stress preparing graduate level nurses for positions in
administration and education, Hassenplug was convinced that clinical
expertise was the key to the advancement of nursing.[90] Peplau wrote a
formal letter to Hassenplug with a personal cover note expressing uncertainty about how to proceed "given the situation at TC."[91] She gave 10
references: two from psychiatrists on the faculty of the William Alanson
White Institute; the two psychiatrists employed on her grants to work
with the students in her graduate program, Joseph Geller and John
Schimel; Dr. Irving Pine, formerly at the Highland Hospital in North
Carolina; Dr. Jay Hoffman, the administrator at the 312th Military
Hospital; plus Dr. Arthur Jersild and the three nurse faculty members at
TC (including again Mrs. R. Louise McManus). What is significant about
this list is that other than the TC faculty members, no nurses were listed
as references, Peplau's growing national reputation and admiration of
her work not withstanding. Clearly, Hilda perceived that physicians and
psychiatrists were more likely to appreciate and understand what she
was trying to accomplish than did most members of her own profession.
This would remain the case for most of her career.

As the word got out that the Maryland offer had fallen through, other universities began to contact Peplau expressing interest. These included Duke, Boston University, the University of Pennsylvania, Vanderbilt, and the University of North Carolina. Things progressed furthest at North Carolina, where Hilda visited late in the fall 1953. On January 26, 1954, the Dean of the College of Nursing, Elizabeth Kemble, wrote Hilda, informing her that she had been asked to "request assurance from you that, if you joined us, it would be with the understanding that you were making a fresh start here and that you would not take any action connected with past experiences at TC . . . Consider the past over and done with and concentrate on the job to be done here."[92] Hilda was in fact very interested in returning to North Carolina, but she had not been comfortable during her visit to Chapel Hill. The nurse faculty had asked few questions about what she would do in regard to developing graduate work in nursing and many questions about which church she planned to attend.[93] By this time she had been in discussions with Ella B. Stonsby, who was developing a new nursing program at Rutgers. There were several things that Hilda found very attractive about the Rutgers possibility. For one thing, Dr. Louis Webster Jones was president of Rutgers and had been very supportive of her. Second, although she found her work with private patients in New York truly interesting and challenging, she had begun to worry that Manhattan was not the best place for Tish, who was now attending a public school and was not finding the challenge she needed. Third, Ella Stonsby was something of a visionary, and she had already implemented at Rutgers a program McManus was only exploring at TC. So, early in 1954, she accepted a part-time position at Rutgers, teaching three credits of theoretical instruction and two credits of clinical supervision. The next fall she would accept a full-time position at Rutgers with the understanding that she could apply for an NIMH grant to design and develop a graduate program there.

Hence, it was easy for her to respond to Dean Kemble's letter of concern about the North Carolina possibility by replying that she would be teaching at Rutgers on a part-time basis in order to assess the situation and to "appraise what is open to me in nursing education without the great financial risk involved in moving to another section of the country." She concluded by remarking that "the situation at Columbia is not so easy to put behind me, but with fortunate experiences it will become something from which I learn a great deal."[94] For her part, Dean Kemble responded that she and the nursing faculty were sorry that Peplau had chosen to go to Rutgers, while assuring her that they would keep open the possibility at North Carolina. She also offered a piece of personal advice:

> Hilda, I believe you have much to contribute to our work here at UNC. I feel confident, too, that in this environment you would find many

satisfactions both personal and professional which would speed your recovery from the recent unhappiness you have experienced. We have faith and confidence in you . . . Let bygones be bygones.[95]

Throughout that spring of 1954 there were notes from nursing leaders and others assuring Hilda that she had more friends than she knew. As deans at Vanderbilt, Boston, and Pennsylvania continued to send inquiries about her plans, Peplau began to regain her confidence and to look forward to the future.[96]

In the end, Peplau was scarred, but not defeated. She learned that rumors are not harmless, but can be powerful weapons. For this reason, she could never again tolerate idle gossip and felt strongly that ruinous gossip must be dealt with aggressively. For a time, her own self-esteem had been seriously compromised. With painful effort, she would repair it.

The Teachers College story reached a conclusion 30 years after Hilda's resignation when, on May 17, 1983, Columbia University conferred the degree of Doctor of Science, *honoris causa*, on Hildegard E. Peplau. Such sweet revenge! As the university's guest, Hilda stayed in an elegant hotel on Central Park South and was feted at a grand dinner at the home of Columbia's president at the time, Dr. Michael I. Sovern. She and the writer Isaac Asimov were paired, limousines zipped them around New York, and a grand time was had by all. The dinner at the president's home was elegant, the conversation intelligent and genteel, everything was done in style and with taste. Some of Hilda's nephews and nieces came to the ceremony, as did three generations of Rutgers students, one of whom organized a lovely catered party in her home in Greenwich Village after the ceremony. Graduation day was beautiful, warm, and sunny. New York seemed to sparkle. The dark days of 1953 were now truly part of another life. No one connected with these Columbia events in 1983 seemed to have any recollection or knowledge of how Peplau's prior association with Columbia University had ended 30 years earlier. As the citation was read in May, 1983, Hildegard Peplau knew there could not be a better end to her "Columbia Story." The citation read,

> Pioneer in the development of the theory and practice of psychiatric mental health nursing, you have had a profound effect on health care . . . In recognition of your distinguished achievements in blending humanistic intervention and scientific formulation, Columbia University is honored to confer upon you the degree of Doctor of Science, *honoris causa*.[97]

The hood was bestowed, she was hugged by the president, and finally the TC story was truly behind her. Indeed, it was literally behind her, for the Teachers College Division of Nursing Education held its own graduation ceremony at a location behind the university's main commencement arena, and was thus out of view. At the Columbia event it was the nurses from the Columbia Presbyterian Hospital School of Nursing who celebrated, toasting the first nurse to be presented the honorary doctorate by Columbia University.

ENDNOTES

1. In October, 1952, Peplau had accepted an invitation from Dr. Dan Stienhoff, Dean of the Evening Education Division of the University of Miami, to lecture in a special Nursing Institute on December 22, 23, 29, and 30, 1952. She was invited to bring Tish: "We have arranged for you and your ward to have a room in our Koubek guest house. The honorarium will be $100.00 plus airfare." See Dan Stienhoff to Hildegard Peplau, October 31, 1952, in Box 18, #636.
2. These events are reconstructed from notes made January 29, 1953, found in Box 14, #484, and also recounted in a letter from Hildegard Peplau to Maurice Greenhill, MD, September 9, 1953, found in Box 14, #483.
3. Ibid.
4. Interview, Hildegard Peplau, March 21, 1994.
5. Most of the reconstruction of these events was pieced together by the author after reading notes, memos, and minutes of faculty meetings in the Teachers College Archives at Columbia University; material saved by Hildegard Peplau and found in Box 14, #483–386 in the Schlesinger Collection; and in discussion with Peplau over a 2-year period as the author worked on this chapter, seeking to understand the events of 1953.
6. R. Louise Metcalf met John McManus, "a very successful business man," and his six children on a Mediterranean cruise in 1929. She married him shortly thereafter; but the marriage was a short one, as John McManus passed away in 1934. Interview, R. Louise McManus, May 28, 1992, in Natick, Massachusetts.
7. Interviews with Hildegard Peplau, March 21, 1994; Catharine Norris, April 10, 1994, in Tucson, Arizona; and Louise Fitzpatrick, March 14, 1994, in Philadelphia, Pennsylvania.
8. In 1952, a psychology graduate student completing an assignment at the Agnes Russell School gave Tish an I.Q. test. The child went off the scale at 180. "Letitia has a high I.Q. and this places her in the Very Superior Group, in fact she exceeds 99 per cent of the standardization population," the report stated. "Report on Letitia Peplau's Performance on the Stanford-Binet Scale," October, 1952, Schlesinger Library, Box 3, #111.
9. In 1980 Peplau wrote a 15-page analysis of the 1952–1953 events and tried to understand them within a broader psychoanalytical/social science context. This paper may also be found in Box 14, #482.
10. Untitled story, Box 14, #482.
11. Letter from Hildegard Peplau to Maurice Greenhill, September 9, 1953.
12. These materials have been deposited in Box 14, #485.
13. Hilda Peplau saved a great deal of material recording her experience of the "TC Incident," as she referred to it. Most of this material is in Box 14 at the Schlesinger Library, in files #482–486. This record includes Peplau's own analyses, written in 1953 and 1980, her long letter to Maurice Greenhill, her notes, copies of letters and notes from her students of the time, annotated copies of faculty meeting minutes, correspondence with Louise McManus, and letters received from colleagues during 1953–1954. In addition to this written record, the author discussed these events with Hildegard Peplau in four interviews in 1992 and one interview in 1994.

Finally, the author contacted 15 individuals, including Louise McManus, who had been at TC at the time, in an effort to verify and/or elaborate on this crisis in Peplau's career—a crisis that in fact could have ended her academic career. Three of the women contacted were on the faculty at the time, 2 were on the staff (McManus's and Peplau's secretaries), and 10 were students whose names were listed on Peplau's rosters and whose notes to her are a part of the written record. Several of these former students claimed they were not in fact at TC in 1953 and thus knew nothing of what had happened that year, others declined to comment, and still others cautioned that such material did not belong in a biography! All asked not to be cited. Louise McManus stated that Hilda Peplau had left TC because she wanted to go into private practice in order to earn more money, which she needed for Tish. Interview, Louise McManus, May 28, 1992.

14. Recounted in the letter to Maurice Greenhill, ibid.
15. This account was given by the student in a meeting with Peplau, McManus, and the TC Dean of Students, Beulah Von Wagonen, on October 29, 1952, Box 14, #484. See also notes found in #483.
16. The telephone bill was found in Box 14, #486.
17. These summations were made after a reconstruction of events from materials in Box 14, reading the record, and interviews with several of Peplau's contemporaries at TC who wish to remain anonymous.
18. See annotated minutes of the October 29, 1952, meeting in Box 14, #484.
19. Memo to staff from R. Louise McManus, November 20, 1952, Box 14, #484.
20. Undated memos between Peplau and McManus, Box 14, #484.
21. Memo from Hildegard E. Peplau to R. Louise McManus, November 24, 1952, Box 14, #484.
22. Minutes, Faculty Meeting, December 5, 1952, Teachers College Archives.
23. Memo from M. C. Del Manzo, Provost, to R. Louise McManus, Director, December 14, 1952, Box 14, #484.
24. See the September 1953 letter from Hildegard Peplau to Maurice Greenhill.
25. Interview, Earl G. Witenberg, January 19, 1993, in New York City. According to Dr. Witenberg, "Frieda and her men were always a problem."
26. See Program, American Psychiatric Association Annual Meeting, May 12–16, 1952, Panel presentation on this project entitled "Conditioning Emotions Under Hypnosis: Measurement of the Intensity of Emotional Force," a research report on a PHS grant with Frieda Fromm Reichman. Peplau presented a paper at this same convention and among the many notations on her copy of the program is one cryptic note of the dentist's panel, "very intense and controversial." Archives, Box 18, File #644.
27. Interview, Hildegard Peplau, January 22 and 25, 1992, and written correspondence from a former student, to Barbara Callaway, November 17, 1996. Also discussed in the letter to Greenhill cited above.
28. Mrs. McManus was on the advisory panel for the dentist/Fromm Reichman project and in November, 1950, invited Peplau, along with several other faculty members, to go to the dentist's office in the evening to see films made of the project. This account is found in the Greenhill letter, cited above.
29. Letter from Edna to Hildegard Peplau, August 20, 1952, Box 14, #484.
30. See the exchange of notes between Edna and Peplau in Box 14, #484.
31. Interview, Earl Witenberg, January 19, 1994.
32. Letter from one of Paplau's students to Barbara Callaway, November 17, 1996, and interview, Fran Martucci, April 10, 1992, in Santa Monica, California.
33. In her letter to Dr. Greenhill, Peplau stated that 3 staff members and 32 students attended this party at which "spaghetti and hamburgers and wine were served and one bottle of scotch."

34. Confirmed in an interview with Evelyn Zimmerman, April 28, 1993, in Spring Valley, New Jersey.
35. Letter from Tom to Hildegard Peplau, August 24, 1957, Box 14, #485.
36. This account is found in the Greenhill letter. The author sought to interview this former student, but she declined an oral interview. In written correspondence, she stated that although she recalls being dissatisfied with her therapy with the dentist, she does not recall any of the specific events related to Peplau's resignation.
37. Notation of phone call, January 5, 1953, Peplau file, William Alanson White Institute, New York City, and as recorded by Peplau in her September 9, 1953 letter to Dr. Greenhill.
38. Peplau File, William Alanson White Institute. Peplau never saw this file, so she never saw the notation regarding "Letitia."
39. Interview, Dr. Earl Witenberg, December 15, 1993.
40. In fact, according to Dr. Witenberg, this man claimed to have been asked by Mac to look after Peplau while she was at the 312th during the last month of 1944. In an interview in March, 1994, Peplau expressed serious doubt that this could be true. First of all, Mac was not at the 312th when she became aware of her pregnancy, and would not have confided in anyone who was there without informing her. Secondly, she is quite certain no one other than her hut-mates and the doctor she saw in Manchester early in January, 1945, knew of her condition. Finally, it would have been "completely out of character" for Mac to have confided such information to anyone. Peplau is certain that the dentist made this story up for his own reasons. She assumes the physicians who did finally learn of her condition early in January, treated the information confidentially. It is possible that he knew or learned of the relationship between Peplau and Mac because during 1944 the two were recognized as a couple by officers at the 312th Military Hospital. He may have simply put two and two together once his path crossed Peplau's in New York City 8 years later.
41. Peplau, for her part, although totally ignorant of the dentist's claim to have been at the 312th Military Hospital, felt that he was particularly hostile to her. In 1992, Peplau reflected, "I always had the feeling that [he] had sized me up, and set her [McManus] against me." She was right, but she did not know how right. Peplau at the time had no idea that he claimed any knowledge whatsoever of her personal life. One can only speculate as to where he'd gotten his information and what made him carry it to Mrs. McManus. It is certainly likely that he'd learned a great deal about Peplau and Tish from her students, who were his patients. Peplau was an imposing woman, and he well might have felt both intimidated and angered by her.
42. All of this information was discussed in an interview with Dr. Earl G. Witenberg on January 19, 1994.
43. From notes found in Box 14, #484.
44. Letter from Hildegard Peplau to R. Louise McManus, January 10, 1953, in Box 14, #485.
45. Interview, Hildegard Peplau, January 22, 1992.
46. Most of the following scenario has been reconstructed from memos, letters, notes, jottings, and other fragments of information found in the archives, Box 14. As noted previously, 10 women contacted for this study who were students at the time refused to comment on these events.
47. Two of these women were contacted by the author, and both claimed to have no memories of these events. They asked that their names not be used. Notes about these events written by all three to Peplau, however, are found in the archives, Box 14, #484.

48. Ibid.

49. Peplau's handwritten notes of this meeting were found in Box 14, #485.

50. Ibid.

51. Memo from R. Louise McManus to Dean Caswell, January 26, 1953, Box 14, #484. On January 30, 1953, Peplau wrote a memo to McManus, but did not send it (Box 14, #484). It is a succinct outline of her thinking on the points at issue. Peplau stated that she did not send the memo because by that time it was evident to her that it would not change anything. (Interview, February 16, 1995.) It nonetheless is a clear statement of her position:

> You have proposed a restrictive discriminatory policy in response to unchecked rumors for one person and her students. Regardless of intent, since it is based on rumors, the inference is: a) the rumors are considered true, thus a policy is necessary or b) the sources cannot be revealed for face to face confrontation because: the bearer must be protected more than the instructor and students involved *or* the methods used for securing information was so unorthodox that greater ethical problems will be revealed . . . Administrative discussions were held, plans laid, action proposed, and the instructor was summoned and told to cooperate in an established individualized policy. Under these circumstances, I had to resign. There was no investigation, no identifying of the problem . . . I cannot accede to anything discriminatory for one individual and group, most especially when based on heresay gathered by persons who cannot be identified from sources that cannot be identified . . . this has been a devastatingly personal experience, and at a university I loved.

52. Note in Peplau's handwriting dated December 19, 1952—"Phone call—Mrs. McManus," Box 14, #484.

53. Note in the file from Edith Roberts to Hildegard Peplau summarizing the meeting with the part-time instructional staff, Box 14, #484.

54. From notes made by Hilda Peplau after a visit from Edith Roberts and Margaret Adams, instructors at the time who were present at the meeting with Dean Caswell, Box 14, #484.

55. Letter from Hilda Peplau to Bertha and Byron Reppert, February 6, 1953, Box 14, #485.

56. Ibid.

57. Walter Peplau to Hilda Peplau, February 11, 1953, Box 14, #485.

58. Handwritten notes to and from students, and notes recording meetings with students and their conversations are found in Box 14, #485.

59. The period known as the McCarthy era was born out of postwar fear of a largely unseen Communist menace, but became characterized by the activities of Wisconsin Senator Joseph McCarthy, a political demagogue who preached that conspiracy and subversion were rampant throughout American institutions—including particularly the U.S. State Department, the entertainment industry, and the faculty of east coast universities. Vigilantism and smear campaigns became commonplace through the medium of televised senate hearings designed to ferret out and punish Communists and "pinko sympathizers." In 1952 and 1953 there were blatant public models of the strategies of the witch-hunt in action. Many hundreds of reputations, careers, and lives in these years were ruined by rumor and innuendo. The charges that McManus leveled against Hilda seemed to Peplau eerily imitative of the targets of McCarthy-style persecutions, that came to include not only presumed Communists, but also homosexuals, alcoholics, and the mentally ill. Again and again in her efforts to understand these events, Peplau referred to "McCarthyism" as having had an impact.

60. Peplau was so concerned about this rumor and how it might harm her students that she attempted on her own to find its source. In a letter to Maurice Greenhill on September 9, 1953, she claimed that Mrs. Gibbs, the Director of Whittier Hall, where most of the psychiatric nursing students lived, had been heard to say that "all psychiatric students are lesbians." Peplau had gotten a floor plan of Whittier Hall to determine where the students lived. She feared that if they lived together, they might provide fodder for the rumors. When she checked the room numbers, however, she found that the students did not live with each other, but were spread out between the third and eighth floors. See map and chart found in Box 14, #482.

61. In an interview on January 19, 1994, Dr. Witenberg told the author that they'd had quite a few discussions at the White Institute about what to do, and had decided that only personal intervention could counter the false charges. There is also a written transcript of a phone call from Dr. Witenberg to Hildegard Peplau on February 13, 1953, in Box 14, #485.

62. Interview, Earl G. Witenberg, January 19, 1994, and notations in Peplau's file at the White Institute.

63. Interview, Earl G. Witenberg, January 19, 1994.

64. Peplau's note of a phone call from Dean Caswell to her was found in Box 14, #484.

65. Peplau's notes of a meeting with Dean Caswell found in Box 14, #484.

66. A copy of Peplau's notes of the March 2, 1953 meeting with Dean Caswell along with a note, dated March 3, 1953, thanking Dr. Harry Bone for arranging the meeting, may be found in Box 14, #885.

67. Typed transcript of meeting with Dean Harold Caswell, March 23, 1953, Box 14, #485. Source not identified.

68. Ibid.

69. Ibid.

70. See letters from Esther Garrison, Dean Elizabeth Kemble, and Dean Lulu Hassenplug, in Box 14, #485. Hilda had some warning that the TC episode was not over and done with. Esther Garrison, a good friend and the nurse consultant at the National Institute of Mental Health (NIMH), wrote her that September that "there are three versions (at least) all over the country. You must lie low, and let it pass" (letter from Esther Garrison to Hildegard Peplau, September 19, 1953, Box 14, #485). This was not easy advice to follow. Garrison, in spite of her earlier advice, wrote again in October with more specific information. In a 12-page letter she warned Peplau to be *very* careful about what she said and wrote about TC. In reference to the dentist, she cautioned: "I'd never mention the non-physician medical person in this connection to anyone . . . It isn't safe, believe me, it isn't!" Several pages later, she urged Peplau to stay far away from former students too, particularly Edna: "You'd be a fool to get within 1000 miles of her or anyone else enrolled at TC" (letter from Esther Garrison to Hildegard Peplau, October 25, 1953, Box 14, #485).

71. Most of this material is in Box 14, #485.

72. *TC Today* (January 1995), 8.

73. Box 11 contains the dissertation and related materials.

74. Letter from Dean Harold Caswell to Hildegard Peplau, April 24, 1953, found in Box 14, #485.

75. From a typescript of a meeting held May 25, 1953, found in Box 14, #483. It is clear in this typescript that the students were fairly inarticulate, but were most concerned that the rumors as to why Miss Peplau resigned not reflect on them, and by the fact that they might "go out under a cloud." After all, by this time Peplau was one of the best known psychiatric nurse educators in the country, and her resignation must have caused a great deal of national speculation in nursing circles.

76. Ibid.

77. Letter from Hildegard Peplau to R. Louise McManus, June 30, 1953, Box 18, #653.

78. Interview, Hildegard Peplau, January 25, 1992. For a discussion of ideas developed during this time, see William E. Field, *The Psychotherapy of Hildegard Peplau* (New Brunfels, Texas: PSF Publications, 1979). There are also extensive case notes made by Peplau that summer in Box 19, #656–673.

79. Letter from Mrs. Lloyd Merrill, Registrar, William Alanson White Institute, to Hildegard E. Peplau, June 30, 1954, Box 18, #651. Peplau was only the second nurse to earn this certificate. The other, Jane Schmall, married a physician and soon moved to Boston, where she dropped out of the field.

80. Interview, Hildegard Peplau, March 21, 1994.

81. Interview, Dr. Earl G. Witenberg, December 19, 1993.

82. See letters from Hildegard E. Peplau to Dr. Ewald W. Busse at the University of Colorado, June 19, 1953; to Dean Elizabeth Kemble at the University of North Carolina, June 22, 1953; and to Dean Florence Gipe at the University of Maryland, June 21, 1953, in Box 14, #483.

83. Letter from Florence Gipe to Hildegard Peplau, July 10, 1953, Box 14, #483.

84. Letter from Maurice Greenhill, MD, to Mae Oster, College of Medicine, University of Maryland, August 3, 1953, Box 14, #483.

85. Letter from Florence Gipe to Hildegard Peplau, August 21, 1953, Box 14, #483.

86. See letter from Florence Gipe to Hildegard Peplau, August 21, 1953; Hildegard Peplau to Florence Gipe, August 24, 1953; and telegram from Florence Gipe to Hildegard Peplau, August 27, 1953; all in Box 14, #483.

87. Letter from Maurice Greenhill, MD, to Hildegard Peplau, August 25, 1953, in Box 14, #483, and interview, Catherine Norris, April 10, 1994.

88. Letter from Hildegard Peplau to Maurice Greenhill, MD, September 9, 1953, Box 14, File #483. Peplau concluded her letter by requesting, "When you have read this, please return it to me. I trust you completely, but I have named people other than myself. I would rest better if this were in my hands again."

89. Letter from Greenhill to Peplau, January 14, 1954, Box 14, #483. Five days later, though, on January 19, he wrote again to say that in a meeting with the new president, the earlier decision was confirmed. "The matter is closed, it has set nursing back a generation or two. I, for one, will not do any more work with nurses." (Box 14, #483). Peplau responded immediately, thanking him for his help, urging him not to abandon nursing, and assuring him that in her private practice she was continuing to evolve clinical insights. Of her situation she wrote that although "nursing leaders forced it upon me, it is entirely satisfying. The test of time will show that any risk any institution takes in employing me is more mythical than real, for I know the quality of my own living and now understand something of the dynamics of the nonsensical business in which I am currently caught." Her letter was signed "Hildegard E. Peplau, Private Practitioner" (Box 14, #485).

90. Interview, Lulu Hassenplug, March, 1991, in Palm Desert, California.

91. Letter from Hildegard Peplau to Lulu Hassenplug, September 18, 1953, Box 14, #486.

92. Letter from Dean Elizabeth Kemble to Hildegard Peplau, January 26, 1954, Box 14, #485.

93. Interview, Hildegard Peplau, January 22, 1992.

94. Letter from Hildegard Peplau to Elizabeth Kemble, January 29, 1954, Box 14, #485.

95. Letter from Elizabeth Kemble to Hildegard Peplau, February 5, 1954, Box 14, #485.

96. See letters in Box 14, #485.

97. Columbia University Commencement Program, May 17, 1983, Box 39, #1428.

Rutgers: "A Formidable Woman" 9

I know there is a shortage of these [nurses with doctoral degrees], having now tried for three years to capture one; you can be sure I will redouble my efforts to preach to nurses the urgency of more of them going on rather quickly [to earn higher degrees] . . . This is a dream I wish could be realized.

—Hildegard Peplau
March 14, 1963

Hilda could not believe it. They stayed huddled in the car. They would not get out. She had worked so hard on this accreditation, spent so many hundreds of hours producing the information they wanted: goals, themes, objectives, measurements, time studies. She had put so much into it, and now they were here, the accreditors from the National League for Nursing. The year was 1957, Hilda Peplau's third year at Rutgers University College of Nursing. It appeared that the accreditors were as unhappy as she was with the situation on this particular day. They had come to review the new graduate program designed to create nurse "specialists"—whatever *that* was. Peplau was now insisting that they visit the New Jersey State Psychiatric Hospital at Greystone Park where her students were working—but the accreditors were not to meet in the medical director's office as they would have expected. No. They were to go into the back wards and down into the locked cages where Dr. Peplau had her students working. Well, they were not going to do it. This was outrageous! They could see patients peering out of the barred windows, they could hear the screams and cries from the locked wards, they could smell, even from the distance of the car, the stench coming from the unwashed bodies in those basement wards. Or at least they thought they could.[1]

In the end, although the accreditors never did go into the hospital—in fact they never even got out of the car—they did award the Rutgers program in advanced psychiatric nursing the accreditation that Hilda had worked so hard to attain. Peplau had completed hundreds of pages of seemingly mindless exercises in order to give the National League for Nursing accreditors what they required.[2] She had jumped through the necessary hoops for the sake of her students. Her program was difficult, and her first class of students would graduate that year. She wanted them to graduate from an accredited program. It was an impressive accomplishment, and it had not been easy. The result justified every effort: This was the first graduate program in the country accredited to train clinical nurse specialists in psychiatric nursing (or any other nursing field)!

RUTGERS: A NEW BEGINNING

When Ella V. Stonsby approached her in 1953 about joining the faculty of Rutgers University's new program in nursing education, Hilda had been cautious. Her private-duty practice was going very well in New York City, but because she was gaining confidence in her therapeutic approaches, she all but ached to put her new therapeutic insights into an academic context. She wanted students to try them, to test them, to experiment, and revise as appropriate. Since her own experience as an undergraduate student at Bennington College, she had held an idealistic notion of the academic life, a dream that, in spite of everything, had not been entirely lost during the last year at Teachers College. She had been excited about Miss Stonsby's desire to start a graduate program and her promise to let Hilda develop a psychiatric nursing program without interference. Nonetheless, Hilda approached the offer carefully. Nursing education as an undergraduate program was new to the Newark campus and Stonsby was new in her position as director. Hilda agreed to a compromise: She would teach part-time for the 1954 spring semester, while continuing her private psychotherapy practice in Manhattan. At the end of the semester both parties could then evaluate their positions and reach agreement concerning the 1954–1955 academic year.

That semester did go surprisingly well, and in fact exceeded Hilda's hopes and expectations. In these months she commuted to Rutgers from New York to conduct her lecture class on Friday mornings at the downtown campus of the Newark College of Arts and Sciences. On Mondays and Wednesdays, she spent the day with students at the state psychiatric hospital at Greystone Park west of Newark. Miss Stonsby arranged for a taxi to meet Hilda at the train station in Newark and take her to Greystone, where she supervised the students in their clinical assignments. The days at Greystone were long, though: She arose at 5:30 a.m. in order to be in Newark by 8:30 and was seldom home before 8:00 in the evening.[3] For these three units of theoretical instruction and two units of clinical supervision, she received a salary of $875.[4]

In order to gain access for her students, Hilda had to go through some of the same routine at Greystone Park that she had perfected at Brooklyn State Hospital in her first year as an instructor at Teachers College (TC). She met with the director of the hospital, Dr. Archie Crandall, and the director of nursing, Miss Letitia Roe, to get permission for her students to talk with patients. Dr. Crandall was most reluctant to give such permission without consulting his board. In the end, Peplau herself met with the board, assuring its members that her students just needed to learn and better understand how difficult it was for doctors to work with the chronically mentally ill and that to do this, they needed to be able to "talk" with patients.[5] Once into the hospital, each student was expected to spend 3 hours a week for 12 weeks with one patient.[6]

By the end of that first semester of part-time teaching, Peplau had a vision and a plan. She longed to take her work a step further: She wanted to prepare nurse clinical specialists at the graduate level who could offer *direct care* to psychiatric patients, thus helping to close the gap between psychiatric theory and nursing practice. Peplau began to share some of her ideas about graduate education and the preparation of clinical specialists with Stonsby. Stonsby was interested in Hilda's ideas and continued to urge her to come to Rutgers full time. Hilda was grateful. Shortly after beginning that first semester's work, Hilda expressed her appreciation in these words: "I particularly appreciate your equanimity in the face of my recent harassing experience [at TC] and feel that this more fortunate one with you will be most valuable for me."[7] In April 1954 she again wrote Stonsby, assuring her that "the experience at Greystone is going better than can be expected" and informing her that she would be in Washington, D.C., the first week in April for the meetings of the National Institute of Mental Heath (NIMH) training committee on psychiatric nursing. She urged Stonsby at that time to apply for an NIMH grant to support "a program of interest to your school of nursing and needed in New Jersey."[8] Soon afterward, with Stonsby's agreement and blessing, Peplau applied to the NIMH for a nurse-training grant to establish a full-time graduate program at Rutgers the following September.[9] That first grant proposal was funded—the wheels were now in motion. Peplau's salary, and much of her program at Rutgers, would be supported by government grants for the next 20 years.[10]

Although only a part-time undergraduate instructor that first spring semester, Hilda was determined her students would receive a "full-time" education. In May, Peplau sent a final comprehensive examination to the undergraduate nursing secretary at Rutgers to be typed and administered to the students. In it, she explained to the secretary,

> The enclosed test is most difficult and I will discuss this aspect of it with the students . . . The students should be instructed to answer what

they can, moving on from question to question to those which come easiest to them and then returning to those questions which were left unanswered. I am not at all sure that any of the students can complete the entire test in the 3-hour period, but the time should not be extended.[11]

Indeed the students could not complete the test. They were, after all, undergraduate students and nothing in their experience prepared them for Hilda Peplau. The exam consisted of 15 exceedingly dense paragraphs, full of complicated concepts and ideas used in both clinical and educational settings. It was preceded by instructions to the students, requesting that for each of the described situations they

> State the purpose of these interrelated educative situations, noting the time arrangements, including sequence and placement, subjective participants, the general form of participation of a teacher and of students including orientation to the situation initially, clusters of methods and ideas which form the subject matter, contents of the events, the educational activities through which the student comes to understand the methods and ideas and to use them—including forms used by the student, aids used by the teacher, etc. Indicate where possible the overlapping relationships between them.[12]

The students were so traumatized by this exam that many of them wondered then and there whether university work was possible for them after all.[13] Hilda, for her part, was apparently so starved for academic exercise, or so excited by it, that she was inclined to demand in one examination everything she had imparted. In spite of this rather sobering experiment, however, things were going well, and Hilda looked forward to the fall with great anticipation. She so informed Miss Stonsby.

An indication of things to come, however, is found in a letter Peplau sent to Ella Stonsby on August 29, 1954, just before the start of the fall semester. In it she informed Stonsby that "in the course of waiting for clearance on this appointment, I have been asked to participate in a number of nursing affairs and have made some commitments which I would like to clear with you . . . They are as follows."[14] She listed three dates in September and three dates in October when participation in seminars, conferences, or state or national committee meetings would take her away from her responsibilities at Rutgers. Stonsby sanctioned all this activity, but later would come to question and then to oppose Peplau's heavy travel and conference schedule. In the beginning, however, Hilda Peplau's broad-based involvement on the national level was seen as a great asset for nursing education at Rutgers.

In addition to her enjoyment of the work, Hilda knew that the time had come to get Tish out of New York. When she ended her affiliation with Teachers College in June 1953, she was required to take her daughter out of TC's experimental Agnes Russell School. Tish was then enrolled for the 1953–1954 school year in the third grade at P.S. 165, a dreary urban school at 109th and Amsterdam. Tish began the year with a wonderful teacher and made a new friend, Marian. She had come home excited about school. Shortly after the opening day, however, the principal sent around a memo announcing that there would be funding for a new class for "special students" and asking teachers to identify candidates for that classroom. Tish's teacher, in her first year of teaching, did not understand that "special" was a code for troubled or learning disabled children. Tish and Marian were nominated for the class. After listening to Tish's accounts of activities in the new classroom, Hilda realized that something was drastically wrong. She made an appointment to see the principal, who was immediately unsympathetic. According to Hilda, the principal's response was, "It's high time she learned how the other half lives." "At age 8?" an incredulous Hilda replied, to which he responded, "It can't be too soon." "Well, then it's 'high time' we get out of New York," Hilda thought to herself.[15] It is possible that the principal had decided that no highfalutin self-impressed woman with a doctorate from Columbia University's Teachers College was going to tell *him* how to run *his* school. He refused to move Tish, and Tish did, indeed, spend her third-grade year in a special education class. At about the same time Hilda had a run-in with the school nurse who, during a cursory physical examination of new students, discovered that Tish Peplau was not wearing an undershirt under her blouse. Horrified, the nurse sent a note home to Hilda informing her that Tish had to wear an undershirt. A confrontation ensued. When Hilda asked *why* Tish had to have an undershirt, the nurse could only stammer, "Because children must wear undershirts, that's why."[16] In this, Hilda fared better than she had with the principal. Tish continued to dress as she pleased.

With Tish's schooling in mind, because the spring semester had gone so well, and with the NIMH grant pending, Hilda agreed that Miss Stonsby should proceed to put through a full-time appointment as assistant professor of nursing for the 1954–1955 academic year. Incredibly, R. Louise McManus, Hilda's nemesis from TC, remained on her list of references. Hilda Peplau's continued national prominence and the passage of time, however, seemed to have tempered McManus. To Rutgers she simply wrote that Peplau had excellent command of her subject matter, and was

Usually most cooperative with the administration and her professional associates. During her last semester a situation arose in which she felt herself unable to comply with an administrative and instructional policy and made the decision to resign. I would expect that if all the conditions of employment were made known to her in advance and she accepted an appointment she would live up to them faithfully.[17]

The 1-year appointment was approved. Her salary at Rutgers would be $4,980 for the academic year to begin on July 1, 1954.[18]

Things indeed did go well in Hilda's first semester at Rutgers. Like R. Louise McManus, the director of the TC nursing education program, Ella V. Stonsby was relatively new at her job. Stonsby wanted people around her who would advance nursing education. She herself had a plan, a vision, and, at least initially, she did not feel threatened by her faculty. She welcomed new ideas, and she was determined to make a difference. Under Stonsby's leadership, Rutgers had been offering university level courses to nurses through the University Extension Division from 1946 through 1952. In 1952 Stonsby was promoted to the rank of a tenured associate professor, moved to the faculty of the Newark College of Arts and Sciences, and named director of a new program in nursing education.[19] From then on things moved ahead quickly, and on July 1, 1956, Ella Stonsby was named the first dean of the new Rutgers University College of Nursing.[20] Hilda Peplau was the first faculty member she hired for the new program when it was moved from the University Extension Division into the Faculty of Arts and Sciences. This was an expression of confidence for which Hilda would always be grateful. Hilda understood that Stonsby was really "putting her head on the chopping block by employing me."[21]

Soon after her promotion to dean, Stonsby put forward an 8-year master plan outlining her vision of nursing education as a continuum beginning with the elevation of hospital diploma programs into college-level 2-year associate degree preprofessional programs. After completing an associate degree, in Stonsby's vision, a nurse could continue on to a 2-year baccalaureate program, then to a 2-year master's program, followed by an additional 2 years leading to a doctorate in nursing education or nursing science.[22] This proposal would have unified nursing education, while providing for different stopping points for the individual nurse. In this, Stonsby, like Peplau, was far ahead of her field. The 8-year model she envisioned would be discussed by the faculty at Rutgers for a number of years, but never adopted. Typical of nursing, the faculty soon bogged down in an endless debate about definitions, content, goals, objectives, and so forth for each level and never agreed on the final design.

For her part, in her first 2 years at Rutgers, Peplau developed a 19-month master's program that prepared *only* clinical specialists in psychiatric nursing. This was in deliberate contrast to the Teachers College program, which prepared nurses for advanced practice, teaching, and supervision, all in a 10-month program. Peplau's program was particularly rigorous because she felt that her students would have much to overcome in order to win respect in nursing. Prior to the passage of the National Mental Health Act in 1946 there was no such field as psychiatric nursing. It was a field in the process of inventing itself, and it wasn't getting any encouragement from the two major nursing organizations, the NLN (National League for Nursing) and the ANA (American Nurses Association). Hilda would later note, "We were highly stigmatized. Any nurse who worked in it was considered almost certifiable . . . We were thoroughly unpopular, we were considered queer enough to be avoided."[23]

The 1946 Mental Health Act provided funds for training programs, but even with generous funding there were fewer than a dozen graduate programs in psychiatric nursing in the entire country in the early 1950s, and none of them were producing nurses who could work directly with patients on a one-to-one basis. Each of these psychiatric nursing programs had a nurse director, but only two of the early directors held a doctorate.[24] Doctorates or not, these directors had the formidable task of developing graduate programs that met university standards when most of them did not have the credentials expected of faculty members in other disciplines. Moreover, the pool of baccalaureate graduates in nursing eligible for and interested in graduate study of any sort was almost nonexistent. Peplau had set out not just to develop a master's level program, but to train "clinical specialists." At that time, it was almost inconceivable that any nurse, under any circumstances, could become a "specialist."

FINDING A HOME

Early in the 1955 spring semester, more security was added to Hilda's life when the dean of the Newark College of Arts and Sciences informed her that her initial 1-year appointment as assistant professor of nursing had been extended to June 30, 1957, at which time she would be considered for promotion to associate professor with tenure.[25] While she was appreciative of the 2-year appointment as assistant professor, Hilda could not help but feel some degree of pique over the delayed promotion to associate professor. By this time she had published a major book and many articles in professional journals, she offered 5 years teaching experience, and she served on more than her share of national and international nursing committees. In most disciplines at Rutgers at this time, this would be sufficient for an immediate promotion if not initial appointment as a full professor. Because this was to be her second chance in academe, Peplau did not object. Instead, she made up her mind to be "nice, good, and obedient" and to continue to work as hard as possible in order to receive tenure as early as possible.[26] That academic milestone was passed in the spring of 1957, shortly after the visit of the accreditors. With little fanfare, and skipping entirely over the associate status after all, Dr. Peplau was promoted to the rank of full professor with tenure, effective July 1, 1957.[27]

By the time Hilda accepted the full-time appointment for 1954–1955 school year, she had begun to pay attention to the towns through which her taxi took her on the way to the Greystone psychiatric hospital. She often passed through Madison, a very attractive town in the northern part of New Jersey. Upon investigation, she learned that the Madison public schools were among the best in the state. She began to imagine that someday she might bring Tish to this nice town where she could have a safe and more secure childhood. Shortly after the renewal of her contract in the spring of 1955, Hilda spotted a house for sale on the outskirts of Madison. Because the house looked to be in need of repairs and because it was located some distance from the fashionable and affluent downtown residential district, she decided to inquire. Two months later, knowing that her position was secure and that tenure could well follow, she bought the house at 118 Shunpike Road, signing the mortgage in June 1955.[28] This would be her home for the next 30 years.

With its church steeples set against rolling hills, beautiful homes with manicured lawns, and the campuses of Fairleigh Dickinson and Drew universities, Madison offered the white picket fence charm of everyone's fantasy of the perfect American town. Madison calls itself the Rose City. Italian and Irish immigrants, who had come to the area to work on the large estates of commuting New York millionaires, started growing greenhouse roses in 1856. At the local industry's peak, Madison had the largest commercial rose-growing operation in the country, sending 50,000 roses a day to New York City.[29] Madison's excellent school system meant that Tish could attend public school without worry. The two university campuses offered regular lecture and concert series, and the New Jersey Shakespeare Festival was held there every summer. An outdoor swimming pool in the summer and community ice pond in the winter provided community gathering space for the town's teenagers. Importantly for Hilda and Tish, it had a wonderful public library as well. One of the first things they did after moving to Madison was to get library cards. The main library was an old stone building with spiral metal stairs leading to the second floor galleries where Hilda loved to read and Tish loved to climb. She soon became a familiar figure, often going to the library after school to read and to wait for Hilda to pick her up on her way home from Rutgers. There was, and is, a closeness to the community that Hilda found very reassuring.

When Hilda bought the house Tish had just completed her second year at P.S. 165 in Manhattan. The fourth grade had gone better for her than her third-grade year, spent as it had been in "special ed." She enjoyed her fourth-grade class, she liked her teacher, and she was involved in activities. True to form, Tish again was back in the news. At Halloween, 1954, the P.S. 165 fourth graders collected money for UNICEF. In February, the class went to the United Nations headquarters to deliver their $53.52 donation. A newspaper photo featured Tish Peplau presenting the check to a UNICEF representative. Hilda and Tish would leave New York City with mixed emotions.

Hilda knew almost immediately, however, that she had made a good choice in buying the house in Madison, which would be Tish's home until she graduated from high school and entered college in 1963—and Hilda's alone for some 20 more years. The schools were, as Hilda had learned, indeed excellent, and the neighbors were wonderful. Hilda and Tish moved into their new house in September, 1955. In November, a huge snowstorm deposited snow almost up to the windows, and Hilda had no shovel. Just as she was considering calling the equivalent of 911, a brigade of neighborhood men showed up to shovel the new neighbors out. Several of these neighbors would become lifelong friends. Mrs. Wendeborn brought over a cake on their first weekend in the house, and her husband mowed the lawn until the Peplaus could afford a lawn-mower. John and Gwen Eager, across the street, watched out for them, shoveled the snow when needed, and brought gifts of fresh strawberries in the early summer. The house itself had great features. It had beautiful hardwood floors, a magnificent fieldstone fireplace, a sensible floor plan, an attic, and a basement. It was situated on a large lot with room for veg-etable and flower gardens and surrounded by mature trees. At the same time it had an aged furnace that provided only intermittent heat and hot water, old plumbing, little or no insulation, a leaky roof, and was badly in need of paint inside and out. Part of the charm of living in the country was the presence of field mice who occasionally made their way into the house. Although Hilda understood the potential of the house and had no qualms about the work that needed to be done, her colleagues at the College of Nursing were more doubtful, and sometimes their disdain showed. In those days colleagues who visited were horrified to see the mice scurrying across the floor. Once, shortly after they had moved to Madison, a colleague from Rutgers in Newark came to stay with Tish for a week while Hilda was away at a conference. The house was not yet ren-ovated and the kitchen still had a laundry tub for a sink. When Hilda returned from the conference, she realized immediately something was definitely wrong. The house smelled—very badly. She discovered a week's worth of dirty dishes piled in the laundry tub. Hilda was not an obsessive housekeeper, but she was very finicky about cleanliness in the kitchen. She attacked the dishes with vigor, discovering, much to her hor-ror, a drowned mouse at the bottom of the tub, hence the smell. After much scouring, more scouring, and rinsing and re-rinsing with boiling water, the tub and the dishes were deemed useable once again. Hilda began to use the money she earned on her ever-widening lecture circuit to fix the house. First, get rid of the critters, then fix the roof, then insu-late, then redo the bathroom, put in a new tub, hot water heater, and updated fixtures. Gradually the house was renovated. In 1958 a study in which she could see private patients was added, and in 1959 an enclosed patio. Eventually, although money would always be tight, the house became quite a comfortable home.

Madison offered the kind of secure, suburban lifestyle that Hilda wanted to provide for Tish. In the first months after the move Tish missed Mary Alameda, her friend from the apartment building in Manhattan, but she soon found another best friend in a classmate, Jeanne Dinsmore. Tish often stayed with the Dinsmore family while Hilda was traveling to workshops and conferences, as she had stayed with the Alameda family in New York. Tish soon became active in the Girl Scouts and later in Tri Hi Y.

Earlier, while still at the Agnes Russell School, Tish had stopped calling her mother "Mummy." At the Midtown Children's Center and at experimental Agnes Russell School it was customary for the children to call their teachers by their first names. This was atypical for the time, when children were expected to address adults with the respectful honorific "Miss," "Mrs.," or "Mr." Tish, however, chose from that time to address adults who were closest to her, including her mother, by their first names. When Hilda and Tish made the move to a new home and a new school in 1955, Tish chose to drop her childhood name and adopt her middle name, "Anne." Thereafter, this was the name she was known by at school and by friends and professional colleagues ever since, although "Tisha" was the affectionate name Hilda continued to use.

A PERIOD OF UNEASY STABILIZATION

Although Peplau's career at Rutgers began on a high note in the 1950s, her 20-year sojourn there would have its ups and downs, and would end problematically in 1974. Clearly the TC experience would always be a factor in how she experienced and responded to the inevitable vicissitudes of academe. Academic life in nursing is perhaps more contentious and more emotional than in many other fields because nursing has had so much trouble defining itself as a profession, and because its place in the university was, and is, less established than that of older disciplines. These factors illuminate the problem of nursing leadership in general and of nursing deans in particular. While Stonsby was a visionary, she lacked a doctorate, making her insecure and somewhat a misfit in the university hierarchy. Peplau soon would be once again in the forefront of new trends, doing original and highly controversial work in the classroom, and serving in a myriad of national capacities. As time went on, she had less and less patience for nursing "nonsense" at Rutgers, which made her an increasingly unaccommodating faculty member. Though for the first few years at least, from 1954 to 1960, Peplau received support and encouragement from Ella Stonsby and from the university administration.

In the first years of her deanship, Stonsby asked a small group to meet with her once a week at 7:30 in the morning to brainstorm, to think through issues in nursing education, and to help plan for discussions at faculty meetings. Initially, Hilda Peplau was in this group.[30] Peplau was full of ideas, and she was gratified to be working with someone who seemed to appreciate her energy and dedication and who encouraged her in developing a graduate program based on a research foundation and clinical expertise. Soon, however, a problem surfaced. Because Peplau had good ideas and constructive suggestions, and perhaps because Ella Stonsby lived alone in a hotel and was most likely lonely, she began to call Hilda at home at night just to "talk things over." The conversations seemed to get longer and longer, but evenings were Tish's time. Tish was now 10 years old, and Hilda had promised her that when they moved to New Jersey, she would be home most evenings, and those evenings would belong to Tish. There were to be no more evening jobs, no more 12–14-hour days—at least for a while. Tish grew less and less tolerant of those hours of long telephone conversations. She began to pester, to pull on the telephone line, to remind Hilda of her promise.[31] And, she was right. In the spring of 1956, toward the end of her second year as a full-time faculty member, Hilda asked Ella Stonsby to please not call her at home, explaining that this time belonged to Tish. Stonsby continued to call, so Hilda started cutting her off rather abruptly, explaining she could not talk now.

Stonsby did not take the rejection with equanimity. The previous year, the College of Nursing had moved from its home in an old brewery on Rector Street in Newark to a brownstone at 18 James Street. Stonsby had assigned Hilda a front office with a bay window and bought her new furniture for it, from Hilda's NIMH grant. At the beginning of the 1956–1957 academic year, following Hilda's possibly less-than-tactful termination of the long evening phone calls, Stonsby moved Hilda from her lovely office up into the attic, where the new furniture would not fit. Peplau now had a scarred desk, a creaky chair, and battered file cabinets instead of the beautiful furniture paid for by her grant. It was hot in the attic and there was no air-conditioning. Things were becoming uncomfortable.

Peplau's single-minded determination to develop the country's best graduate program, while also reforming psychiatric nursing across the country, became another source of tension after 1957. Hilda, characteristically, worked like a woman possessed. She allowed herself no free time. When she wasn't at Rutgers, she was off to national committee meetings, or to conferences, or to visit state mental hospitals. When she *was* at Rutgers, she fleshed out the sequence and content of each course for a major master's degree program, put together voluminous course materials, wrote papers and gave presentations on what she was doing, worked with the clinical agencies where her students would do their clinical training, hired assistants, and began developing the library collection.

The graduate-level Psychiatric Nursing Program was very faculty intensive, and thus the envy of other programs in the College of Nursing. A

2-year renewal of her grant in 1957 allowed Peplau to hire three additional faculty members on NIMH money. There was constant pressure for the psychiatric nursing faculty to help out in the growing undergraduate program, but Peplau was adamant that since these faculty members were supported entirely on her grants, they would do only the work specified in the grants. To some extent, this kept the faculty in psychiatric nursing insulated from the politics of the college. The same, however, could not be said for the graduate program's director. It was perhaps inevitable that Peplau would increasingly be at odds with the rest of the faculty. It was an undistinguished faculty, at best, and Hilda's increasing national visibility rankled in the most fundamental ways. Hilda tried to ignore the growing tension and stay focused on her own agenda. She did, however, write a grant proposal to fund the development of courses to integrate psychosocial concepts into the undergraduate curriculum. Having served on the national committee that developed these concepts to begin with, she had a clear idea of what was needed, and subsequently secured the grant for Rutgers. As a general rule, though, she defended her own program while trying to remain uninvolved in the undergraduate program which was fraught with unresolved tension. Such aloofness did not sit well with her faculty colleagues.

In spite of tensions at the College of Nursing, Hilda Peplau's work outside of Rutgers progressed very well. In order to improve patient care in New Jersey's mental hospitals, Peplau began to conduct in-house clinical workshops for the nursing staff at these hospitals. The state agencies in the mental health field were grateful for this service, and each new workshop began with an opening ceremony attended by the hospital administration and appropriate state officials. Ella Stonsby appreciated these events and made an effort to attend each opening session—and it was indeed an effort on her part because Stonsby did not drive and had to take a train or a taxi to each ceremony.

On one occasion, Hilda asked Stonsby if she'd like to ride home to Madison with her and stay for dinner. Hilda would then drive her back into Newark to her hotel. Stonsby accepted. When they arrived at the house, however, Hilda discovered that Tish had invited her own friend to dinner. In those days, Hilda still lived hand to mouth and was barely making ends meet on her Rutgers salary. That night she had only three pieces of frozen fish and three potatoes in the house, a house that was generally quite cool because Hilda kept the heat low to save money. Stonsby must have sensed Hilda's tension and must have been cold to boot, because she sat in the living room without taking off her coat or hat. After eating the inadequate meal, she insisted on taking everyone out for dessert. Tish thought this unexpected treat was wonderful, and let Miss Stonsby know how appreciative she was. For her part, Stonsby's attitude toward Hilda softened somewhat after this modest show of hospitality, at least for a while. She recommended a small raise and let up on her demands to help in the undergraduate program.

Although by 1958 Hilda felt more secure, having won the protection of academic tenure, the context of the times was such that she simply could not relax. The TC experience had left her unnerved, and she felt unremitting pressure to accomplish everything she could before something happened to derail her. Relative postwar prosperity, sprawling suburbs, TV sitcoms, and Elvis Presley's famous swinging hips form an idyllic portrait of the times. This was not lost on the Peplaus. Hilda and Tish at last had a home of their own in a lovely, small town; they watched television news and documentaries; and they even had a cat named Elvis. For Hilda, though, the 1950s remained an uneasy time. The spirit of McCarthyism was still abroad in the land. The victim of rumor and innuendo herself, Peplau did not forget the icy feel of a stab in the back, the loneliness of the victimized, and the ensuing disillusionment with one's fellows. By the end of the 1950s, the national mood was changing. A young John F. Kennedy was elected President in 1960. Hilda loved the new sense of optimism that he evoked, his call to citizens to "give" to their country, the landing on the moon, the Peace Corps and all the "new frontiers." The 1960s was a decade punctuated by idealism, social change, technological breakthroughs. Mid-decade a counterculture emerged, challenging the "establishment" and overturning conventional hierarchies of authority. Unlike the rest of the university world, though, nursing education, which continued to cling to its "traditional values," would be hardly affected.

THE GRADUATE PROGRAM IN PSYCHIATRIC NURSING

Although small, the Rutgers College of Nursing graduate-level Psychiatric Nursing Program was quite distinctive. Focused exclusively on the preparation of clinical specialists, the Rutgers program was unlike any other then or now. All undergraduate, and most graduate programs, in nursing prepared generalists rather than specialists. Graduate programs might focus on nursing education, or nursing administration, or in later years perhaps on nursing research. With the exception of Peplau's at Rutgers and one or two others, however, they did not focus on the clinical content of nursing such as psychiatric nursing, maternal/child nursing, or medical/surgical nursing. At the undergraduate level students had clinical rotations and as college graduates were expected to be able to function in any clinical situation.

Peplau had become passionate in her belief that clinical specialization would enrich nursing practice and education. She increasingly believed that the future of nursing education at the graduate level would lie in the development of clinical specialties that would have the potential to define and distinguish what nurses did from what physicians did. Peplau's program required 19 months of clinical and academic study for students, and required faculty members to continue their own clinical practice, to do clinical research, and to publish the results.[31] At Rutgers, she was preparing nurses at the graduate level to explore clinical interventions on a one-to-one basis with patients before, during, and after the onset of mental illness. In this pursuit, she was opposed by the majority of nurses who continued to follow the axiom that "a nurse is a nurse is a nurse," opposing any differentiation between who was doing what among them. Except for a few of her students and other nurses in academic settings, Peplau's challenge was not taken up by her colleagues.

While the College of Nursing at Rutgers in many ways seemed to stall soon after its establishment, the graduate Program in Psychiatric Nursing was making great strides. Peplau's NIMH training grants made it possible for her to move forward rapidly and gave students an entre into other schools and colleges within the university. Peplau realized that if her students were to receive a true graduate level education, they must have access to courses beyond those available in what remained basically an undergraduate program in the College of Nursing. Stonsby's vision notwithstanding, psychiatric nursing was the only graduate program to be developed in the College of Nursing during these years. To flesh out her students' program, Peplau sought and received university sanction for students to take the research design and statistics graduate courses in psychology and sociology taught in the Graduate School on the university's research campus in New Brunswick. In their first venture into the Graduate School, eight of Peplau's students took a research design course in psychology on the New Brunswick campus. All eight failed it. Peplau was alarmed and thought the situation so serious that she went to see the professor herself. She requested that he go over the students' exams with her in order that she might better understand where the problems were. The professor informed her that he hadn't bothered to read the exams—he knew from class discussion, he said, that none of the nursing students were prepared to pass his course. The unfairness of this drove an irate Peplau to see the dean of the Graduate School, Dr. Marion Johnson. Johnson was sympathetic, but the only remedy for the students was to retake the course—which they did. The second time around, with a different instructor, all the students easily passed.

This altercation served to introduce Peplau to Dean Johnson, who soon agreed with her that the graduate Program in Psychiatric Nursing would be better served by being under the academic jurisdiction of the Graduate School in New Brunswick, the university's research campus, rather than remain solely a freestanding program in the College of Nursing on the university's Newark campus, 20 miles away from the university's main libraries and other research facilities. He helped guide her through the procedures as she prepared the various documents needed to effect this change. To Peplau's surprise, Stonsby agreed with Dean Johnson, and endorsed the effort. She even accompanied Peplau to New Brunswick the day the matter was on the agenda of the Graduate School faculty meeting. As Hilda later put it, "All our grey cells were ticking."[33] All the questions were answered, and the Graduate Program in Psychiatric Nursing, in spite of some initial skepticism, was approved unanimously by the faculty. Dean Johnson immediately appointed Peplau to the executive council of the graduate school, and thus she began to learn firsthand what graduate education was like in the rest of the university.[34]

As appreciation of her talents grew, together with her stature in the university, Hilda withdrew somewhat from the strain of life in the College of Nursing. Relocating the focus of her graduate program in New Brunswick got her out of many of the endless debates over curriculum in the College of Nursing, but not all of them. When it seemed important to the future of the college, or to the future of nursing education in general, she was there. For some time there was a debate about whether to develop a doctorate, and if so, what kind of doctorate. Peplau felt strongly that only a PhD would give nurses the skills they needed to do research, particularly that of a clinical nature. She was convinced that only a doctorate based on in-depth clinical research would produce the kind of credibility needed to give nursing recognition as a serious discipline within the university. In time this debate became a national one, but it was not resolved at Rutgers until the 1990s, when the faculty finally developed a PhD in nursing.[35]

In part because the nursing faculty never made the commitment to develop doctoral level work during Peplau's time at Rutgers, the master's degree in psychiatric nursing grew to become a 64-credit, 2-year master's program—that number of credits alone being sufficient for most PhD programs. Students were so staggered by their course load upon entering the program that it did not occur to them to question the sense or logic of a 64-credit program leading only to the master's degree, not a doctorate.[36] The renewal of Peplau's NIMH grant in 1957 not only supported the hiring of three faculty members for the program, it also provided stipend support for students in the program to remain at Rutgers as assistant instructors for 2 years after completing their degrees. Thus, the 2 years of coursework and clinical work could be followed by 1 year of clinical research and a thesis project, and that could be followed by 2 years of "instructoring." In this way, a 2-year master's program became a 5-year educational experience.

In 1958–1959, Peplau applied to the NIMH for special funds to create faculty positions in other disciplines important to the nursing program, specifically in psychology and sociology. While these departments welcomed the new faculty resources, they did not welcome participation of

the nursing faculty in the selection process. In fact, the faculty members
of the two departments decided they would turn down the positions
unless they were given total control of the hiring process. As a result of
her membership on the Graduate School Executive Council, Peplau had
gained a better understanding of faculty prerogatives, and none, she knew,
was more sacred than that of hiring departmental colleagues. Thus, she
prevailed upon Ella Stonsby and her nurse colleagues to back off the hiring process, as she herself did. The end result was that the two departments hired faculty on nursing money who had an obligation to offer
research courses for nursing students but who had no knowledge of, little sympathy for, and almost no interest in nursing as a discipline.[37]

This experience led Peplau to work with Esther Garrison and Seymour
Vestermark at the NIMH to include "nurse/scientist grants" in the NIMH
training program to enable nursing graduate students to earn PhDs in
fields cognate to nursing such as anthropology, chemistry, or biological
sciences. Nursing literally bought two to three fellowships for nursing
graduate students in selected PhD programs. The result would be a cadre
of nurse faculty members holding PhDs in fields other than nursing
available to fill faculty positions in colleges of nursing. Peplau immediately began to urge graduates of her own program to pursue these
stipends, and about half of them did.[38] Thus, within 5 years of its incep-
tion, the Rutgers graduate program in psychiatric nursing had become
nationally visible and highly regarded. By this time, too, Peplau was on
the lecture circuit, and her workshop schedule was becoming increasingly national in scope. Competition for admission to her program increased
enormously, but over the objections of both Dean Stonsby and leaders in
nursing in New Jersey, she kept it small. At its largest, in 1973, there were
only 28 students in the program. It was highly selective, highly competitive, and nationally recognized as the best such program in the country.[39]
Because of this, and because of the relatively large amount of federal
money that supported it, the program had its critics, several of whom
served on the New Jersey State Board for Nursing or on committees of the
National League for Nursing.[40] Mostly, the Rutgers program was faulted
for remaining too small, being too intense, and producing nurses who
were proud of their difference in a profession that valued sameness.[41]

A DIFFERENT KIND OF STUDENT

For the students accepted into the program, the experience was profound. Peplau truly wanted them to be scholars and researchers and to
contribute to the profession. Thus she drove them to be all that they
could be, to develop all their capabilities. She was a wonderful mentor,
but she kept her distance. Many students professed to feel "scared to

death" in her presence.[42] Others felt Peplau was almost seductive in her intensity, her focus, and her belief that they could do it.[43] Students felt it was a privilege to know and work with Peplau, but that they did not know her on a personal level. They sensed there were boundaries that could not be crossed, that Peplau would draw the line and step away.[44] She was a "personage," but the comment that "I never think of her as warm," was a common one among students who did not become friends with her in later life.[45] Her students understood she had immense faith in them and they felt fortunate to be in such an intense life-changing environment, but many of them also felt she was a remote, "godlike" figure. As intense as it was, and as small as the student cohorts were, Peplau maintained the boundaries. Her personal life did not spill over into her professional life, at least not with students. This was quite in contrast to the experience at TC where students and faculty members were very much a part of her life with Tish, and Tish a part of her life at school. This was not so at Rutgers. Each year she did invite all her students to a party in her home, but the discussion at these events was almost always professional, not personal.[46] Several former students did in fact become good friends in later years, but during the years of graduate study, Peplau gave evidence of having learned her lessons at TC well. Thus, she was truly very lonely for most of her career. It was not until after her retirement, when she was able to establish a "community of practice," sharing ideas and intellectual insights with many of her former students and a few professional friends, that she felt she had true friendships.[47]

Because the classes were small, each student admitted to the program received intensive personal attention. No student dropped out unless the decision to do so was mutual and then not until suggestions about what to do next were discussed. Nonetheless, fully half of those who entered did drop out before graduation. They either found the work too overwhelming, or they discovered they were not as committed to psychiatric nursing as they thought, or they did not have the personal psychological strength to endure the course of study. There is no doubt this was an anxiety producing program. Not surprisingly, those who stayed and completed the program formed exceedingly strong bonds with their professor and mentor, as well as with one another. If they succeeded in this program, they did not doubt that they were among the best.[48] Peplau's students were easily recognized—they spoke out, they were assertive, and they never doubted they had something to contribute. They had confidence in themselves and their work. Peplau herself was always proud that no one who completed the program experienced failure later in his or her career.[49]

After their initial coursework in New Brunswick which focused on Sullivanian interpersonal relations theory, Peplau's students began intense clinical work with patients. Peplau believed that psychiatric patients made progress through intense person-to-person work with a nurse. Peplau would give students the basic structure of an interview, and then immediately assign them a patient. They would meet with the same patient 1 hour a day, 3 days a week during the academic year. Students' clinical experiences were centered in two New Jersey mental hospitals, Greystone Park and Overbrook State Psychiatric Hospital. Three days a week students would be at one of the two hospitals at 8:00 in the morning to meet for an hour with their assigned patients, all of whom were chronically psychotic—in many instances, schizophrenic. Students carried tape recorders to capture these conversations verbatim. At 9:00 they met in the supervision room with Peplau, or, as time went on, with one of the other instructors. From 9:00 a.m. until 4:00 p.m. they would engage in nonstop analysis of their data. Each student would present her material, the tapes would be played, and every interaction would be analyzed. The purpose was to recognize and make nursing diagnoses of patient illnesses and to recognize and record therapeutic progress. In this review of the data, the individual attention and attention to detail were incredible. Peplau's focus never wandered. There was no small talk. She commented throughout each presentation, hammering and hammering on the concepts being dealt with through the data. She talked about the conceptual content, she took the students' notes and wrote on them throughout the discussion, and at the end of the day she returned to each student a notebook covered with her red-penned notes and comments on every page. The goal was to make students acutely aware of how their interactions with patients contributed to progress and understanding. One student once decided to count the number of negative comments on her 1-hour's work as recorded in her notebook: The number was 93.[50] Many students kept those notebooks for the rest of their lives.[51]

Hilda was always supportive, but was an incredible taskmaster. "You could always see that she was working twice as hard as you were, and you felt you were working so hard you could drop."[52] Her expectation was that graduate school would be the most intense and exhilarating time of the students' lives, and they'd better not miss a minute of it. She wanted to recreate her own Bennington experience for her students. Students often felt they didn't have time even to eat, so intense was the work.[53] The program required 18 months of coursework, or 2 academic years.

The academic year ended in May, but no student in the graduate Psychiatric Nursing Program assumed this meant their time was their own. Peplau had become convinced that in addition to one-on-one work with a single patient, students needed exposure to families in order to develop an understanding of how families contributed to or coped with mental illness. Beginning in 1956, students spent the month of June working with indigent families in Red Bank, New Jersey. An 18-month program quickly became a 19-month program. The Red Bank experience was a requirement, and it never occurred to the Peplau students to object to this rather arbitrary extension of their academic year. Working with the Monmouth Country Office of Social Services each summer to identify families where mental illness or psychiatric stress was a factor in their problems, Peplau selected a family with whom each student would work. Each student spent 2 hours every weekday morning for 4 weeks with the family or a subset of it, and the afternoon analyzing, in minute detail, the data collected. The students worked with families with drug and alcohol problems, families with schizophrenic children, families with psychotic mothers, and families experiencing incest or sexual abuse. In these encounters, they were feeling their way, discovering what worked and what did not, trying to understand why. At the end of the month, a summary of their work would be given to the social worker assigned to the family in the hope that appropriate interventions would be arranged. It was exceedingly interesting, challenging, and absorbing work.[54] The culture that Peplau created was so intense and the work so engrossing that those who survived the rigors of the program never questioned its demands.

From the very beginning of their graduate work, it was taken for granted that Peplau's students would go to professional meetings, present papers, and ask questions. Students were never asked whether they wished to attend such extracurricular meetings. Rather, they were told when and where the meetings were. At a time when few nurses engaged in research, and fewer still ever published their findings, Peplau made sure that each graduate, before completing the program, had published at least one paper based on clinical research in a professional journal. In the first 5 years of the program, 13 had published two or more papers in the journal of record for nurses, *The American Journal of Nursing,* as well as in other professional journals such as *Nursing Research* or *Mental Hygiene.* Four of the first 19 graduates published a book before graduating, 2 had books in preparation, and a seventh was author of a copyrighted manual for nursing practice.[55] This would be a formidable record in any discipline.

DISINTEGRATION OF A DEANSHIP

At Rutgers, Peplau's success and incredible productivity eventually provoked the very envy and hostility she tried hard to avoid. At first, Peplau's coming to Rutgers was regarded by Dean Stonsby as a great coup. Peplau added luster and energy to the school, she was unfailingly helpful in its early development, and she was supportive of Stonsby's ideas. As time went on, however, Peplau's reputation began to outstrip that of the school, and as the reputation of the College of Nursing stalled and then sank, Peplau's program gained in national standing. Stonsby was unable to lead the faculty in the direction she wanted to take it, and

Peplau was less and less available to help her out. By 1960, Stonsby was becoming physically ill, and as her health deteriorated, she complained to the university's central administration that Peplau was a source of dissent and trouble in the faculty. Fortunately, by this time, Peplau's position in the faculty was safeguarded by academic tenure.

Beginning in the 1960–1961 academic year, tensions between Stonsby and Peplau began to increase. First, Stonsby was indeed sick. She lived alone in a hotel, and after the Christmas holidays in 1961, came into the college looking more and more haggard, often suffering vaginal hemorrhages during the day. Second, perhaps because of her physical condition, she was not able to function efficiently.[56] Third, her vision of the 8-year plan for nursing education was floundering. Fundamentally, the faculty did not accept it. Because both the 2-year and 4-year students were on campus at the same time, there were endless discussions about how to differentiate between the courses for each. By this time, too, community colleges were being established across the country and were offering 2-year associate degrees in nursing. These degrees were regarded as "terminal" by the profession at large, and were not to be equated with the first 2 years of college or university education, nor were they equivalent to the last 2 years of baccalaureate nursing education. Peplau was in fact quite sympathetic to the Stonsby proposal, believing it incumbent upon nursing leaders to move nursing education out of hospitals and into institutions of higher education while making an educational continuum possible, associate degree through to the PhD.[57] While she thought Stonsby right in concept, however, she did not believe it was her responsibility to make it happen. She had her own goals to achieve.

The faculty for its part could see no way to reconcile Stonsby's 8-year design with the emerging junior college associate degree movement. Stonsby did not want to give up her continuum idea, however, and the faculty's only solution was to ask the university to hire additional faculty members to offer separate courses for the 2-year students, and awarding them the associate degree. The university had no patience for any of this, little interest in the associate degree, and no interest in providing the extra funding requested by the faculty. Stonsby clearly felt frustrated.

Then there was Hilda Peplau, with her well-funded graduate program, her "extra" faculty, and few students. Peplau wanted only that the college be run efficiently, and to be left alone to develop her own program. The Graduate Program in Psychiatric Nursing was, after all, the only program based in the College of Nursing with national visibility and standing. She did not regard the undergraduate program as her responsibility, and did not want to engage in the faculty turmoil surrounding it. This, of course, only added to Stonsby's frustration. For her part, Peplau was willing to help, but she was most definitely not interested in the endless "nonsense" that passed for faculty meetings. Indeed, if one reads through the faculty minutes for those years, it is easy to see how the continual circling around the issues with no resolution reached would be most distressing to someone of Peplau's single-minded determination to get things done. The end result was that despite its one strong program, the college of nursing as a whole was perceived by the university as marginal.[58]

In December 1961, Stonsby, hoping to goad the faculty into adopting her ideas and programs, brought matters to a head by informing the faculty that the university was considering closing the college if it could not move on in developing its curriculum and programs. Taking the challenge seriously, Peplau and her colleagues in psychiatric nursing proposed developing a PhD program built around clinical specialties—the first would be in psychiatric nursing. This plan too was doomed, for the already demoralized faculty was not interested in committing itself to this hard road. In fact, the faculty would not take this step for another 15 years. What the faculty did do in December 1961 was to write a long letter to President Mason Gross extolling the virtue of the College of Nursing and expressing dismay at any plans to close the college.[59] The letter was from "The Faculty of the College of Nursing" but carried no signatures. There were no signatures because the psychiatric nursing faculty members refused to sign the letter, and rather than reveal dissension in the ranks, the letter was simply sent unsigned. An immediate reply came from the university's chief academic officer, John Swink, dean of the faculty. He assured the nursing faculty that there are "no facts to substantiate such a statement" (plans to close the college), but then went on to state that there was in fact a study under way to evaluate "the status of the college."[60]

If the 1960–1961 academic year was a tense and unsettled one, 1961–1962 would be even more so. The faculty was mired in endless debates about rules of procedure, faculty governance, and the "role of department chairs," which was a euphemism for disagreements among Hilda Peplau, the rest of the faculty, and Ella Stonsby. Disagreements centered around Stonsby's efforts to impose a "philosophy" and curriculum, absent faculty agreement.[61] As Stonsby's frustration centered more on Peplau, Peplau took to documenting everything, no matter how minor, and writing long, dense and exceedingly detailed notes to Stonsby, including notes she took to reconstruct even the most casual conversation between them.[62] There were memos about the budget, about grant expenditures, about meetings to be attended and meetings to be missed, and about personnel matters. The tone of this exchange is captured by the following example of a Stonsby response to a Peplau memo: "I call your attention to your memo of October 11, in which you quote from my memo of October 9 . . . You should not have used the word 'concluded' . . . nor should you have omitted 'is this so . . .'[63]

In addition to this, the paperwork alone involved in administering Peplau's grants was voluminous, and Stonsby began questioning more and more details. Peplau thus began to take every detail to Stonsby, being sure to dot every i and cross every t. Soon the memo war between them escalated out of control. Any meeting with Stonsby was followed by long, five- or six-page single-spaced memos recording every word exchanged and the "content of any agreements reached."[64] They are dense, tight, formal—and probably excessive.

The deteriorating relationship with Peplau was actually the lesser of Stonsby's problems that semester. During the spring of 1962, the college was due for reaccreditation by the National League for Nursing. The League required that a voluminous self-study precede its visit for purposes of reaccreditation, but, during the fall semester the faculty was in such disarray that it could not agree on any of the prerequisites for a successful self-study. The faculty appeared ready to abandon the 2-year associate degree program, but Dean Stonsby opposed this strategy. At the other extreme, Peplau was urging an expansion of graduate work and the development of a PhD program, also resisted by the faculty. The result was that no self-study was prepared.

On a cold Friday night early in February, Dean Stonsby called Peplau asking for help. It was the weekend before the external review team was to visit. She wanted to come out to Madison that night to put together a report, which, given the nature of the required self-study outline, would have been an impossibility. Hilda told her as much, but did promise to come in early on Monday to see what she could do. Trekking into Newark at 5:30 on Monday morning, Peplau was appalled at the state of disorder in Stonsby's office. She saw immediately that there was nothing to be done but to allow the League to witness the disarray. Hopefully, they would make constructive recommendations. While Peplau was accused in some quarters of being primarily responsible for the disastrous external review that year, the record makes clear that such was not the case.[65] The visit was indeed a disaster, but the report itself makes clear that the problems the visitors described were endemic to the college, and not a reflection on one member of the faculty. In its report to Rutgers's President Mason Gross, on March 2, 1962, the team strongly urged that the dean and faculty reexamine what they were doing while expressing the opinion that "in the present environment of tension and suspicion neither is capable of examining the question clearly or developing a plan for transition."[66]

On June 2, 1962, President Gross wrote a long letter to the faculty in which he challenged them to address and resolve their differences in the next academic year, 1962–1963. After reiterating and summarizing the conclusions of the external review team, he stated,

> I am unwilling to accept at this time the conclusion implicit in the above statements that the situation is so bad that it cannot be resolved.

I therefore call upon the dean and the faculty to work together to resolve these issues . . . The attempt should be made in the confidence that the university desires to have a strong and flourishing College of Nursing, and has no desire to discontinue a program that in many ways merits high praise. Yet the fact remains that it is an expensive program and that the expense partially at least stems from the particular curricular design.[67]

Gross asked the faculty to work to resolve their differences with the dean, and in any event to present him with a progress report on or about December 1, 1962, with an interim report due in March 1963 and a final report due on or about May 1, 1963. He concluded by warning that

Unless within the academic year 1962–1963 there is a prompt, harmonious, and reasonably successful attack upon the issues presently dividing and impeding the progress of the College of Nursing, the university will be obliged to make a drastic reappraisal of its attitude.[68]

The faculty response to the June 2 letter from President Gross was to seek an audience with him, which was granted on June 27, 1962. Peplau was among the seven faculty members who met with him on that date. In this meeting, College of Nursing faculty members found the president condescending toward them. Basically, he lectured the senior faculty members that they needed to take charge of their own house, take charge of the curriculum, and make decisions about academic matters, leaving personalities aside. He suggested that perhaps College of Nursing faculty members could gain by attending meetings of the Douglass College faculty as visitor-observers in order to see "an active, verbal and responsible faculty at work."[69] He also reiterated his support for Dean Stonsby, expressing his belief that she would cooperate with the faculty in resolving difficult issues in regard to the curriculum.

This pressure made the fall of 1962 chaotic. For Peplau the tragedy was that "This continued turmoil is killing any intellectual potential there might be in the faculty."[70] Peplau's response to the rising frustration and tension was quite mixed. On the one hand, her own program was running well, her national commitments were at full tilt, and she did not want to be drawn into all the turmoil at the College of Nursing. She felt the problems were with the undergraduate program and that the faculty teaching in that program should resolve them. On the other hand, she did care about the college and certainly did not want to see it disbanded. Also, on a personal level she felt an allegiance to Stonsby and concern for her well-being. She knew that Stonsby was physically sick and mentally exhausted. Fundamentally, Peplau was angry and frustrated that the university seemed oblivious to Stonsby's situation. She felt strongly it was the university's obligation and responsibility to see to it that one of its administrators received the help she needed. In her view, it was simply not the faculty's responsibility, and most particularly, it was not the responsibility of one member of said faculty, namely herself. To her, any such expectation was highly unprofessional.[71]

If Peplau had been the clear leader of faculty opinion, it might have been a different story—but the fact was that this was not the case either. The faculty had as much trouble with Peplau as it did with Stonsby. The last thing in the world they wanted was Hilda Peplau, with her high standards and little tolerance for those who did not meet them, to be in a position of authority over their professional lives. Peplau's efforts to provide leadership were quite simply resisted.

In November 1962, Dean Stonsby called Hilda into her office. Stonsby was angry, and accused Peplau of going to New Brunswick to discuss college matters without informing her. The accusation was in fact true. Stonsby's behavior had become increasingly erratic, and Peplau felt that the essential work of the college wasn't getting done: grant vouchers were not being signed, faculty meetings were out of control, appointment letters were not being written, and day-to-day life at the college was chaotic. Peplau feared the college was in danger of losing its accreditation. Hence, Peplau, together with several other faculty members, requested a meeting with the Rutgers University's new provost, Dr. Richard Schlatter. Schlatter had arrived in New Brunswick just that semester, and the senior faculty hoped he would hear their concerns with an open mind. He agreed to meet with them on November 7, 1962. This was the meeting to which Stonsby referred.

Unfortunately, the meeting had not been a success. Notes taken by Peplau make clear that Schlatter was not interested in the details the faculty wanted to present. His response to their concerns was essentially that a college full of nurses ought to be able to take care of one sick nurse.[72] He stated that he was interested only in how the faculty and the dean were going to work out their differences and cooperate. Furious at what she considered to be an unprofessional response, Peplau had stomped out of the provost's office. Ella Stonsby told Hilda that upon learning that a group of faculty headed by Dr. Peplau had been to New Brunswick, she had gone home and was so sick she had almost died, which was literally true. She had hemorrhaged so badly that night that she had been hospitalized and given a blood transfusion.[73]

Peplau's response to the meeting with Schlatter, the confrontation with Stonsby, and the growing disarray in the college was to become even more obsessive about protecting herself, putting everything in writing, and taking down verbatim every word exchanged with Stonsby. This war of memos would continue for the next 3 years. The archives are packed with exceedingly detailed, dense, single-spaced memos on every item of faculty concern, typed by Peplau in her effort to defend her positions.

There are very formal, long, and detailed memos to Dean Stonsby on courses, on grant expenditures, on stipend allocations, and on her professional activities.[74] These also record profound disagreements on faculty appointments, reappointments, duties, and responsibilities.

In the months following the meeting with Provost Schlatter, Peplau joined with others on the faculty in sending very long memos to him and to President Gross, detailing the faculty's frustration and trying to illustrate and demonstrate why they could not "get along" with the dean. They sent detailed curriculum reports, details of the efforts of faculty chairs to engage the dean, and minutes of long and disorderly faculty meetings.[75] This deluge of material was not welcomed in the president's office. It succeeded only in reinforcing the perception that this college was troublesome, and the faculty, as well as the dean, not too competent.

A BREAKING POINT

Things came to a head in February 1963. This "nursing thing" was taking up too much of Provost Schlatter's time, and he decided to put an end to it. He had been provost for only a few months when the College of Nursing problem came to his attention. He wanted to move on to bigger issues. After reading through the voluminous material received in the president's office in just 1 month from the college and its faculty, he decided that Stonsby was right: Peplau was the problem. She was an eminent psychiatric nurse, and if she would help the dean instead of harassing her, things would be a lot better.[76] So, on an impulse he picked up the phone and called Hilda at home, asking her to come in the next morning. Peplau was excited. She thought that the provost had looked into the matter, determined that something must be done, and wanted her help in getting the college to move on. She actually believed that Schlatter might be interested in the psychiatric nursing graduate program, and was calling her in to talk about that too.[77] She was partially right in her initial assumption, but ultimately that assumption proved to be quite the wrong one.

In another setting and under different circumstances, Richard Schlatter and Hilda Peplau would undoubtedly have formed a mutual admiration society. Schlatter's journey from a small town in Ohio to Harvard and Oxford universities, a Rhodes scholarship, and prominence in his field as a historian were not unlike Peplau's own trajectory in nursing. He was as impatient with foolishness as she. He could not understand this "nonsense" going on at the College of Nursing. Why couldn't they sort it out and get about their business? He understood that Peplau was the one member of the faculty with true national prominence. Why then, if she was such a national figure in psychiatric nursing, could not she deal

constructively with Dean Stonsby?[78] Be this as it may, however, he realized that action must be taken. Things could not continue as they were.
When he telephoned Peplau, he had actually intended to size her up and
possibly talk with her about assuming the leadership of the college in the
event that they needed to ask Stonsby to resign. Before doing that,
though, he decided to check with a few members of the faculty. He called
the most senior member of the faculty first. In doing that, he had gotten
an earful. The faculty member was aghast at the suggestion that Peplau's
views might prevail and made it clear that this was simply not a tolerable
solution.[79] Schlatter thought he had a convenient solution to the faculty
problem, and it just fallen apart in the course of one phone call. He was
not in a good mood when Hilda arrived for her appointment.

Schlatter kept Peplau waiting for 20 minutes before seeing her. By that
time she, too, was most decidedly not in a good mood.[80] The meeting
was a disaster. Hilda began by expressing her displeasure at being kept
waiting, as she had rearranged an already tight schedule to be in New
Brunswick that morning.[81] Schlatter asked her about the situation at the
college. After about 5 minutes, he had heard enough. He decided that
Stonsby and his senior faculty consultant were right. According to
Peplau's recollection, about 5 minutes into the session, he said, "Why
don't you just resign and leave? *You're* not helping. I'm sick of troubles
from that school."[82] Peplau was unprepared for this and she was angry.
She began shouting at Schlatter, and as her voiced carried down the halls
of the university's old administration building, her reputation was
forged. She told the provost in no uncertain terms that she thought him a
weasel on the Stonsby matter, that it was *his* responsibility to sort out the
troubles, that *her* career was her own responsibility, not his, and she again
stormed out of his office. Later that day, in the faculty club, Schlatter
remarked to his lunch companions, "That Hilda Peplau is one formidable
woman!"[83] Hilda never saw him again.

By March 1963 Dean Stonsby had reached the breaking point. She
wrote an astonishing letter to President Gross. Academic tenure is one of
the most sacred traditions in academia. For Peplau, it was a particularly
meaningful protection given her experience at TC 10 years earlier. Schlatter's
suggestion that she resign had shaken her to the core. Thus, when she
received a copy of the following letter to President Gross, she became
truly upset. Stonsby wrote,

> As you know, the proper administration of the College of Nursing has
> been made increasingly difficult by the personal opposition and unneces-
> sary obstruction of one person, namely Miss Hilda Peplau . . . Therefore,
> it is my request that Miss Hilda Peplau be relieved of her tenure as a
> member of this faculty at the end of the current academic year.[84]

This letter upset Hilda so much that she broke one of her cardinal rules and confided her distress to a younger colleague and former student, Sheila Rouslin. Unannounced, Peplau dropped in on Rouslin in her office, something she seldom if ever did. Peplau was obviously very, very upset—so distressed that she began to cry. She then related some of her fears, discussing for the first time some of the events of 1953. To Rouslin, this was both very moving and very unsettling. Until that time, she had thought of Dr. Peplau as "a goddess," someone above emotion or normal feelings of vulnerability.[85] At this point, it was clear to Rouslin, however, that something just had to be done.[86]

Soon thereafter, Rouslin and Anita Werner, graduates of Peplau's program and both serving their first year as assistant instructors supported on grants awarded by the NIMH, decided to try to take action. They felt they were the graduates of the most avant-garde, exciting nursing graduate program in the country, and here they found themselves on a faculty that was about to destroy itself. They could not understand how the university could be so oblivious, both to the national prominence of the Psychiatric Nursing Program and to what was happening to the College of Nursing.[87] They made an appointment to see President Gross. Gross, gentleman though he was, decided he'd really heard all he wanted to hear about the College of Nursing and its troubles. He asked that the university's senior vice president, John Swink, meet with the nurses, which he did.[88] Werner and Rouslin told Swink that things could not go on like this, that the college was at a standstill, and no one could do any work. Swink, as had President Gross and Provost Schlatter earlier, suggested that instead of the university interfering, the nurses should help the dean. He asserted that they, of all the faculty, should understand that the dean had problems. "After all, aren't you in fact psychiatric nurses?" he asked. "Can't you help Miss Stonsby?" Swink then assured them the university was aware of the situation, that it was doing all that it could, but the process was a slow one. He urged them to be constructive, and, above all, to be patient.[89]

Frustrated by the lack of action on the part of the university administration, the younger faculty members decided to take matters into their own hands. They took the first step toward passing a motion of no confidence in the dean. As is typical of many nurses, however, they wanted to be as protective of her as possible while expressing no confidence. In a special faculty meeting they introduced a rather vague resolution to the faculty to this effect: "That each faculty member express her opinion regarding the mutual good will between faculty and dean, and that a three-member committee be appointed to abstract material to express faculty opinion."[90] A committee was established, but Peplau declined to serve on it. It was an exceedingly busy and active time in her professional life, and the troubles at Rutgers were a major distraction, one she felt she did not need. On the national level, she was then chairing the Committee on Intergroup Relations for the American Nurses Association and was serving as a member of the Southern Regional Council, a semigovernmental group dealing with a host of higher education issues in 11 southern states. Of greater importance were the facts that Hilda had been profoundly shaken by the suggestions that she resign or be de-tenured and that she had lost confidence in the university's central administration.

Apparently, however, the central administration was looking into matters more closely, for in that very same month, March of 1963, several things happened. The president requested Stonsby's resignation and she obliged. She was put on a leave of absence on March 30, 1963, with her resignation to become effective on March 31, 1964.[91] Then, unrequested, the university gave Peplau a $5,000 raise (which did not actually cost the university anything, since Peplau's salary was paid by her grants).[92] Finally, one of the quieter senior faculty members, the only one other than Hilda who possessed a doctorate, a quiet and dignified woman, Dorothy Smith, was named acting dean of the College of Nursing.

Although recognizing that Stonsby was ill and that a new dean needed to be found, the university's senior administrative officers remained convinced that Hilda Peplau had not helped the situation—in fact, they speculated that Stonsby's physical and mental problems were exacerbated by Peplau's continuous confrontation on nearly every issue. Instead of confronting, the administrators continued to believe that she could have used her expertise in psychiatric nursing to help rather than hasten the decline of Stonsby's health. Further, the provost and other university administrators thought that the young faculty members in psychiatric nursing had joined their mentor to harass the dean, causing her behavior to become all the more erratic.[93]

This was a rather simple-minded, easy, unfair, and wrong analysis of the situation. Because this was a college of nursing, that is, a women's college, and moreover because the "troublemakers" appeared to be psychiatric nurses who presumably could have used their skill and training to "save" the situation rather than exacerbate it, university administrators wanted them to solve an administrative problem no faculty members in other disciplines would have been urged to undertake. The central administrators decided that not only must Stonsby be relieved of her responsibilities, but that Peplau and her supporters should be held accountable.

A PERSONAL DISAPPOINTMENT

The Stonsby problem was not the only source of Peplau's dismay in 1963, however. One of the most disappointing incidents of her life occurred that spring semester. In January 1963, Florence Wald, dean of the Yale

University School of Nursing, invited Peplau to accept the Annie W. Goodrich Visiting Professorship for the academic year 1963–1964. The Goodrich Professorship would have freed Peplau from her administrative and teaching responsibilities at Rutgers, while providing her residence in and access to a truly great research university. Tish was graduating from high school in June and would be away at college by fall. This would be the first time since before the Second World War that Hilda would be free to accept such a position. Furthermore, a year at Yale would not only get her out of the troubled situation at Rutgers but would offer her a challenging academic environment for the first time since graduating from Bennington. She was excited beyond dreaming, but knew that it would be tricky from the Rutgers standpoint. She was now in the position of having to ask the University for permission to take a leave of absence, and she had thoroughly alienated its principal officers. Nonetheless, she wrote to Dean Stonsby on January 22, 1963, asking for the leave and providing an outline of how all her programmatic responsibilities would be covered by the members of her departmental faculty. Provost Schlatter was sent a copy.[94]

It was Schlatter who responded. On Valentine's Day 1963 he offered congratulations "on this distinguished appointment which honors both you and the school," but also wrote that "if you can get a suitable person with the PhD degree in nursing to join the staff next year and help with the graduate program in your absence, I see no difficulty about authorizing your leave."[95] He very likely did not realize that this was a precondition almost impossible to meet. Stonsby certainly did know this, and she well might have suggested the precondition to Schlatter, as he would have consulted with her before approving the request. She would have known that most nurse faculty in the country, as at Rutgers, held the master's, not the PhD degree. Five Peplau graduates had entered PhD programs, but none of them could possibly complete their degrees in time for the fall 1963 semester. In addition, they were all committed to positions elsewhere once they did complete their degrees. Nurses who held the doctorate, as was the case with Hilda Peplau herself, held them in fields other than nursing.[96] Thus, while the requirement that she replace herself, for 1 year only, with a nurse who had earned the PhD degree, may have seemed a logical precondition from the point of view of the university, it was in fact an extremely difficult one to meet.

Although Peplau had hired five additional instructors by this time, none held the doctorate. In addition to the need to find and lure to Rutgers a psychiatric nurse with a doctorate, she also wanted assurances from the NIMH that her grants would not be jeopardized should she take a year's leave. She wanted to guarantee her students' continued support. Reassurance was not forthcoming from this source either. As her old friend, Esther Garrison, wrote, "It is not within my jurisdiction to give you any assurances that your being away from the Rutgers program would not jeopardize the training grant."[97] Garrison did, nonetheless, urge her to accept the Yale professorship.

In March, Peplau reluctantly wrote to Dean Wald at Yale:

> I am giving up the dream of the Annie Goodrich Professorship and a year at Yale. First, I couldn't find a proper replacement and feared losing the grants . . . The official letter of regret is attached. Now, I am off to Idaho and Minnesota. It is not fair to keep you waiting . . . Florence, I cannot tell you how dreadfully sorry I am; I know there is a shortage of these doctoral people, having now tried for three years to capture one; you can be sure I will redouble my efforts to preach to nurses the urgency of more of them going on rather quickly . . . This was a dream I wish could be realized. Surely Tisha will weep with me, too, for she wanted so much for me to have the year at Yale, also.[98]

This would have been Peplau's only leave in a 20-year career at Rutgers. She declined the Yale offer, and would remain at Rutgers another 10 years without a sabbatical.

ENDNOTES

1. Interviews, Hildegard Peplau, March 4, 1992, in Sherman Oaks, California, and Shirley Smoyak, April 2, 1994, in New Brunswick, New Jersey.
2. See materials in Box 1, Folders 1–4, "Graduate Psychiatric Program" in Special Collections and Archives, Rutgers University Libraries.
3. See handwritten account in Box 2, #38, in the Schlesinger collection.
4. These details are outlined in letters from Ella V. Stonsby to Miss Hilda Peplau, February 2, 1954, and to Dean Herbert P. Woodward on February 5, 1954. These letters are in Hildegard Peplau's Personnel File in the Rutgers University Personnel Archives in the University Library.
5. See Minutes, Board of Directors, New Jersey State Psychiatric Hospital at Greystone Park, February 1954, 3, in Box 2, #40.
6. Interview, Hildegard Peplau, February 2, 1992.
7. Letter from Hildegard E. Peplau to Miss Ella V. Stonsby, February 3, 1954, Peplau Personnel File, Rutgers University.
8. Letter from Hildegard Peplau to Ella Stonsby, April 1, 1954, Peplau Personnel File.
9. That she did apply for federal funds that first year is noted in her letter of acceptance to a 2-year reappointment as Assistant Professor. See letter from Hilda E. Peplau to Herbert P. Woodward, March 5, 1955: ". . . I look forward to continuing the relationship with a particular interest in the program outlined in the 1954 application for funds under the Mental Health Act" (Peplau Personnel File).
10. In the 1960s Mary Margaret Schmidt, with whom Peplau had worked at the NLN in the 1940s, began to refer to Peplau as "the kept woman of the government." As Peplau noted wryly, "I was." Not until her last year at Rutgers, 1974, did the University actually pay her salary. See Salary History, Peplau Personnel File.
11. Letter from Hilda E. Peplau to Mrs. Gordon, May 20, 1954, found in Peplau Personnel File.

12. Ibid.

13. Interview, Sandra Gauker, March 21, 1993.

14. Letter from Hilda Peplau to Miss Ella Stonsby, August 29, 1954, Peplau Personnel File.

15. Interview, Hildegard Peplau, March 16, 1992.

16. Letter from Anne Peplau to Barbara Callaway, Feb. 26, 1999.

17. Letter from R. Louise McManus, to "Whom It May Concern," n.d., Peplau Personnel File. When asked about this, Peplau responded that she thought it appropriate that McManus be asked to write because of her position. In addition to McManus, the Rutgers file included four more letters of recommendation, all very strong. They were from Seymour D. Vestermark, MD, Chief of the Training Branch of the National Institutes of Mental Health; Lucille Petry Leon, Chief Nurse Officer at the NIMH; Jay Hoffman, MD of St. Elizabeth's Hospital in Washington, D.C., who had been Chief of Staff at the 312 Hospital; and Spafford Ackerly of the University of Louisville, who wrote,

> I have rarely met a person who could see a problem so clearly and be so objective, analytic and tactful in discussion of the problem with the principals. Some constructive move in regard to the problem or situation usually resulted . . . With it all she showed skill as a teacher, relegating herself to the background in favor of drawing out the other person. She has a warm and ready smile that attracts and instills confidence.

    See letter from Spafford Ackerly, MD, "To Whom it May Concern," January 26, 1954, in Peplau Personnel File.

18. Letter from Ella V. Stonsby to Dr. Herbert P. Woodward, June 29, 1954, and from Herbert P. Woodward to Ella V. Stonsby, July 1, 1954 in Peplau Personnel File.

19. Letter from Dean Herbert P. Woodward to Miss Ella V. Stonsby, December 1, 1951; Herbert P. Woodward to Ella V. Stonsby, July 1, 1952 (letter of reappointment and promotion effective July 1, 1952); Rutgers Personnel files, "Ella V. Stonsby Employment/Salary History Form," Division of Personnel Archives.

20. See list of title changes accompanying the salary history of Ella V. Stonsby, Rutgers University Personnel Archives and letter of appointment from Albert E. Meder, Dean of Administration, to Miss Ella V. Stonsby of June 18, 1956, informing Miss Stonsby that she had been appointed Dean of the College of Nursing and Professor of Nursing Education, effective July 1, 1956. Her salary was to be $8,760. (Rutgers University Personnel Archives, Ella V. Stonsby file.)

21. Interview, Hildegard Peplau, January 27, 1992.

22. Ella V. Stonsby, "The Eight Year Model of Nursing Education," College of Nursing Archives, Rutgers University Library, 1954.

23. From an abstract of a panel discussion in 1983 on "mentoring" found in Box 2, #36, in the Schlesinger Library collection.

24. See Archives of Psychiatric Nursing X, (1) (1996): 14–15.

25. Letter from Herbert P. Woodward to Hilda E. Peplau, February 2, 1955, Peplau Personnel File.

26. Interview, Hildegard Peplau, January 27, 1992. Tenure was a very important matter to Peplau given the capricious and flimsy nature of the allegations made against her in 1953 and her own lack of job protection at that time.

27. Letter from President Louis Webster Jones to Hilda Peplau, May 25, 1957, Peplau Personnel File.

28. The deed and mortgage for 118 Shunpike Road are in Box 2, #46. Peplau made a down payment of $2,000 on the $14,000 house. While money in the early years

was always in short supply, Hilda had formed the habit from the day that Tish was born of putting aside a small amount from each paycheck to buy bonds as an education fund for Tish. When the budget permitted, she conservatively invested any money left after the bare essentials had been covered in the stock market. She explained that profit from her stock investments provided the money for the down payment of the house, for the purchase of a car, and to cover moving costs.

29. From the *Madison Gazetteer*, published by the Chamber of Commerce, 1993.
30. Interview, Hildegard Peplau, January 27, 1992.
31. Ibid.
32. In her own research, Peplau's major focus was on clarification of clinical phenomena and appropriate nursing interventions. Her thinking is laid out in a series of clinical papers dealing with major concepts in her work—see, for example, "Loneliness," *American Journal of Nursing 55*, (Dec. 1955): 1476–1481; "Anxiety/Panic" in Shirley Burd and F. Marshall, eds., *Some Clinical Approaches to Psychiatric Nursing* (New York: Macmillan, 1963), 78–93; "Hallucinations, Interpersonal Relations and the Process of Adaptation," in *Nursing Science 1*, (Oct–Nov. 1963): 272–279; "Learning and Cognition" in Burd and Marshall, 103–110. During her 20 years at Rutgers, her publications also addressed psychosocial and psychiatric aspects of nursing care for patients recovering from cardiac surgery, for nurses working in operating rooms, for nurses dealing with cancer patients, with the aging, with mother-infant relationships, and working in industrial settings as well as mental health challenges in public health nursing. In other papers Peplau analyzed processes and techniques related to individual, group, and family psychotherapy. There are also publications on theory development (11), on nursing research (12), and on doctoral education for nurses (15). And finally, Peplau shared her observations on innumerable audio and videotapes, as well as in a major motion picture (see bibliography).
33. Interview, Hildegard Peplau, January 27, 1992.
34. Letter from Marion Johnson to Hilda Peplau, April 7, 1958, Peplau Personnel File.
35. The Rutgers PhD did focus on nursing research, but not necessarily on clinical problems and was not organized around clinical specialties.
36. Interviews, Suzy Lego and Anita O'Toole, September 14, 1996, in Sewickley, Pennsylvania.
37. Interview, Matilda Riley, November 1977, in Washington, D.C. At this time, the author of this book was Acting Dean at the Rutgers College of Nursing and interviewed Riley in regard to personnel issues involving both the College of Nursing and the Rutgers Department of Sociology, which Riley had chaired during the 1960s.
38. One result is that to this day there are Peplau graduates in faculty positions across the country. In her first 5-year review of the program in 1962, Peplau noted that of the 19 graduates to that date, 6 had been granted career-teacher awards from the PHS and were on the academic track, another 5 had been awarded career clinician post-master's education fellowships, and 5 had applied for the NIMH "nurse/scientist grants" for direct admission into PhD programs. Thus, 16 of her first 19 students continued their education, and would join that elite small number of nurses who earned advanced degrees beyond the master's. In addition to their academic pursuits, the 19 graduates were beginning to have an impact on the profession of nursing at large. Eight had conducted clinical workshops of their own or run institutes for professional nurses. In the archives there are many letters from physicians and directors of nursing across the country commenting on the extraordinary competence of these early Peplau graduates. See Hilda Peplau, "Graduate Program in Psychiatric Nursing, Five Year Review," and related letters in Box 15, #498.
39. Interviews, Lucille Joel, November 18, 1992; Jessie Scott, November 10, 1992; Grayce Sills, October 29, 1992; Martha Rogers, March 14, 1993; Lulu Hassenplug, March, 1991; and Gwen Tudor Will, October 8, 1994.

40. Interview, Sara Erickson, September 12, 1996, in Washington, D.C.
41. For a report on Rutgers graduates and their affiliations across the country see "Brief Summary of Accomplishments of Graduates of the Rutgers Graduate Psychiatric Nursing Program, 1957–1974" in Box 17, #603. For a detailed list of graduates, showing year of graduation and current positions in 1978, see a report prepared by Shirley A. Smoyak, also in Box 17, #604. The program at Rutgers had remained small, partly at least because of the fact that Peplau would agree to hire only PhD nurses and there simply were not very many of them. In her 20 years at Rutgers, her program had produced only 128 advanced clinical specialists. These 128 nurses, however, had an enormous impact on their profession. Her legacy from the Rutgers years was not so much to the College of Nursing, but to the profession at large, as her Rutgers students fanned out across the country making major contributions in a wide variety of settings. They defined themselves as clinical nurse specialists and were very clear that they wanted to work directly with patients. They assumed leadership roles across the country as clinical practitioners, administrators, consultants, educators, and researchers. They worked in community, VA, state, and county hospitals, community mental health centers, colleges and universities, federal and state policy planning and regulatory offices, national and state nursing associations, publishing companies, and in private and group psychotherapy practices in 30 different states. 21 of them continued their education, earning their doctorates and assuming posts in universities across the land. Thus, although small in number, their impact was widespread. They became leaders within the health and education institutions within which they practiced, and carried Peplau's influence to institutions and organizations across the country.
42. Interview, Wendy King and Sandy DeLeu, November 18, 1992.
43. Interviews, Sheila Rouslin Welt, October 14, 1994, and Elizabeth Carter, August 27, 1994, in Lake Hapatong, New Jersey.
44. Interview, Lucille Joel, November 30, 1992.
45. Interview, Fern Kumler, August 27, 1994, in Lake Hapatong, New Jersey.
46. Interview, Suzy Lego, September 14, 1996, in Sewickley, Pennsylvania.
47. Interview, Hildegard Peplau, February 18, 1992.
48. Interviews, Sandy DeLeu, November 18, 1992, in Edison, New Jersey, and Bruce Mericle, September 1995, in St. Louis.
49. Interview, Hildegard Peplau, February 18, 1992.
50. Interview, Wendy King, November 18, 1992.
51. Interviews, Bruce Mericle, October 29, 1992, in St. Louis; Evelyn Zimmerman, April 28, 1993, in Spring Valley, New Jersey; and Ildaura Murillo-Rhode, March 2, 1993, in New York City. Ruth Southard, Kay Delaney, and Evelyn Zimmerman actually sent their notebooks to the author of this book, who has deposited them in the Schlesinger collection.
52. Interview, Suzy Lego, September 14, 1996.
53. Interviews, Anita O'Toole, September 15, 1996, Sheila Rouslin, October 14, 1994, Bruce Mericle, October 29, 1992, Shirley Smoyak, November 18, 1992, and Suzy Lego, September 14, 1996, ibid.
54. Interviews, Shirley Smoyak, October 29, 1992, in New Brunswick, New Jersey; Peggy Marshall, November 14, 1992, on the telephone; Liz Carter, August 27, 1994, in Lake Hapatong; Anita O'Toole and Suzy Lego, September 14, 1996, in Sewickley, Pennsylvania.
55. For a report on Rutgers graduates and their affiliations across the country see "Brief Summary of Accomplishments of Graduates of the Rutgers Graduate Psychiatric Nursing Program, 1957–1974" in Box 17, #603. For a detailed list of graduates, showing year of graduation and current positions in 1978, see a report prepared by Shirley A. Smoyak, also in Box 17, #604.

56. Interviews, Dorothy Smith, January 1993; Elizabeth Fenlason, October 1976; and Isabel Duetcher and Ann Clark, May 1997.

57. Interview, Hildegard Peplau, February 17, 1992.

58. Interview, Richard Schlatter, June 12, 1977.

59. Letter from the Faculty of the College of Nursing to President Mason Gross, December 12, 1961, in Box 15, #506.

60. Letter from John Swink to the Faculty of the College of Nursing, December 15, 1961, in Box 15, #506.

61. See notes of faculty meetings in Box 15, #517.

62. Examples of such notes, with carbon copies, may be found in the Peplau archives, Box 15, #515.

63. Note from Ella V. Stonsby to Hilda E. Peplau, October 12, 1962, Box 15, #517.

64. See memos in Box 15, #509–513. See also the exchange of memos in regard to Peplau's annual reports to the College Committee of Review in November and December, 1962, in the Peplau Personnel File in the University achieves. Every statement of fact in Peplau's report is challenged by Stonsby, asking for the "evidence." Peplau answered with bitingly terse comments while providing the requested documentation.

65. Peplau's diaries and notes express her concerns about the external review, and record the events leading up to it. See Box 15, #508 and #510. In addition, the author interviewed Elizabeth Fenlason and Dorothy Smith, both of whom were on the faculty at the time; Richard Schlatter and Malcolm Talbott, university administrators at the time with whom the author spoke in 1976, made clear that Peplau and not Stonsby was nonetheless generally blamed by university personnel. This would lead to difficulties for the rest of Peplau's years at Rutgers.

66. "Report of the National League for Nursing/Middle States Association Team to President Mason Gross at the Rutgers University College of Nursing, March 2, 1962" found in Box 15, #507.

67. Letter from President Mason W. Gross to the Faculty of the College of Nursing, June 2, 1962, Box 15, #510.

68. Ibid.

69. Minutes from a meeting with President Gross, June 27, 1962, found in Box 15, #511, no author cited. Douglass College was an undergraduate women's liberal arts college located on the University's New Brunswick campus.

70. Peplau's notes, Box 15, #508 and #510.

71. Interview, Hildegard Peplau, January 28, 1992. Also, see Peplau's notes made in 1962 and 1963 found in Box 15, #508.

72. See notes from a meeting with Provost Schlatter in Box 15, #509.

73. See Peplau's personal notes about this meeting in Box 15, #506.

74. See memos June–December, 1962, in the personnel file at Rutgers and in Box 15, #506 at the Schlesinger Library. The memos are invariably polite and proper, but it's clear that the tension is running near the surface.

75. Examples of this material may be found in Box 15, #518.

76. Interview, Richard Schlatter, June 12, 1977.

77. Interview, Hildegard Peplau, January 27, 1992.

78. Interview, Richard Schlatter, June 12, 1977, in Princeton, New Jersey.

79. Ibid.

80. Interview, Hildegard Peplau, January 27, 1992.

81. Peplau notes in Box 15, #508.

82. This is the conversation as reconstructed by Hilda Peplau in an interview on January 27, 1992.

83. As recalled by Shirley Smoyak in an interview, November 10, 1993.

84. Letter from Ella V. Stonsby to Mason W. Gross, March 6, 1963, Rutgers University Personnel file.

85. Interview, Sheila Rouslin Welt, October 14, 1994, in Morristown, New Jersey.

86. Ibid.

87. Interviews, Sheila Rouslin Welt, October 14, 1994, and Anita Werner O'Toole, September 14, 1996.

88. Interview, Sheila Rouslin Welt, October 14, 1992.

89. Ibid.

90. A copy of this resolution was found in Box 15, #508.

91. Stonsby Personnel File, salary chronology, Rutgers personnel archives.

92. See Peplau salary history in her University Personnel File.

93. Interviews, Vice President Malcolm Talbott, Dean and Acting Provost Horace dePodwin, Associate Dean Eleanor Gersman, and Provost Richard Schlatter in 1976 prior to assuming the acting deanship of the College of Nursing, and in later discussions with Provost James E. Young in 1976, 1992, and 1999.

94. Letter from Hilda Peplau to Ella V. Stonsby, January 22, 1963, Peplau Personnel File.

95. Letter from Richard Schlatter to Professor Hilda E. Peplau, February 14, 1963, Peplau Personnel File.

96. NYU, for example, offered a doctorate in nursing education in the College of Education, not a PhD from the Graduate School.

97. Letter from Esther Garrison to Hilda Peplau, January 7, 1963, Box 23, #789.

98. Letter from Hilda Peplau to Florence Wald, March 14, 1963, Box 23, #792.

Summers on the Road ── 10

If you had worked with the mentally ill as long as I have, you would know that one of the most tragic aspects of mental care today is that our mental institutions, the very places to which these tormented people turn for help, often provide a scene for the day by day, week by week, year by year reinforcement of a patient's illness until [s]he is virtually incurable. That this tragedy is the result of ignorance rather than malice, does not make it less a tragedy.

—Hildegard Peplau
1964

Beginning in 1954–1955, after classes ended for the spring and grades were submitted, Hilda locked her office door, asked the secretary to hold her mail until the fall, and cheerfully headed home to prepare for a summer on the road. Her faculty appointment at Rutgers was for 9 months a year, and the summers belonged to her. She and Tish hurriedly cleaned the house, packed the car, asked the neighbors to watch the house, and headed west. Hilda loved to travel and the summer was a time for exploration and adventure.

Summer was also a time when Hilda, like a modern day Johnny Appleseed, spread the seeds of her ideas about psychiatric nursing across the United States. For more than a decade, she traveled to state after state, holding workshops in public mental hospitals to teach nurses more humane and effective ways to treat the patients in their care. Her travels eventually took her along the legendary old Route 66 all the way from New Jersey to California, and from Michigan in the north to North Carolina in the south. Her basic message was simple but revolutionary: The lives of patients warehoused in dreary state hospitals were not hopeless—they could change and get better, and nurses could play a pivotal role in that recovery process. These summer workshops constitute one of the most important and little known chapters of Peplau's long career.

In early 1955, Dorris O. Stewart, a nurse consultant from Indiana, attended a clinical workshop Hilda conducted for staff nurses at Overbrook Hospital in New Jersey. Stewart was so impressed with what she learned that she invited Peplau to come to Indiana and give the same workshop at the state hospital in Madison.[1] Hilda went to Madison in the summer of 1955 and returned the following year to repeat the program. In 1956–1957, in addition to Madison State Hospital, and Indiana Central State Hospital in Indianapolis, Hilda conducted workshops in Ohio, Illinois, and North Carolina. From that point on, the word spread quickly. Nurse consultants in the several state departments of health or mental health met regularly, and they soon were abuzz about this most unusual nurse who was having a dramatic impact conducting intense workshops in the public mental hospitals—and at almost no cost to the institution or the state.[2]

A SENSE OF MISSION

From the time her Teachers College students began working on the back wards of the Brooklyn State Hospital in the late 1940s and early 1950s, Hilda had argued that the nursing staff in state mental hospitals had a therapeutic role to play in introducing more humane treatment of patients and in promoting patients' return to mental balance. It was by then clear to her that there were two standards of care for the mentally ill in this country. At Chestnut Lodge in Maryland and at Highland Hospital in North Carolina, Hilda had experienced the care given to a few highly select patients in private hospitals. These patients were affluent, generally well educated, and were treated by the ablest, most experienced, and often most innovative psychiatrists. When she sought sites for her Teachers College (TC) students to gain experience in clinical practice, however, she was thrust into the world of the public mental hospitals, where over 90% of the mentally ill were "cared for." The challenge in these hospitals was immense. From the 1940s through the 1960s most of the nation's institutionalized mentally ill were warehoused in huge hospitals where they received minimal care and virtually no individual attention. This was before the development of psychotropic drugs, and patients were cuffed, held in restraints, and subjected to ice packs, electroshock treatments, and lobotomies. They were deprived of their eyeglasses, shoelaces, belts, dentures, toothbrushes, combs, mirrors, and jewelry. They were lined up and marched to a cafeteria where they ate off tin plates and carried tin cups to water fountains, standing in line to fill them up. In these hospitals there was no dignity, no encouragement, and no hope. There was the constant smell of the insulin used to induce deep sleep and of paraldehyde, a sedative with a powerful odor, all mingled with the acrid fumes of the disinfectants used to clean the ward.

There were calls for reform in public hospitals, but these went largely unheeded. *The Snake Pit*, Mary Jane Ward's thinly veiled fictional look inside a mental institution was published in 1946; Olivia deHavilland played a patient in the 1948 movie classic based on the book. *The Shame of the States*, by Albert Deutsch, was published in 1948.[3] Its photographs of naked patients in restraints or lying about in deadly idleness was a clarion call for reform, but the harsh publicity did not arouse enough anger or concern to bring about significant change. This was due, in part, to the fact that by the 1950s, most psychiatrists were abandoning the public hospitals and going into private practice. Publicity revealing the horrors of mental hospitals only assured that psychiatrists would increase their efforts to avoid them. At a time when the population of such hospitals was increasing (in 1955 over 818,000 patients were institutionalized), psychiatrists were turning their attention to the problems of the middle and upper classes.[4] Peplau saw not only a crying need but also an opportunity for trained psychiatric nurses to step into the vacuum left by psychiatrists and make a difference in the environment of the public mental hospital—the "insane asylum" depicted in *The Snake Pit.*

The workshops Hilda conducted were of 1- to 3-weeks' duration. They were planned in such a way that Hilda and Tish would arrive at the scheduled hospital on a Sunday afternoon. While Tish settled into whatever quarters were provided for them, Hilda met with the hospital's nursing director to select patients, the number depending on the number of nurses who had signed up for the workshop. She asked that patients be verbal, and not be scheduled for electroshock therapy or lobotomies during the course of the workshop. Such requests were not always honored, and she adapted accordingly. She always left on Friday, after 4:30, to go on to the next site. She didn't work Saturdays—this was the day for sightseeing with Tish.

Hilda requested that any nurse working in the hospitals she visited be allowed to participate. Through these workshops Peplau exposed hundreds of general duty nurses to the theories and practices being developed in her graduate program at Rutgers. In her workshops she would demonstrate that any nurse could learn to work more effectively with patients in even the most difficult settings. The concentrated, meticulous attention given to every detail of nurse-patient interactions in these intense workshops helped nurses in these institutions understand the importance of their work and develop confidence that they could contribute to a patient's recovery.

A further goal in all of Peplau's workshops was not only to help nurses interact with and relate to patients, but in so doing come to understand nursing's contribution to patient care as distinct from that of medicine or other health care professions. Hilda understood that if nursing was to be appreciated as a profession, it had to define its unique scope of practice and contribution to the total system. Hence, the constant exhortation to take notes, to record, to articulate, and understand the dynamics of every nurse-patient interaction. In the workshops each nurse was encouraged to build upon her own personal strengths in order to perform therapeutically. Students and faculty were urged to share these results through conferences and publications. The essence of nursing care as Peplau outlined it was not only communication between nurse and patient but the integration of theory into practice and the development of self-understanding on the part of both the nurse and the patient. These goals gave structure to the summer experiences. Hilda hoped that participants in the summer workshops would help nurses in general make appropriate assessments of patients' needs and give them guidelines for making appropriate interventions in their care. Hilda believed that if nurses played an appropriate role in each phase of a patient's illness and recovery, the experience for both nurses and patients would be both educational and therapeutic and would lead to growth and healthy change.

To understand the significance of this contribution, it is important to know the context of 1950s nursing as well as the milieu of the public (and private) mental hospitals. Nurses working in mental institutions were involved for the most part in custodial care, not in therapeutic care. As Peplau saw it, nurses dealt with patients only when they had something in their hands—a thermometer, a lunch tray, medications, or a bedpan. They had to have an identifiable *task*. Talking to patients in any substantial way was discouraged for fear that a nurse would say the "wrong" thing. Nurses were taught to report observations related to a patient to the doctor whose duty it was to care for the patient. There was no recognition that nurse-patient interactions themselves could be therapeutic. Nursing was about rules, regulations, and carrying out the doctors' orders.[5] In contrast, Peplau began with the Sullivanian theory of interpersonal relations and techniques of psychotherapy based on the principle that people are influenced by their relationships with others. Observations of the communications and patterns of behavior between patient and the nurse were the heart of interpersonal relations in the psychiatric nurse-patient relationship she advocated in her classes and in her workshops. It was no small challenge for nurses who had been trained as custodial caretakers to develop the confidence and the ability to see themselves as *a part of* the patients' world rather than seeing themselves as *apart from* it—to see themselves as playing a crucial role in influencing how patients behaved and how they perceived themselves. Workshop days were structured in much the same pattern as the clinical experience segments of Hilda's graduate courses. The first hour of the day, from 8:00 until 9:00 in the morning, was dedicated to nurse one-on-one interviews with a selected patient. The remainder of the morning was spent reviewing the participants' interview notes and relating observations to clinical theory. The afternoons were spent in meetings with hospital staff, in lecture and seminar sessions, and in some sites in conducting group and family therapy.

Students of that time tell of the excitement of working intensely with a patient for the first time and beginning to make sense of patients' hallucinations and of the joy of discovering that delusions could often be controlled or mediated through effective verbal work.[6] Peplau's focus was always on the nurse and her role in this process. Most nurses participating in these workshops experienced a dramatic change in their perception of the role the nurse might play in patient care. Participants' language changed, their body language changed, and their ability to appreciate their own potential effect grew as they analyzed each segment of their clinical work. As a nurse's awareness of her (or occasionally his) own behavior became heightened, the focus of discussion shifted to the patient's behavior, and then to the nurse-patient relationship itself. Throughout the workshop, concepts such as anxiety, loneliness, shame or rage, never heard of in nursing school, were introduced to the participants, who began to see and respond to the therapeutic potential of this new vision of their role as nurses.

State funding was so inadequate for these institutions that there was no question of psychiatrists or physicians actually working in them on a one-to-one basis with patients. State budgets provided funds for custodial care only. Through her workshop work with nurses in the public mental hospitals, Peplau opened up the possibility of a new day in these depressing institutions. Nurses working in this vacuum, she believed, could truly make a difference. Moreover, the workshop experience inspired many nurses not only to go back to school for a baccalaureate degree but also, in many cases, to pursue graduate degrees.[7] As a result, many made career changes that brought them onto faculties in colleges of nursing where they too taught the "Peplau method."

At Rutgers, Peplau had been criticized for accepting too few students into her graduate program. Early on in her work in the state hospitals she was similarly criticized for spending so much time on a few selected patients while "ignoring" all the others. Her response was, "It's better to do something real with one patient than pat ninety-eight on the head and do nothing."[8] In fact, her students' work in the state hospitals had a ripple effect. Other patients watched warily as a patient was being interviewed, and over time it would become apparent that the interviewed patient was benefiting from the exchange. Just as they had at Brooklyn State Hospital back in 1949–1952, patients would begin to look forward to "talking" with the nurse each morning. They would begin to comb their hair, watch their grooming, respond more appropriately, and to get better. Seeing this, other patients would then begin to volunteer, and other nurses would want to become involved. In most of the hospitals in which Hilda worked, patient care improved, sometimes dramatically. Once nurses could see that changes could be made, that what they did could make a difference, they began to take an interest and, consequently, make an impact on the overall health and well-being of the patients.[9]

The summer workshops represented a commitment to a special mission, a vision of a different kind of nursing profession, but these experiences also had a synergistic impact on Peplau's teaching and writing. During the summer, Peplau was constantly testing her concepts and clinical skills in the crucible of the state mental hospitals. Then, back at Rutgers, working with her graduate students, she would search the literature for reinforcement or elaboration of what she had observed or tried. Some of this work was captured in her 1964 book, *Basic Principles of Patient Counseling*.[10] During these years, her primary commitment was to Rutgers, where she held academic tenure and a professorship, and to her constantly reaffirmed belief that a university degree was essential for nursing practice. In addition, as the years went by, she was more and more certain that the future of nursing depended upon the development of clinically based graduate programs. The point of such programs, and the mission of nursing itself, was to have an impact on patient care. Nowhere could this be better demonstrated than in the nation's mental hospitals.

ON THE ROAD

Hilda had not forgotten the pledge she made to Tish when she was born— that she would see to it that her daughter saw the world. Tish's world travels began with seeing America—and from a rather unusual vantage point at that. From 1957, the summer when Tish was 12 years old, until 1963 when she entered college, Tish accompanied Hilda on these annual cross-country road trips. A great comfort to Hilda in this period of simmering faculty dissention at Rutgers was to see Tish, who was now known by her middle name, Anne, proceed happily through her junior high and high school years in Madison, growing into a thoughtful, serious, bright, and engaging young woman. Throughout Tish's teen years, Hilda's sister and brother-in-law, Bertha and Byron Reppert, lived close to Hilda's home in Madison, first about 10 miles away in Green Brook, and then in Mechanicsburg, Pennsylvania. The Repperts eventually had four daughters. The cousins were close and the families spent most holidays together.

Tish flourished in the excellent Madison school system. She was placed in honors classes and accelerated groups and had a wide circle of friends. Many of her high school friends, including her first serious boyfriend, were members of the Methodist Youth Fellowship she joined in high school after abandoning the Presbyterian youth group in which she had been active in junior high school. Tish's disillusionment with the

Presbyterians was precipitated by a falling out with the assistant pastor in charge of youth programs. A rigid man who took the Presbyterian doctrine of predetermination literally, he assured the young people that God helped him select his new refrigerator at Sears. More distressing to Letitia Anne Peplau, independent thinker that she was, he insisted that the "heathens" in Africa who did not accept Jesus as their savior would be consigned to hell. At that point, Tish and most of her friends abruptly stopped attending the Presbyterian Church. Tish was editor of the high school yearbook, a National Merit Finalist, winner of the local DAR (Daughters of the American Revolution) award, and, not surprisingly, valedictorian of her graduating class. More surprising—at least to Hilda who claimed that her daughter "couldn't boil water"—Tish was also the winner of the Betty Crocker Good Homemaker Award. The explanation of this particular honor, however, may relate more to Hilda's own influence than to Tish's skills in the kitchen. The school required all girls to take the "Good Homemaker" test, believing perhaps that students in the non-college preparatory track would do best on questions related to matters such as the proper temperature for washing colored versus white clothing. As luck would have it, the essay portion of the test that year asked the young women to comment on the emerging pattern of "working mothers." Having been raised by a working mom, Tish was in an excellent position to write on this topic.

Hilda had always nurtured her daughter's independent spirit, supporting, even in her early grade-school years, such choices as Tish's personal style of dress. As Tish matured through junior high and high school, the relationship between mother and daughter more and more came to resemble a close friendship between friends in different disciplines whose lives constantly intersected and were deeply interwoven. Partly for this reason, in the years in which Tish accompanied Hilda on the workshop circuit, both looked forward to the summer adventure. For Tish, the summer travels were a grown-up alternative to the eastern summer camps customarily attended by her friends in Madison. For Hilda, they were a satisfying respite, albeit an exhausting one, from the stress of her academic year at Rutgers. For both, these trips meant cherished time to be together.

In May, during the last week of classes at Rutgers, the house would be thoroughly cleaned. The two scoured the bathroom, scrubbed down the kitchen, washing all the linens, and vacuumed every room. Ottylie's influence on Hilda was thus instilled in her daughter. The thorough housecleaning was nonnegotiable, and Tish, always tidy herself, learned not to argue about it. Finally, after Hilda's last class, Tish would load up a summer's worth of books from the library, and the two would hit the road. On a typical summer journey, 1-week workshops would be conducted in hospitals in Ohio, Indiana, Illinois, and/or Michigan during the month of June. Then mother and daughter would drive pell-mell across the country, bound for California where they would spend the month of July. At the end of July, they would head back east, making stops in Arizona and New Mexico, then moving on, again at a pell-mell pace, to North Carolina and the east coast. California, Indiana, Ohio, New Mexico, and North Carolina were almost always in the summer loop. Other states and other hospitals would be added and dropped, so the cross-country route would vary from year to year. Hilda usually made these exhausting cross-country trips without compensation other than expenses.[11] On their return to New Jersey, Hilda often made a stop at the Wernersville State Hospital in Pennsylvania where her sister Clara remained a patient. There is little doubt that Clara's life in a state institution played a part in focusing Hilda's interest on these hospitals. She would return to Rutgers just in time for the first day of the fall semester inspired, but tired.

The first of the mother-daughter cross-country trips was made in 1957. This trip was special and somewhat atypical of the trips that were to follow. This was also the year that Hilda's brother Walter retired from the army, and that Walter and Anne and their two children briefly stayed with Hilda and Tish in Madison while they relocated. Walter and Anne were there to take care of the house while Tish and Hilda made their summer trip. When they returned, many repairs had been made, the yard was immaculate, and the house was fresh and clean.

That first long trip was indeed cross-country: A 2,930-mile dash from New Jersey to California and an equally long return trip to North Carolina and back to Madison. The summer was full of adventure. Mary Alameda, Tish's friend from New York City, was invited to come along. The day after school was over, Mary arrived in Madison. Hilda and the girls loaded up Hilda's (non-air-conditioned) white Ford with books, maps, and supplies of food for the road; and they set off, heading due west. The destination was Fresno, where Hilda would conduct a 2-week workshop followed by a period as a visiting instructor at California State College. As always Hilda had little money, but she had a gasoline credit card and for once wasn't worried about the limited cash in her pocketbook. The two girls were excited, as was Hilda, who had never lost her love of driving. The three hit the road full of confidence and a spirit of adventure. California, here we come!

The first day they drove all the way through to Ohio, where the adventure really began. As it was getting dark, and this was their second night on the road, they were looking for a place to stop when, with a loud clang, the muffler fell off the car. Unable to seek emergency help, the three travelers spent the night at the side of the highway. Hilda stretched out on the ground on a blanket beside the car, and the girls slept inside on the blue upholstered, plastic covered seats. The next morning, a kind motorist drove them to the nearest garage, and using her plastic card, Hilda purchased a new muffler. Now humming along, they almost literally flew across the country, crossing the wheat fields and endless plains, over the awesome Rocky Mountains, skirting the Great Salt Lake, and then dropping down into the scorching desert, and on into the fertile valleys of central California.

Peplau came at the invitation of Dr. Helen Nahm, the dean of the College of Nursing at the University of California, San Francisco. In Fresno, Hilda would be working with public health nurses who in turn were working with the migrant families of the San Joaquin Valley. Hilda alternated lecturing between all-morning or all-afternoon sessions, and when she wasn't teaching, she and the girls took in as much sightseeing as they could. In the late afternoons, in the evenings, and on the weekends, Hilda took the two girls into San Francisco or to Yosemite National Park or to explore other California sights. When she taught in the afternoons, they used the cool mornings to explore the surrounding wine country.[12] At other times, the public health nurses took Tish and Mary to visit the orchards of the San Joaquin Valley, where they observed how the fruit was picked, handled, and packed for shipping.

Somehow Hilda, Tish, and Mary managed to see a significant cross section of the western states in the course of this summer. Photos show the girls at Snowy Range Pass outside Laramie, at the Great Salt Lake, Donner Pass, Chinatown in San Francisco, Sequoia National Park, Yosemite, driving down the coast to Monterey and Carmel, and visiting Disneyland shortly after the park opened.

At the conclusion of that summer program, Hilda and the girls reloaded the Ford and struck out to see the Grand Canyon in Arizona. Driving through the night, they made it in one day. They were astonished by the grandeur and the beauty of the countryside. Accustomed as they were to the dense cityscapes and verdant fields and leafy forests of the eastern states, they were awed by great expanses of land and sky of the American southwest. After a night spent at the Grand Canyon, Hilda decided to drive through Monument Valley, Arizona, to Four Corners, where Arizona, Utah, New Mexico, and Colorado meet. Unfortunately she didn't look too carefully at the map of the Indian country they would cross and thus failed to note the distinction between paved and unpaved roads. Leaving the Grand Canyon in the morning, they drove onto the vast lands of the Navajo reservation about 10 a.m. The paved road turned into a sandy track, too deeply rutted to risk trying to turn around. They had brought no food or water with them. Traveling at a snail's pace, they slipped and slid across the reservation land, arriving at Four Corners late in the afternoon—hot, thirsty, and hungry, but also inspired by the majesty of that deeply spiritual place. After drinking their fill of fresh water and eating sandwiches at a little restaurant, they discovered the car could go no further; it was out of gas. After a long walk to the only gas station for miles around, Hilda discovered that not only was the tank empty, but all four tires had huge heat blisters, just on the verge of bursting. Once again the plastic card proved a lifesaver. With four new tires and an almost new muffler, the white Ford, mercifully, got the travelers on their way south again to Gallup, New Mexico, for the annual Indian dance festival, and on to North Carolina and then home—and the trusty white Ford still had many more years of travel ahead of it.[13]

A FILM IS MADE

It was not long before the demand for Peplau's summer workshops began to outstrip even her considerable energy. Part of this demand can be attributed to an award-winning film. After her return from the first California trip with Tish, Hilda was back at her desk at Rutgers in September 1957, when Helen Arnold, the nurse consultant at Smith, Kline and French Laboratories, telephoned. Smith, Kline and French (SKF), which had developed a new psychotropic drug, Thorazine, wanted to finance the making of a film showcasing Peplau's students talking with patients. A writer from SKF had attended a workshop Peplau conducted at the Pennsylvania State Hospital in Erie and had made a transcript that he proposed developing into a pamphlet. The transcript had ended up with Peter Hickman, director of the medical film center at SKF, who was impressed with what he read. He had asked Helen Arnold to contact Peplau to inquire whether she would be interested in such a project. Hilda was intrigued and asked for more information. The film would present a vignette demonstrating the Peplau method—a nurse interacting with a patient and examining her reactions to the patient, keeping a detailed diary, talking to the patient, constantly analyzing and trying to understand that patient's reality. The movie would be filmed at Greystone Park State Hospital in New Jersey using professional actors. Peplau verbally endorsed the proposal, and in October Hickman wrote to inform her that the proposed director, Lee Bobker, and two scriptwriters would be attending her classes at Greystone as they worked on the script.[14]

When Hilda read the first version of the script in February 1958, she was disappointed. Its focus seemed to be on how nice the hospital was; completely missing, she believed, was the point of the nurse-patient relationship. She immediately began to suggest revisions, and kept on revising until in the end she had *her* script! She was obsessive about getting it all right, knowing that the SKF marketing department now intended to distribute the film to all hospital schools of nursing, to all colleges of nursing, to physicians, to nursing organizations, to every graduate program in psychiatric nursing, and throughout the mental hospital system, as well as to the Public Broadcasting System (PBS). Peplau felt that the film would "serve as a blueprint for the further advancement of psychiatric nursing" and therefore had to be exactly right.[15] As she explained in a letter to Bobker, in setting the tone for the film,

> The mentally ill patient needs his sickness. It enables him to feel safe. A world of his own making offers him comfort—comfort that he cannot find in the real world. Therapy consists in finding the bridge that exists between the two worlds, and leading the patient back over to reality. It is also the careful search for the lacks in skill or information which prevent the patient from using the real world and which make it necessary for the patient to create a world subject to his exclusive control.
>
> However extreme his behavior may be, the patient must feel that he, himself, is not disapproved of. This is a basic principle in psychiatric nursing. And the nurse learns to apply it through her experience with patient after patient. The therapeutic relationship is a process through which two people grow stronger—the patient and the nurse . . . She will learn to adapt to the needs of each individual patient; she will develop inventiveness—finding ways to bring her patients closer to reality; she will look upon her patient, first of all, as a human being—and think always in terms of what is best for him.[16]

Lee Bobker was most grateful for her obsessive attention to each detail of the film. In turn, Hilda believed that Bobker grasped what the film should be, and made it that. *Psychiatric Nursing—The Nurse Patient Relationship* almost immediately became a hit. It was filmed on location at Greystone Park and was sensitively and movingly acted, with a touching and convincing script. It caught Peplau at her best, talking with patients, talking with nurses, counseling both, and then lecturing on the whole process. Before the film's release, Peter Hickman asked Hilda to write a discussion guide. The guide, which because of the color of its cover became known as "The Purple Pamphlet," was distributed with the film.

Exhausted but exhilarated by the experience, Hilda wrote to Hickman in October 1958 urging a second film showing the continuity of the Peplau method as the patient returned home and received follow-up care from a public health nurse—something that she had not been able to do in her classes. Hickman replied that although SKF was interested in such a project,

> Our present plans and commitment do not leave room for an additional film for the nurse-mental patient area in the immediate future. However, we will certainly keep your proposal very much in mind and let you know if we can handle such a project at a future date.[17]

It was the classic brush-off, and Hilda was devastated. Although she had completely rewritten the script for *The Nurse Patient Relationship*, she had not asked for, nor received, any credit or fee. She had just wanted to make it as good as possible in order that it might help nurses, and she had spent hours and hours doing so. She wondered if her efforts had been appreciated.

Her spirits improved in December 1958 when Hickman wrote again, this time to thank her for the "Purple Pamphlet" and to inform her that demand for the film was heavy:

All 160 prints are in constant use. Within eighteen weeks of the film's release, we had arranged 830 showings, and this is in addition to those handled by ANA [American Nurses Association] and NLN [National League for Nursing]. It is by far the most widely used film in our history.[18]

Hilda's spirits improved still more 3 months later when she again heard from Hickman. In a letter dated March 3, 1959, he informed her that

The film has been nominated for an Academy Award by the Academy of Motion Picture Arts in Hollywood . . . It has been nominated in the feature-length documentary category together with three other films which include Disney's feature-release, *White Wilderness* . . . Because of the strong competition from Hollywood, I am not optimistic about our chances of winning an "Oscar"; but the nomination itself is a significant recognition not commonly given to this type of motion picture . . . In the seven months from the film's release in June to the end of December, we recorded 1,208 showings to an audience of 58,550 . . . Many hospitals and schools of nursing are now using it routinely in their teaching programs . . . We thank you again for your very great contribution to the success of this film.[19]

Initially the film was distributed by Dynamic Films, Inc., the film division of SKF. After the first year, the ANA-NLN Film Service was also given distribution rights. The film service notified Peplau in December 1958 that "the film has been booked three to four months in advance ever since its release date."[20] Hilda received more news of the film's success from Kathryn Linden, the director of the ANA-NLN Film Service:

By now you will have heard that *our* film [emphasis added] *Psychiatric Nursing—The Nurse Patient Relationship* has been nominated by the Academy of Motion Pictures for the Oscar . . . The other features nominated are *Antarctic Crossing, The Hidden World,* and *White Wilderness.*

The letter went on to list other honors accorded *The Nurse Patient Relationship,* including "acceptance by the Edinburgh Film Festival Council, the Vancouver International Film Festival, and the Festival of Contemporary Arts" as well as "an award as best in the sociological film category at the Yorktown International Film Festival in Canada." It noted that the

American Medical Association had recommended the film to "resident physicians in psychiatry as well as for basic and advanced nursing at the graduate level." In closing, the director added that *The Nurse Patient Relationship* had become the most popular of the ANA-NLN training films "in terms of requested reshowings."[21] Hilda herself was accorded personal recognition in May when the Board of Managers of the New Jersey State Hospital at Greystone Park organized a testimonial dinner at the elegant Far Hills Inn in Sommerville, New Jersey, to celebrate the Oscar nomination.[22]

After this, it is fair to say that Peplau's fame spread far and near. From this date forward, she would be under constant pressure to add one more workshop to her schedule, to attend one more conference, or to give one more lecture. She coped as best she could, seeking desperately to respond as fully as possible to all the requests. Coinciding as it did with Tish's teenage years, the effort to respond was remarkable.

THE WORKSHOPS

Peplau's summer workshop tour followed a basic route from east to west with stops in the midwest and back again to New Jersey with stops along a southern route. Each summer one or two new sites would be added or dropped. Working with colleagues and patients during the summer workshops, Peplau constantly revised her own thinking and subsequently her teaching when back at Rutgers. As she moved back and forth across the country, each new hospital presented new challenges and illuminated changes taking place in the public mental hospital system, as the following accounts help to illustrate.

Indiana

Following the invitation and arrangements made by Indiana nurse consultant Dorris Stewart for the first of the summer workshops in 1955, Hilda returned to Indiana every summer for 12 consecutive years to conduct workshops at the Indiana Central State Hospital in Indianapolis. The Indiana group over the years proved to be strong supporters of Hilda's work and her goals. In fact, to Hilda's great satisfaction, the Indiana State Hospital hired a Rutgers graduate as its first clinical specialist.[23]

An early highlight of the annual Indiana visits was a courtesy call Peplau and Dorris Stewart made to Emily Holmquist, the first dean of the University of Indiana's College of Nursing in Indianapolis. Holmquist was one of the few deans of colleges of nursing who understood from an early date what Peplau was doing and was enthusiastic about her work. She always offered hospitality, encouragement, and looked forward to the visits and the wide-ranging discussions of nursing that ensued over the years. In the midwest Peplau often found the intellectual stimulation she so lacked at Rutgers, and Emily Holmquist in Indiana became a close friend. With Peplau's encouragement, Holmquist founded one of nursing's first research journals, *Nursing Research*. The first areas of nursing "research" had been in the use of procedures and the economical use of equipment, time, and supplies. In the 1950s nurses began to conduct research in such areas as teaching, administration, curriculum, recruitment, and careers. It was not until the 1960s, however, with Peplau's encouragement and Emily Holmquist's editorial control, that the emphasis shifted to clinical research.[24] In 1965, the ANA, with a grant from the U.S. Public Health Service, held the first of four annual invitational nursing research conferences. These conferences were a direct result of Hilda's pleading and urging, and of the fact that her students were now scattered across the country, supporting the view that nurses, through research, could make a difference in patient care. It was not until 1986, however, that a National Institute for Nursing Research was established within the National Institutes of Health.[25]

After the first few years of the Indiana workshops, a slight variation in the established routine was made: Each day, from 2:00 to 4:00 in the afternoon, Hilda Peplau would meet with directors of nursing from around the state.[26] The purpose of these sessions was to encourage the directors to use clinical specialists to develop programs to assist staff nurses in their work with patients. The goal was to break the "illness maintaining systems" that always seemed to develop in the state hospitals. Peplau's only requirement for these afternoon sessions was that a pitcher of ice water be placed on the table with a glass, so that she could sip through these hot afternoons in the days before the hall was air-conditioned. About her eighth year there, the pitcher held a surprise, much to Hilda's delight. It held not ice water, but martinis! The workshop must have been a hit. The Indiana State Hospital director of nursing, Martha Rogers, who had always been quite reserved, usually put in only short appearances. After *this* workshop, she became an enthusiastic participant.[27] For the final 2 years of Hilda's Indiana odyssey, Martha Rogers made sure all the arrangements were meticulous and that all the patient participants were selected with thought and care. Rogers, like Stewart, became a strong advocate for Peplau's efforts in Indiana.[28]

One indicator of Hilda's growing acceptance at the Indiana State Hospital was in the accommodations offered her and Dorris Stewart on the hospital grounds. The first year, they were assigned "not totally pleasant" rooms; the next year the rooms were larger and more comfortable; finally rooms with private baths were assigned. During the last years of her visits Hilda was given lovely doctors' quarters facing the river, fully stocked with food and beverages. In the final year, a daily maid was provided.[29] Over time, also, the hospital superintendent began to consult with her during her visits. Peplau convinced him to put the more qualified and more sensitive RNs in the admissions wards and to give them a chance to counsel with patients before assigning them to a ward. The objective was to cut down on the movement of patients toward and into the back wards, where they were destined to become chronic patients. Finally, in Hilda's tenth year in Indiana, the superintendent took her advice and assigned the best, most competent nurses to admissions, thus stemming the seemingly endless flow of patients directly to the back wards.[30]

Hilda's experiences in Indiana were not, however, all easy ones. While Hilda was conducting a workshop at Logansport State Hospital, a very verbal doctor began to attend the afternoon lectures. The lectures were open to anyone, but Hilda always made it clear that only the nurse participants could ask questions. She felt that the workshops belonged to them and she did not want them intimidated by supervisors or physicians taking over the discussions. While nurse supervisors often attended these lectures, it was most unusual for physicians to do so. After the first afternoon, when the doctor had raised a number of questions, Hilda took him aside and again explained that he was welcome to attend, but not to ask questions. She assured him she would be pleased to have lunch with him to respond to his specific questions, if he liked. Or, she would talk with him about the work in general for as long as he liked after 4:00 p.m. when the workshop day ended. He nodded curtly and walked off. The next day he was back. He interrupted often, tried to lecture the students, and constantly assumed an air of authority. Each time, without responding to his questions or to the points he was trying to make, Hilda would simply point out the rules and continue the discussions. The third day he was back again, and again began to interrupt. This time, Hilda asked him to leave if he could not observe the rules of the session. He left very angrily, got into his car, and drove right into the path of an oncoming train.[31] The accident was fatal. Peplau felt very guilty that she had not perceived that this physician needed help, and that she had reacted primarily to his position and his inappropriate claim to special prerogatives. Never again would she let status or position blind her to the individual. After this sad experience, she paused to assess analytically not only the nurses but also the doctors with whom she interacted.[32]

Michigan

Hilda made her first trip to Michigan in 1958. It was a difficult one. She had been invited by Luther Christman, the mental health nurse consultant in Michigan, to give a workshop for nurses at a hospital for the mentally retarded. In accepting the invitation, Hilda had not realized this was a hospital for children, many of whom suffered from either hydrocephalus or Down's syndrome.[33] Hilda arrived with Tish, and as would become the norm, they were housed on the hospital grounds. Hilda's mission was to work with the nurses and families to assist them in appreciating the psychosocial needs of these patients. The hospital itself was immaculate, and the patients were well cared for, but only in a purely custodial way. Although she was moved, and convinced that nurses working with families could make a difference in the lives of these patients, Hilda found the work too depressing to want to continue to do it herself. Her feelings in this regard were not helped by the fact that one of the retarded patients had attached himself to Tish and followed her incessantly during the 5 days Tish and Hilda were there. One day this patient took Tish into the hydrocephalic ward, a very depressing experience. Tish was sympathetic and seemed to bear it well, but Hilda was not comfortable. Her own discomfort on encountering these patients, together with her concern about the impact of the week here on Tish, helped her decide, reluctantly, that this was one hospital to which she could not return. This decision was not typical of her. Usually she took all in stride, but deformed and retarded children were too much even for Hilda Peplau to bear. She did return to Michigan, but not to this particular hospital. She also lost touch with Luther Christman, clearly a dedicated nurse with whom she had much in common.[34]

New Mexico

The New Mexico stop on the way from California back east was always a welcome one. For Hilda, New Mexico was truly the Land of Enchantment. She loved the desert, the mountains, the old Spanish culture, and the clear air of the high mountain plains. She conducted her first New Mexico workshop in 1958 at the invitation of Katherine Norris, who had been an early student of Hilda's at TC and later became the nurse consultant at the New Mexico State Hospital in Las Vegas, New Mexico. The following year, Kay Norris and Josephine van der Meer, then an instructor of nursing at the University of New Mexico (UNM) in Albuquerque, convinced the dean of the College of Nursing at UNM, Virginia Crenshaw, to seek an NIMH grant for clinical workshops. In 1959, a 5-year grant was awarded for a week-long workshop in psychiatric nursing, to be held in the month of July each year, at the state hospital at Las Vegas.[35] Thus, from 1958 on, Hilda would stop in Las Vegas where she was housed in a dormitory on the campus of Highlands University while she conducted workshops at the hospital. The students came from the University of New Mexico, and from across the country. The first class was limited to 16 RNs, 5 from UNM and 11 from around the country.[36]

Hilda soon came to love New Mexico and to look forward to the summer experience there. Las Vegas, New Mexico, is 40 miles northeast of the state capital in Santa Fe. Lying at 6,470 feet in the foothills of the Sangre de Cristo Mountains, it was a sleepy, unpretentious place, cool in the summers and seemingly remote from the hectic modern world. Off the beaten track, Las Vegas has long played a kind of Sienna to Santa Fe's Florence. Home to gunslingers and bandits in the 19th century, the town fell into genteel desuetude for most of the 20th century. The historic, authentic plaza offered a few good cafes and coffee shops, but no other diversions. Over a hundred of its lovely Queen Anne, Romanesque, and Victorian homes are on the National Register of Historic Places. At twilight, the mountains glow a blood-red color, and the sky seems to reach to infinity. For Hilda, Las Vegas, New Mexico was a special place. The summer workshops there were just as intense as anywhere else, but the mountain air and breath-taking vistas added solace for the soul.

Hilda loved nothing more than to drive into the hills overlooking the Pecos River Valley with Tish, to watch the sunsets and feel the healing power of the high desert air. For several summers a male nurse from Oklahoma drove down in a 2-ton flatbed truck in which he kept a prodigious array of camping equipment, cooking utensils, and an ample supply of spirits. Several times during the workshop he would take Hilda and a few students into the lovely Gallinas Canyon, just 6 miles south of town. The road from Las Vegas crosses a flat prairie until it suddenly drops below an horizon of swells on the landscape. Here the headwaters of the Gallinas River, fed by spring runoff, have created a startlingly narrow, rocky canyon. In the ribbon of the Gallinas Canyon the spring water and the cooler air that sinks to such naturally low places have brought about diverse changes in the habitat, the most striking aspect of which is a string of pools dammed up behind slabs of sandstone that have toppled from the canyon walls. Biologists describe such zones of unexpected, sudden, and surprising change as microclimates. Hikers, artists, and poets see such treasures as miracles to be enjoyed, and so did Hilda Peplau.

Once the truck stopped, out came the camp stove and picnic food while the bottle of martinis cooled in the nearest pond. While supper cooked over an open fire, Hilda often talked about her visions for nursing. Here, in this pristine place, full of beauty and peace, with only the grumpy croaking of frogs echoing up and down this cool oasis, anything seemed possible. Here, students could envision all of which she spoke—and, from here, many a new nursing leader in fact did emerge.[37]

Kansas

In 1960 Hilda stopped for the first time on her cross-country circuit in Kansas, at the Parsons State Hospital and Training Center. It was after conducting a workshop at Parsons that Peplau decided she needed assistance in conducting some of these workshops. Parsons, like the hospital in Michigan, was a hospital for mentally retarded children, who were basically warehoused in custodial care. In spite of the name on the hospital, very little training was provided, and in spite of the presence of behavioral psychologists, little behavioral modification was done to help mentally retarded children to use or develop whatever skills or abilities they possessed. In fairness, not much was known about rehabilitation for the mentally retarded in the late 1950s and early 1960s. Peplau found the work itself very, very discouraging, but the desire of the staff to be positive and helpful was very encouraging. Thus, she invited Shirley Smoyak to join her in this work the following year.[38] Smoyak had been in Peplau's first class in psychiatric nursing at Rutgers, earning her MS in 1959. She later returned to Rutgers to teach in the graduate program and work on her PhD in sociology. For the next several years, Peplau worked directly with the staff and children at Parsons, and Smoyak worked with the families. Because she felt that this was indeed helpful and useful work, she began to go back in the winter to follow up with the families, and encourage them in their commitment to these children. The superintendent at Parsons, Dr. Howard Baer, was so impressed with the results that he eventually agreed to let nurses carry their own caseload of families. The psychologists and social workers were none too happy to have the nurses treading on their turf, but it was clear to Dr. Baer that the nurses were making an impact with the families, whereas the psychologists were focused on testing and the social workers on providing family services and financial support.[39] Here was an example of psychiatry appreciating the work of psychiatric nurses, and encouraging them to pursue it. Hilda treasured the Parsons experience, because it gave her a clear sense of having made a difference in the lives of patients. She therefore tried to make a return trip every winter, both to do follow-up work with the families and to encourage the nurses in their work.[40]

California

Hilda returned to California in 1958 to spend 3 weeks at the Napa State Hospital and continued to make the California trip every year until 1969. The Napa Valley, whose name in a local Indian dialect means valley of plenty, is just that—a long, flat stretch of land with neatly ordered grape rows marching up to the mountainsides that flank the valley. The Mayacamas Mountains to the west and the Vaca range to the east frame a canvas of vines that change from succulent green to crisp golden yellow with each season. Stone buildings and bridges interrupt the landscape, giving the area the pleasing look of European farm country. When Hilda and Tish made the first of what became annual trips to Napa, however, the region was not the Beverly Hills of agriculture that it later became, with art shows, smart shops, gourmet restaurants, and seemingly endless wineries arrayed in any number of architectural styles. Then, the town of Napa was more likely to be served by the local A & W Root Beer stand and Dairy Queen than wine-tasting boutiques and the tours of the wineries themselves tended to be informal. There were motels, with postage-stamp-sized swimming pools, but no elegant little bed and breakfasts as there are now. The quality of Napa accommodations, however, was not a consideration for Hilda and Tish. They would be staying on the grounds of the Napa State Hospital. In 1960 Helen Nahm, dean of the College of Nursing at the University of California, San Francisco (UCSF) applied for and received an National Institute of Mental Health grant to support the work, and to support her own faculty's participation in the workshops. Faculty members from the UCSF College of Nursing participated first as students and then as assistant instructors. Graduate students, supported by stipends, also joined the program. Shirley Smoyak joined Hilda there as a co-instructor in 1962, and often Hilda brought one or two of her current Rutgers graduate students with her to assist in the program. This participatory experience was continued for 7 years, until the entire College of Nursing faculty in San Francisco had received the Peplau workshop training.

With stipend support from the National Institute of Mental Health and the U.S. Public Health Service, the emphasis in California was to introduce the nurse faculty members to the techniques of the nurse-patient relationship so that they might incorporate it into their curriculum while preparing graduate students as clinical specialists.[41] In this way, an important Peplau goal was addressed; namely, upgrading the level of nursing education at the university level.

At Napa State Hospital a new routine gradually emerged. In the mornings, students met in pairs with patient groups. In accord with her conviction that staff's help with the workshops obligated her to offer something in return, Peplau held a 1-hour "staff seminar" every afternoon. Any staff member could attend. At one of these sessions, a staff member asked if Hilda would agree to interview a patient herself. She said she would, but stipulated that she would relay data to the group only if the patient agreed. Another staff member volunteered that the patient they had selected, Lucinda, was "the worst patient in this hospital." Peplau replied that nonetheless, she would see her. The ward on which Lucinda resided was one reserved for patients who were violent and hard to manage. Shirley Smoyak recalls that the staff had selected Lucinda because she had hit, kicked, punched, or bitten every staff member, as well as other patients. She also cursed creatively, starting at the beginning of the alphabet and going forward. In the first interview, the staff huddled about, waiting for Hilda or Shirley to be "belted."[42] Rather, with Peplau leading her, Lucinda related the circumstances of her commitment, which she attributed to anger toward her brother whom she considered to be her mother's favorite. Smoyak took verbatim notes as no tape recorders were allowed in this unit. The staff were dumbfounded when the interview ended peacefully, without any violent or verbal incident.[43]

Hilda then suggested that Shirley continue to see Lucinda daily at a time when the students were engaged in group work. Smoyak recalls that

Most of what Lucinda talked about was her "bad rap" in being hospitalized when she was not sick. She did describe "getting sick" after being at Napa and being unable to control her limbs. One of her many diagnoses was "schizophrenia—catatonic type." One very hot day when I went to see her she was lying on a macadam patio, partly under a bench, with her head resting on her arm.[44]

Smoyak relates that she invited Lucinda to come inside, out of the heat, and that Lucinda refused, until Smoyak herself got up to go inside. Lucinda muttered something about Smoyak being a "wimp," but followed her into the building, asking Smoyak (who was then pregnant) when the baby was due, about her other children, and wondering aloud what kind of mother she was.

She also told me that she was to be the subject of a lecture that afternoon, by a psychiatrist she "hated." At about 1:45, an aide came to get her for the lecture and was appalled that she was speaking to me. The subject of the lecture was "catatonia," and the lecturer was using Lucinda to demonstrate "waxy flexibility." The psychiatrist complained to the administration that I was ruining his "subject material" and tried to get the UCSF program out of the hospital, or at least off his ward. I continued to see Lucinda.[45]

Each year when Peplau and Smoyak returned to Napa, Smoyak would take up the work with Lucinda, who would make great progress only to regress again between summer workshops. Smoyak asked to see the mother, but this meeting never occurred. Instead, the mother wrote letters to the administration demanding that they remove "that stupid, pregnant social worker" from her daughter's treatment team. Smoyak saw the problem as this: Lucinda's mother had a vested interest in keeping her daughter in the hospital; she was seeking vindication for having institutionalized her daughter in the first place. Smoyak notes that

Each year when I returned, Lucinda was still on the same ward. Some years she just stared at me blankly, not hostilely, for a day or two. Then she would begin to speak and delighted in telling me stories about how she had outwitted the staff. When I approached the subject of discharge, her anxiety increased tremendously and she would yell at me to "knock it off." However, she never hit me.[46]

The young woman remained in the hospital until she was deinstitution-alized in the 1980s movement to empty out all mental hospitals.[47] Lucinda's story does illustrate, however, that when a nurse treats a patient with respect and tries to understand the patient's circumstances and world, the patient may well respond and progress can be made.

In 1963, in addition to the workshops at Napa and Fresno, Moffitt University Hospital in San Francisco was added to the itinerary. Here Peplau and Smoyak began to give the first workshops ever on psychoso-matic illnesses funded as a part of a grant awarded UCSF to study migraines, gastric ulcers, colitis, and similar conditions. For the next 5 years, Hilda and Shirley continued to give these workshops, thus open-ing up another area for nurse clinical practice. At Moffitt, each student nurse again worked with one patient. They prepared family histories and worked to help patients in the vacuum left between the doctors' work and that of the nurses. No medications were used, just "talking." The two psychiatrists on the staff understood what was being attempted and were very supportive. The staff nurses, too, although initially resentful and suspicious, eventually became very supportive.[48] As at Napa, UCSF urged all of its College of Nursing faculty to attend these workshops at Moffitt. The work in San Francisco, with the support of the hospital psy-chiatrists, the College of Nursing faculty, and the dean and hospital direc-tor, was a far cry from the early days at Napa, when Hildegard and her workshops were met with great suspicion and outright hostility from the nursing staff.

North Carolina

The Dean of the College of Nursing at the University of North Carolina, Elizabeth Kemble, an early believer in Peplau's theories, was among the first to suggest that she give workshops across the country. North Carolina soon became a part of the regular summer workshop circuit. In 1957, Kemble applied for an NIMH grant to support workshops in North Carolina and to assure that North Carolina colleges of nursing could send their faculty as trainees to these workshops.[49] Two consecutive 5-year grants were received, providing support for 10 years of workshops.

In one state mental institution where workshops were held in 1958, Peplau found that many of the women patients with whom the trainees worked showed unusual signs of shame or sadness. It wasn't until the second week of the 2-week workshop that a patient revealed that these emotions were connected to a fear common among patients that they would be subjected to complete hysterectomies. At that time, it was pos-sible for a North Carolina man to put his wife in a mental hospital and authorize, without her consent, a surgical sterilization. The resulting depression and continued hospitalization then became grounds for divorce.

This had happened to many of the women in this hospital. The women learned that they could trust no one—that physicians accommodated the husbands. Older patients oriented new patients, and all stuck together in a system of silence, covertly supporting one another through this trauma.[50]

Once she had insight into the problem, Hilda began to design appropriate strategies. For this particular situation, she believed the appropriate approach to be group work. Group work, however, got off to a rocky start. The patients seemed abnormally anxious. They paced the floor, only to be chased back to their seats by the male attendants who had posted themselves at the door, reportedly to "protect" the faculty trainee observers. Eventually, on the next to the last day, the superintendent agreed to dispense with the attendant guards at the door. The patients became less anxious. The work could begin. Physically, it was exhausting. The staff continued to watch the faculty trainees closely, the trainees were extra careful to take exceedingly detailed notes, and Hilda went over them in even greater detail than usual. In this case, Peplau was dealing with a particularly difficult *collective* problem: the women patients' (justifiable) fear of sterilization and abandonment by a male-dominated culture—husband, doctor, guard. The behavior of the male attendants in this hospital reinforced the women's feelings of betrayal and heightened their anxiety. Here, as elsewhere, Hilda faced an obstacle to her work that was common to many institutions. It was the attendants, not the psychiatrists, who tried time and again to sabotage her work. Here, the 2-week workshop was not enough to counter an entrenched system in which hospital staff and physicians had a vested interest. The nurse faculty trainees, however, learned firsthand the importance of seeking to understand both the system and group dynamics in order to impact care.

After 1962, Peplau's work centered at the Dorothea Dix Hospital in Raleigh, where Shirley Smoyak would join her. Beginning that summer and continuing for the next 5 years, Peplau and Smoyak would meet up in California to conduct the Napa workshops and open the Moffitt program, after which Peplau would head east to Las Vegas, New Mexico while Smoyak continued with the Moffitt workshops. At the conclusion of the workshop in San Francisco, Smoyak would put her two, then three, then four children into the car and with her husband, Neil, at the wheel, would race back across the country from California to North Carolina. During these summers, Hilda and Tish and the entire Smoyak family became very close friends. It was a family atmosphere. In Raleigh, the Smoyak clan would meet up with Hilda at the Alamo Hotel on U.S. Route 1. While not exactly luxurious, the Alamo did have a pool for the children and a kitchen so that meals could be fixed on site. Shirley did the cooking for everyone, and the girls shared the cleaning-up chores. Cockroaches and even rats were sometimes a challenge, but the Alamo nonetheless suited their purposes—cheap and convenient. Neil provided child care while Shirley and Hilda were working. A local dress shop offered a favorite opportunity for back-to-school shopping for Tish, and Tish and Hilda often took short excursions into the countryside with a picnic basket to enjoy the surroundings. North Carolina always brought back a bit of nostalgia for the good memories of the days in Ashville and picnics with Uncle Walter and Auntie Anne. One summer while Tish went to Ghana with the Experiment in International Living, Hilda continued to bunk in with the Smoyaks, and Aunt Hilda became an important part of the Smoyak children's lives, a relationship that would continue over the decades.

At Dix itself, Peplau and Smoyak were always treated well. Arriving on Sunday night, they would be invited to have dinner with the superintendent and his wife on the porch of their spacious home on the grounds. The superintendent was dubious that nurses could do more than provide custodial care, but he was always gracious. Unlike the basement assignments in hospitals elsewhere, Dix always provided a light and airy classroom, and an effort was made by the staff to select patients according to the criteria set by Peplau. Here as in all state hospitals, however, there was sabotage. Patients were routinely given electroshock treatments or sent elsewhere during the hour scheduled for the nurse-patient interview. Nonetheless, Dix was the last hospital on the summer "tour" and a good experience overall.

Arriving on a Sunday toward the end of August in 1965, however, Hilda knew almost immediately that something was amiss. The superintendent and his wife were tense and barely communicative. Finally, they expressed their dismay and worry about events to occur the next day. That Monday was to be the day of the official integration of the separate Black and White mental hospitals in the state. Dix in Raleigh and the Black hospital in Butner were to exchange patients. Peplau and Smoyak agreed to be in the wards early with the faculty trainees from the University of North Carolina to help ease any tension that might arise when the Black patients arrived, and to intervene if any difficulties arose.

The patients from Butner arrived early on the scheduled morning and as always, Peplau and Smoyak tried to project confidence in order for the faculty trainees to feel secure and to overcome any sense of apprehension that might be communicated by the staff. The staff had predicted riots on the wards, thus raising the tension level considerably. The first day was tense, but seemed to go smoothly enough. On the second day, however, a White patient on the women's ward where Peplau's students were working began shouting. From what Hilda and Shirley could gather, she was upset that a Black patient had stolen her peach. Soon other patients joined in. Hilda sprang into action, wading into the melee and separating the patients into two groups while Shirley Smoyak tried to quiet them down. Peplau kept the quieter patients with her and the trainees while

Smoyak took the more disturbed patients into a separate room. When they got into the room, the shouting about stolen peaches erupted again. Smoyak quickly determined these patients were angry and disturbed, but not psychotic. She reported this to Hilda.[51]

By this time other patients and staff were trying to get into the ward. Hilda suggested that Shirley keep the most disturbed patients in the other room and told the students to begin a group therapy session with the patients in their group. Hilda herself went to stand in the door fending off the staff, who had arrived on the scene prepared to use restraints to carry disturbed patients off into seclusion. Peplau stood stolidly in the door, assuring the staff everything was under control, while in the room with Shirley, patients were threatening one another, shouting, and throwing shoes. The situation there, in fact, seemed quite close to being very out of control. Shirley Smoyak, an energetic 5-foot, 2-inch bundle of energy, first separated two patients on the verge of attacking each other by literally hurling them into different corners of the room, then climbed up onto a chair, loudly whistled, and shouted "STOP THAT!!!" In the moment of shocked silence that ensued, she ordered the patients to *sit down*, and say what they had to say, one by one. By noon each had spoken her piece and calm was restored. Smoyak informed them that they would meet together in that room every morning at 8:00 for the rest of the week, which they did. By the end of the week, speaking with one another normally, they began to sing hymns together, and even to share cigarettes—a sure sign of "sisterhood." Not surprisingly, the upset had nothing to do with "peaches." It had to do with the fact that the Dix patients perceived that the Black patients smelled like "rotten peaches," perhaps due to poor hygiene. Once the newcomers began taking showers and wearing clean clothes, the problems evaporated. The patients realized that they were all in the same boat and that they could help one another.[52] From then on, the work went smoothly. Once again, Peplau had demonstrated that treating patients with respect, urging them to air their concerns, and listening attentively can be effective and more beneficial than using restraints or drugs.

Ohio

Like Indiana and North Carolina, Ohio was one of the first states on the annual summer circuit and one that remained an annual workshop site. Hilda enjoyed the respite in Ohio because one of the stops was the state hospital in Dayton, where Grayce Sills and her husband lived. The Ohio workshops became very special, because it was here her growing friendship with Grayce Sills was nourished. Sills attended Ohio University in Athens, and in 1946, between her sophomore and junior years, had attended a Quaker summer camp that provided an experience in a mental hospital as a part of its program.[53] That summer 90 college students worked as attendants at the Rockland State Hospital in Orangeburg, New York—the hospital about which *The Snake Pit* would later be written. Grayce was among 12 students who, in the Quaker tradition, decided they would enter nursing in order to "do something" about the appalling conditions they witnessed at Rockland. She never returned to Ohio University. Instead, she stayed at Rockland and earned a diploma in its school of nursing. She found herself in 1951–1952 in New York, at Teachers College, where she was baffled by this "weird woman who was just off the wall, who had us running all over the place trying to make connections between what we learned, what we were seeing, and what we were doing."[54] Grayce knew nothing of the drama unfolding around Hilda Peplau that year at TC. She only knew that she herself had not finished college, that she had only a diploma from a state hospital, and that she was taking classes with MA students being taught by a "crazy woman" who truly believed they could either save or change the world. It was all too fast for Grayce. The combination of being in New York City, feeling inadequate in her classes, and the high expectations of her professor, made her feel very uncomfortable. When her brother-in-law called asking her to return to Ohio to help take care of her ailing sister, Grayce gave a huge sigh of relief and fled. Hilda by this time was too immersed in her own problems to do what she normally would have done—inquired as to what had happened to the young woman from Ohio. Grayce married a psychiatrist and stayed in Ohio, where she worked with her husband at the state hospital in Dayton.

By 1957 she began to hear about an incredible nurse from the east who was giving workshops in Indiana. Soon, nurses from Ohio were going to Indiana for these workshops. They came back with the news that "Dr. Peplau said we were lucky to have you in Ohio." Sills was floored. She couldn't believe that Hilda Peplau remembered her at all, let alone believed that she might have something on the ball. In those years, Hilda never lost a chance to affirm any nurse in whom she encountered courage and intelligence. She sent word that she would come to Ohio the next summer—which she did and continued to do every summer after that until 1969. Grayce Sills would go on for her MA and doctorate and become a lifelong friend and traveling companion to Hilda, as well as a highly acclaimed nurse in her own right. Peplau had found a colleague with whom she could share, both intellectually and personally. It was an enduring friendship that would see her through the rest of her career and provide much joy in retirement.

While the summer workshop experiences were generally positive and very affirming, Peplau did encounter her share of snake pits, places where she felt hopeless and helpless, unable to impact patient care one iota. Such experiences were seared into her memory, and acted to assure a deep humility when she herself discussed the summer workshop experience. By far her most distressing experience was in Ohio.

Grayce Sills accompanied her to the Ohio State Hospital in Athens in 1958, and stayed through the first day. Here the contradictions were nearly beyond comprehension. The hospital in appearance was peaceful, even beautiful. During the Great Depression of the early 1930s, the superintendent's wife had scoured the countryside buying up priceless antiques cheaply. All the wards were splendidly furnished—rocking chairs, settees, paintings. The feeling evoked was of a lovely country home, or museum. Grayce warned Hilda not to be taken in by the surroundings, for this lovely museum concealed chambers of horror.[55]

After Grayce left, Hilda knew immediately that something was very wrong, more wrong than in other hospitals where she had worked. The staff was withdrawn, and nothing she did drew them out. The patients were clearly depressed and resigned with a resignation that went far beyond what she had seen in other hospitals. The patients selected by the staff for the nurse-patient interviews were all blind in at least one eye and appeared unreachable. When Hilda inquired about the blindness, she received only blank stares from the staff. While she was used to working with patients deemed hopeless and selected from the back wards, these patients were clearly in a class by themselves. Grayce had left, and she had no one with whom she could discuss the situation. It wasn't until the fourth day when a woman physician on the staff—who had been particularly thoughtful, keeping ice water available on the hot wards and providing a fan for the lectures in the afternoon—told Hilda in private and in confidence that these patients had all been seen by Dr. Walter Freeman, and that she felt so guilty about it that she'd assigned them to Peplau's workshops in the hope that something could be done to help them. She confided that the State of Ohio had a federal grant to experiment with lobotomies, and Dr. Freeman and his partner, Dr. James Watts, had the contract to conduct the "experiments."[56]

Peplau had heard of Dr. Freeman of course (nearly everyone had), but had not seen him in action. She was about to. The next week the doctor arrived, driving his "lobotomobile"—a van equipped with his instruments. He swept through the wards, picking patients at random: "I'll take that one, and that one." The selected patients were taken to a room where they were tied to chairs by the staff. Once the patients were restrained, Freeman breezed in. He read no charts, asked no questions about a patient's history or condition, did not check up on prior patients from earlier forays through the hospital. Patient number one was wheeled before him. He put electrodes on her temples and shocked her into a faint, lifted her left eyelid, and plunged an instrument resembling an ice pick into her head. He pulled it out, dipped the bloody pick into the alcohol emesis basin, and moved on to the next patient. Again he shocked and stabbed, and another, and then again another, and so on, and on, remorselessly, in a production line of controlled, casual violence that left 40 to 50 patients bloodied and blinded.

Hilda, seized by nausea and stunned by the sheer horror of what she had witnessed, left the room. Afterward, she visited the patients in a dark and silent ward, where they lay supine on beds, or cried quietly, their faces disfigured with a questioning blankness. She had no answers for them. The victims were all women, committed and abandoned for the most part by their husbands. Many such patients would be released to drift off into oblivion, many others would spend the rest of their lives quietly in the back wards, forgotten by society and their families. In Athens, Ohio, they would certainly be in no condition to do damage to the priceless antiques among which they shuffled aimlessly.

Dr. Freeman practiced lobotomy with a recklessness that bordered on lunacy. Hilda was sickened and appalled, but there was absolutely nothing she could do. Freeman's work was sanctioned by both the American Medical Association and the American Psychiatric Association. The interest in lobotomy as a means of altering personality began in this country in 1847, when a manual laborer of Irish extraction named Phineas Gage was injured in a mining explosion during which an iron bar was driven through the front of his head.[57] To the surprise of everyone involved, Gage survived the removal of the protruding bar, but his personality was much changed. Once an angry, hostile, and disruptive man, he was now quiet and subdued. As a result of this crude surgery, the extraction of the iron bar, Phineas Gage became the object of immense medical interest.

Walter Freeman went to medical school at the University of Pennsylvania and in the early 1930s was appointed professor of neurology at George Washington University in Washington, D.C. In 1935 he attended a neurological conference in London where a celebrated Portuguese neurosurgeon reported on the results of the first full frontal lobotomy performed on a uncontrollable female asylum patient in Lisbon. After the "surgery," this woman was quiet and accommodating, no trouble at all. Remembering the case of Phineas Gage, Walter Freeman was excited. He vowed he would experiment with lobotomies, and would thereby become famous. Although he was a neurologist, Freeman had no qualifications as a surgeon. He needed a neurosurgeon as a collaborator if he was to experiment with lobotomies, and so enlisted his colleague, Dr. Watts. Freeman and Watts became virtual crusaders for lobotomy as a way of controlling patients in mental hospitals. They traveled the country, seeking out patients on whom to perform the surgery. The procedure drew outraged responses from psychoanalysts and many psychiatrists, but reservations were not voiced to the public for several decades. In

1948 Freeman was elected president of the American Board of Psychiatry and Neurology. He was now a full-fledged celebrity. He gave lectures across the country extolling the amazing potential of lobotomies for controlling society's misfits, specifically schizophrenics, homosexuals, communists, etc. By 1955, over 40,000 men, women, and children in the United States had undergone psychosurgery that damaged their brains and turned them into vegetables to be left in the custody of the state mental hospitals.[58]

By the 1950s, psychiatrists began to raise their reservations in public, but mental hospital populations were soaring and cures were few. Thus the combination of overcrowding and limited budgets persuaded hospital superintendents to adopt lobotomy as a way of controlling agitated patients.[59] By this time, Freeman was operating alone, Watts having abandoned the practice as too extreme. Freeman charged $250 per lobotomy and, according to him, the patient would be left with nothing worse than a black eye and a splitting headache, his or her "anxiety" would be relieved, and he or she could then live "peacefully" for the rest of his or her life. Initially used as a last resort, the lobotomy had now become the *first step* to creating a manageable personality. Freeman crossed and recrossed America on what he called his "head-hunting" expeditions, promoting the ice pick, looking for new patients. Fortunately for Peplau's sense of self and commitment to hope, her path did not again cross his. From that day in Ohio onward, though, she would be a passionate crusader against the practice, shaming her psychiatrist colleagues into speaking out against it.

Astonishingly, there were no reliable sustained studies of the effects of lobotomy on patients, only Freeman's eternally optimistic reports. Again and again, Peplau pleaded with nurses to do such studies themselves, but no one did.[60] In 1952, chlorpromazine, the first of a new generation of revolutionary tranquilizers, was tested in France. It signaled the end for Walter Freeman. His pool of potential victims would begin to diminish, along with his reputation. By 1954, Thorazine was approved for use in the United States. In 1962 Ken Kesey's *One Flew Over the Cuckoo's Nest* was published. The Pulitzer Prize winning novel became a bestseller and was made into an Academy Award winning motion picture. It presented a damning portrayal of a psychiatric hospital and the effects of lobotomy. By the late 1950s and on into the 1960s, the inert, emotionless, inhuman quality of many of the lobotomized, who were now everywhere to be seen, began to revolt the public. Well into the 1960s, however, Freeman was still "head-hunting," and would continue to do so until 1967 when his surgical privileges were finally removed by the AMA. He died in May 1972, at the age of 77, still believing in his methods and motives.[61]

Chicago State Hospital

Peplau's witness to the practice of surgical sterilization of mental patients or to the brutalities inflicted upon them by heartless lobotomies were by no means her only experiences with the regressive, even medieval, practices she found in the nation's public mental hospitals. Some, however, were more benign. Such was the case with the oddly reactionary culture she encountered on her first visit to Chicago State Hospital in 1964.

Chicago was to be Hilda's first workshop stop of the summer. Tish was there working for the summer as a research assistant in social psychology in the research laboratory of Professor Fred Strodtbeck. Hilda had driven straight through from New Jersey, and she was tired. She had driven alone and would meet Tish there. The 2-week workshop for nurses at Chicago State had been arranged by Mary Lohr, who had been a student at TC and was now dean of the College of Nursing at the University of Illinois. Mary met Hilda when she arrived late on a Saturday afternoon and took her to an apartment on the grounds of the hospital where she was to stay. The two sat talking and gossiping for about an hour. Hilda went out to meet Tish for dinner, returning to the apartment after 9:00, collapsing into bed. She had just fallen asleep when the voices started coming through her open window: "Sara, Sara, Saraaaaaaaara—are you in there, Sara??? Sara, oh Sara," the voices pleaded. Hilda was annoyed. The voices continued calling and pleading until she got up and closed the window. As it happened, she was staying in the apartment of the late Sara Abrams, a well-known nursing figure in Chicago circles during the 1940s—but this was 1964! The next morning, slightly uneasy after a fitful night, Hilda had a cup of coffee, moved a vase of plastic flowers into a closet and thus out of view, and set out to find a newspaper. When she returned to the apartment, she was surprised to find the coffee cup washed and put away, and the plastic flowers back on the table. This is strange, she thought.

In spite of a feeling that things were a bit "odd" here, she was nonetheless taken aback when she walked out onto the hospital grounds just before noon and caught sight of dozens of women sitting on camp chairs beside large wicker picnic baskets. They were feeding their grown sons, who sat on the ground at their feet. Hilda walked among them largely unnoticed. After the feeding, out came washcloths, towels, shaving cream, and razors as the mothers washed and shaved the men. She would soon discover that many of the patients here were retarded rather than mentally ill. By 4:00, the visitors were gone and the patients had returned to their wards.

That night over dinner with Mary Lohr, Hilda inquired first about nocturnal voices and reappearing plastic flowers, and then about the afternoon picnic scene. Lohr explained that Sara Abrams had been so revered by both patients and staff here that nothing could be changed. Insofar as possible, all was kept exactly as she had left it, including the innovation of the Sunday picnics for the male patients and their mothers. For Hilda, that night was again full of patients calling for Sara. The next morning the instant cleanup and restoration of the apartment was repeated. It was too disorienting, and Peplau decided to move to a motel on the highway, at her own expense, for the duration of the workshop.[62]

This workshop proved to be a difficult experience. The absentee hand of Sara Abrams still ruled, the conditions on the wards were appalling, and the hospital superintendent was as neurotic as any she had met. He was afraid of the patients. He drove to his office, parked right outside the door, and went in and shut the door, never leaving the office during the day. Clearly Hilda needed help here. The next year she would bring Anita Werner and Sheila Rouslin, two of her students from Rutgers, as assistants.[63] Before she was through, she had convinced this superintendent that he had to break the obsession with Sara Abrams and that to do it he had to begin by demolishing "Sara's" apartment.

MOVING FORWARD

By the early 1960s, Hilda had shifted her focus, both at Rutgers and in the summer workshops from work primarily with individual patients to work with both patients and their families. As she had at PHTS, Bennington, in the army, and at TC, Hilda continued at Rutgers her lifelong habit of voraciously reading. She did her best to incorporate new psychiatric, psychological, and nursing ideas into her teaching and practice. The development of family systems theory interested her very much and seemed a logical extension of her interest in interpersonal relationships. The emphasis in her workshops and teaching shifted from an exclusive focus on individuals, to groups, and then to families. At Rutgers, Peplau's students had worked from the mid-1950s on with families during their summer add-on clinical experiences in Red Bank, New Jersey. There families selected by the Monmouth County Organization of Social Services (MCOSS) met with graduate student nurses in family groups. By 1960, after trying different approaches, a form of family therapy had evolved in which Hilda had great confidence. In this, she emphasized the fundamentals of communication and family dynamics.

Working from this model, Hilda suggested to Rienna Hall, who had become dean of the College of Nursing at the University of New Mexico, that she seek a NIMH grant to support family therapy workshops in Albuquerque to train nurses in family therapy counseling. The grant was funded, and in 1962 the first workshop was conducted in an old Catholic private hospital, Nazareth Psychiatric Hospital, run by Dominican nuns.

During the workshops, the students and faculty were housed on the first floor of the Roman Catholic convent adjacent to the Nazareth Hospital; Hilda herself stayed in a room usually reserved for the bishop when he was visiting, which amused her a great deal. Putting aside her fantasies, Hilda worked with the dean to develop the criteria for selecting the nurse participants. A public health background with experience in the community and in patients' homes was required. Peplau, together with one or two faculty members from the university's mental health center, then met with Veterans Administration officials to select the participant families.[64] The program grew to the extent that Shirley Smoyak from New Jersey and William Field from Texas soon joined the effort. Smoyak had become something an expert on "systems theory" through her training in sociology. Field was more psychodynamic, and complemented Smoyak nicely.

Nurses who participated in these workshops in New Mexico seemed to have a sense that something important was happening. One former participant wrote a general letter to all members of the State Nursing Association in New Mexico in 1966, stating that

> Any course under Peplau is magnificent, but this particular one is of very great value not only to the psychiatric nurse, but also to any nurse who really wants to improve her ability to work in an interpersonal relationship with any patient, physician or family . . . any nurse with any question about what nurses can do should take this workshop . . . When your course is finished, you will realize you have just started to learn . . . it will change your life.[65]

In fact, Hilda was trying to change not just individual lives, but the whole nursing profession. Working with her colleagues and students in the summer workshops, Hilda Peplau continually refined her own conceptual frameworks to explain and examine processes of healthy change, whether within families, between individuals, or in systems of care, while at the same time helping to redefine nursing itself.

Additionally, these conceptual frameworks helped to identify interrelationships not only within the family, but also between patient/family/physician/staff/nurse and their belief systems, and subsequent decisions. Assessments were made through hypothesizing, therapeutic questioning, and engaging family members in discussion to elicit a greater understanding of each member's hopes, fears, and coping styles.[66] Again and again Peplau emphasized that for nurses only knowledge about clinical phenomena and interventions that produced beneficial outcomes would promote the profession.

Each fall when she returned to Rutgers, Peplau was unrelenting in trying to get her students to think analytically and conceptually. Each semester each student had to choose a concept such as anger, conflict, guilt, anxiety, dependence, frustration, or envy; do a literature search on it; and then come up with an original interpretation based on the integration of the literature and his or her own clinical work. Peplau then worked with the students to develop clues that could be observed by any nurse so that she would know that this concept was operational in a specific situation. Then, during the summers, new insights in relation to the concepts studied at Rutgers would again be integrated into the workshop experience.[67] In this way, the academic work at Rutgers was constantly integrated into the summer work in the field. This summer work was used to help all nurses advance professionally. Peplau's unpublished papers in the Schlesinger Library recording this work provide a treasure trove of extensive and intensive theory concerning both student learning and patient care.

In her specialty of psychiatric nursing, it was clear that Hilda was deeply and humanely committed to improvement of nursing practice in public state mental hospitals, for this was where the large majority of the mentally ill were to be found during the years of her professional career. She honored that commitment through extraordinary work in those hospitals year in and year out, and in spite of or in addition to her full-time responsibilities at Rutgers. In her own words,

> If you had worked with the mentally ill as long as I have, you would know that one of the most tragic aspects of mental care today is that our mental institutions, the very places to which these tormented people turn for help, often provide a scene for the day by day, week by week, year by year reinforcement of a patient's illness until [s]he is virtually incurable. That this tragedy is the result of ignorance rather than malice, does not make it less a tragedy.[68]

In 1967, a former student invited Peplau to come north to Mendocino, California to conduct a 3-day "talking workshop" at the Mendocino State Hospital. Tish was now in college and no longer making the cross-country trek with her, so instead of driving, Hilda decided to splurge on a plane ticket. She flew from New Jersey to Ohio and then on to California, in order to have the time to drive up the California coast to Mendocino. The site of this remote and lovely northern California coastal town had been discovered by accident. A shipwrecked sailor washed ashore there in 1850. He was found a year later by the crew of another shipwreck, living happily in a log cabin on a bluff among the giant redwoods, above a small, but usable harbor. Before long, New England loggers came to build new homes and make their fortunes in lumber. On the bluff above the restless, dramatic surf, they built their down east Victorian houses to recreate homes left behind on another shore. A half-day's drive north from San Francisco, along the stunning, sinuous Pacific Coast Highway, the trip to Mendocino provided Peplau a quiet interlude in which to reflect, relax, and regather her strength and spirits for the year ahead. It was a time for transition, a time for reflection. Things looked grim at Rutgers, and Hilda knew it would be a difficult year. Thus, this trip to Mendocino was a conscious inner retreat—a private, special time—a luxury she seldom gave to herself. As it turned out, this solitary trip would conclude her bi-coastal summer workshop travel.[69]

ENDNOTES

1. Dorris O. Stewart to Barbara Callaway, August 31, 1992 (to be deposited in the Schlesinger Library collection).
2. Dorris O. Stewart, the nurse consultant in Indiana, became a one-person publicity machine, and was constantly reporting on the changes made in Indiana as a result of Hildegard Peplau's visits. Letters from Dorris O. Stewart may be found in the Schlesinger Library collection, Box 24, File #853, and interview, Dorris O. Stewart, June 21, 1996, in Washington, D.C.
3. Albert Deutsch, *The Shame of the States* (New York: Ayer Company Publishers, 1948).
4. See Gerald N. Grob, *From Asylum to Community* (Princeton: Princeton University Press, 1991), 260.
5. Interview, Hildegard Peplau, March 22, 1992.
6. Bruce Mericle, November 7, 1996, in New Brunswick, New Jersey. See also Peplau's categorization of "The Hallucinatory Process and Nursing Interventions" as outlined in a chapter entitled "Theoretical Constructs: Anxiety, Self, and Hallucinations" in Anita Werner O'Toole and Sheila Rouslin Welt, *Interpersonal Theory in Nursing Practice: Selected Works of Hilda E. Peplau* (New York: Springer Publishing, 1988), 270–336. It was her practice to work on one concept, or a set of concepts, during the summer workshops and then, based on the clinical data gleaned, to write papers to guide nurses in expanding their nursing practice. Her work on hallucinations is just one example. Others included work on schizophrenia, anxiety, loneliness, and the "Process of Focal Attention," now known as Learning Deficiency Disorder. Many of these working papers may be found in Box 14, #449–467.
7. These workshop experiences were discussed in great detail by Hilda Peplau in an interview on February 4, 1992, and in a long interview with Dr. Lee Spray, videotaped at the Inn at Honeyrun, Ohio, November 4, 1995. This tape is deposited in the Schlesinger Library, Box 45. See also Grayce Sills, "Hilda Peplau: Leader, Practitioner, Academician, Scholar and Theorist," *Perspectives in Psychiatric Care* XVI, (1998): 122–128. It should be noted that Peplau had been instrumental in assuring that the National Mental Health Act of 1946 and the subsequent funding of traineeships by the National Institute of Mental Health (NIMH) in 1948, included funds for psychiatric nursing graduate work. Thus, when a summer workshop nurse showed the ability and the interest to return to school, Peplau would provide the means. Whether nurses went to Rutgers or to another institution, it was often her direct influence and knowledge of programs and resources that sent them on their way. Largely because of these workshops, by the early 1960s, her influence in psychiatric nursing reached far, far beyond Rutgers, both inside and outside the academy.
8. Interview, Hildegard Peplau, February 4, 1992.
9. Sills, 123.
10. Hilda E. Peplau, *Basic Principles of Patient Counseling*, 2nd ed. (Philadelphia: Smith, Kline and French, 1964).

11. According to Peplau, she at first asked for reimbursement for expenses submitted. Beginning in 1959, she asked for $10 per day for expenses, and raised it to $50 per day by 1967. Interview, Hildegard Peplau, February 4, 1992.

12. Interview, Hildegard Peplau, February 4, 1992.

13. Interview, Hildegard Peplau, April 13, 1992.

14. Materials about the film, letters and correspondence, and drafts of the scripts may be found in Box 38, #1394, in the Schlesinger Library.

15. Letter from Hilda Peplau to Lee Bobker, n.d., Box 38, #1394.

16. Ibid.

17. Letters from Hilda Peplau to Peter Hickman, October 13, 1958, and Peter Hickman to Hilda Peplau, October 24, 1958, both in Box 38, #1394.

18. Letter from Peter Hickman to Hilda Peplau, December 2, 1958, in Box 38, #1394.

19. Letter from Peter Hickman to Hilda Peplau, March 3, 1959, Box 38, #1394.

20. Letter from Kathryn Linden to Hilda Peplau, March 10, 1959, Box 21, #736.

21. Ibid.

22. The Program for the Testimonial Dinner is found in Box 22, #742.

23. Letter from Hilda Peplau to Barbara Callaway, September 10, 1998.

24. Interview, Emily Holmquist, June 21, 1996, in Washington, D.C.

25. Interview, Claire Fagin, October 30, 1992.

26. Letter from Dorris O. Stewart to Barbara Callaway, August 31, 1992, and letters and materials in Box 23.

27. Martha Rogers, Director of Nursing at the Indiana Central State Hospital, should not be confused with Martha Rogers, nurse theoretician and professor of nursing at New York University.

28. Interview, Hildegard Peplau, February 5, 1992.

29. Ibid.

30. Ibid.

31. See newspaper clipping regarding this accident in Box 21, #726.

32. Interview, Hildegard Peplau, February 5, 1992.

33. Ibid.

34. Luther Christman later became Dean of the College of Nursing at the Rush Memorial and Roosevelt Hospital, and then at Vanderbilt University. He was widely recognized as a forward-thinking Dean and, like Peplau, emphasized the development of scholarship and research on nurse faculties. He and Hilda's paths, however, did not converge until both were well into retirement. In the early 1990s, they began to correspond with each other, retracing their careers. This wonderful correspondence is now deposited in the Schlesinger Library as a part of the Hilda Peplau collection.

35. Clippings about the grants and the grantees for these workshops may be found in Box 2, #33.

36. Clippings, Box 2, #33.

37. Katherine Norris, Grayce Sills, Josephine van der Meer, Bill Field, Rienna Hall, and Wanda Nations were all "alumni" of these mountain seminars.

38. Shirley Smoyak was in the first MS class in Psychiatric Nursing at Rutgers, earning her MS in 1959. She then went to Perth Amboy General Hospital as its first clinical specialist. They didn't know what to do with her. First of all, she wanted to do research, and no one could imagine what "research" a nurse could possibly do. Smoyak did a study of scopolamine—a drug given to women to produce amnesia of labor and delivery. Using the Apgar scale, Smoyak compared infant vital signs of 50 women who had been given scopalamine during childbirth with 50 women given just Demerol. The vital signs of infants whose mothers had been given scopolamine were much lower than those whose mothers had been given only Demerol. She took the study to the chief of pediatrics in order to get permission to

publish it. He confiscated the data, and Smoyak went to Peplau, asking what she should do. Peplau advised her to return to Rutgers, help teach in the graduate program, and work on her PhD. Smoyak earned her PhD in Sociology in 1970. She joined Peplau in the summer workshops for the first time at Parsons Hospital in Kansas in 1961. Beginning in 1962 and for the next 5 years, she regularly joined Peplau on the summer cross-country junkets. Interviews, Hildegard Peplau and Shirley Smoyak, March 16, 1992.

39. Interview, Hildegard Peplau, February 5, 1992.
40. Unfortunately, in the early 1970s psychologists replaced psychiatrists in administrating this hospital, and as that happened the role of nurses was again restricted to patient care or administering patient care. See letters to Hilda Peplau from Patricia Devine, RN, Director of Nursing, Parsons State Hospital, during the years 1968–1974 in Box 32, Schlesinger Library.
41. See materials related to these workshops in Boxes 21–24, Schlesinger Library. Beginning in 1960, a Rutgers faculty member went with her to help conduct the California workshops. Peg Marshall made the trip in 1960 and 1961, and Shirley Smoyak from 1962–1969.
42. Letter with enclosure from Shirley Smoyak to Barbara Callaway, July 10, 1999.
43. Interviews, Shirley Smoyak and Hildegard Peplau, March 16, 1992.
44. Ibid.
45. Letter from Shirley Smoyak, July 10, 1999.
46. Ibid.
47. Interviews, Shirley Smoyak and Hilda Peplau, op cit.
48. Interview, Shirley Smoyak, March 16, 1992, in Sherman Oaks, California.
49. Interview, Hildegard Peplau, March 16, 1992. Elizabeth Kemble had left TC in the early 1950s, under no illusions about the limitations and vindictiveness of R. Louise McManus. Thus it was that she had tried to encourage Hilda Peplau to accept a position in North Carolina after Hilda's own TC career was disrupted in 1952. Kemble kept up with Hilda's career after she went to Rutgers, and was a warm supporter of Peplau's efforts to make an impact on patient care in the public hospitals.
50. Interview, Hildegard Peplau, February 5, 1992.
51. Interview, Hildegard Peplau and Shirley Smoyak, March 16, 1992.
52. Ibid.
53. Interview, Grayce Sills, October 30, 1992.
54. Ibid.
55. Interview, Hildegard Peplau, February 4, 1992.
56. Interviews, Hildegard Peplau, February 4 and March 17, 1992.
57. Robert Youngston and Ian Schott, *Medical Blunders* (London: Robinson Publishing Company, 1996), 34.
58. Ibid, 35–43.
59. Grob, 128.
60. One of Peplau's great regrets was that she could never engage her students or summer workshop participants in doing follow-up studies. She actually received funding for one of her graduate students to do such a study in 1965, but it was never done.
61. Youngson and Schott, 57. See also the chapter of "Lobotomy" in Ronald Kessler, *The Sins of the Father: Joseph P. Kennedy and the Dynasty He Founded* (New York: Time Warner Books, 1996), 238–258. Joseph Kennedy had his mentally ill daughter, Rosemary, lobotomized by Freeman, with Watts supervising, in 1941.
62. Interview, Hildegard Peplau, February 4, 1992.
63. The next year, Peplau and the two students stayed in a larger motel, with a kitchen and swimming pool where the two students could cool off at night. Anita Werner

drove this year, so Hilda wasn't so exhausted from the trip. By the end of the third year, Dean Lohr and the faculty of the University of Illinois College of Nursing were involved in the workshops. After 3 years of working with Peplau, the faculty took over the effort to improve nursing care there. Interviews, Sheila Rouslin Welt, October 14, 1994; Anita O'Toole, September 14, 1996; and Hildegard Peplau, February 4, 1992.

64. In 1964, these nurse/patient/family interviews conducted in Albuquerque were recorded on tape, and then verbatim transcripts were made. These tapes and transcripts are found in Box 24, #869 in the Schlesinger Library.

65. See this letter and many other letters from former Rutgers students and/or workshop participants working around the world using "the Peplau method" in Box 5, #185–193.

66. See Hilda E. Peplau, "The Art and Science of Nursing: Similarities, Differences, and Relations," *Nursing Science* 1(1), 8–15.

67. Student work, Hilda's notes, and professional papers related to concepts may be found in Box 14, #449–467. A partial lists of "concepts" explored include Interference, Defense Theory, Guilt, Anxiety, Loneliness, Psychosomatic Illness, Motivation, Self Concepts, Frustration, Conflict, and Dependence.

68. Peplau, *Basic Principles of Patient Counseling*, "Introduction."

69. Peplau did return to California and New Mexico the next summer, but the cross-country trips would not be repeated.

Rutgers: The Traveling Years   11

If we can just keep plugging away, this sagging profession may yet be saved.

—Hildegard Peplau
February 14, 1968

The summer workshop tours never failed to revive Peplau's spirit and bring her back with renewed energy to the rigors of the year ahead at Rutgers. The summer of 1963 had been particularly productive. Hilda had been excited by the groundbreaking work that summer at Moffit University Hospital in San Francisco where she and Shirley Smoyak conducted workshops directed toward recognition and treatment of psychosomatic illnesses. Hilda saw the program at Moffit as the first step toward opening an entirely new area for nurse clinical practice. From Napa and San Francisco, Hilda had gone on to New Mexico where the new program in family therapy was being launched, and then proceeded east to the familiar ground of North Carolina and on home to Madison.

The trauma of the previous academic year had culminated with the resignation of College of Nursing Dean Ella V. Stonsby and the appointment of Dorothy Smith as acting dean. Smith labored that spring to introduce calm and sanity to the faculty, and a search committee had been appointed to launch a search for a new dean. As one of only two doctorally prepared nurses on the faculty—Dorothy Smith was the other one—and the only faculty member with a clear national reputation, Peplau should have been regarded a serious candidate for the position. She was reluctant to consider it, but at the urging of colleagues outside the university, Hilda decided that she would accept the challenge of putting the chaotic College of Nursing back on track and so agreed to submit her credentials for consideration. On May 22, 1963, she officially put herself forward as a candidate in a letter to the chair of the search committee.[1]

The timing of the search could not have been worse. Within a week of submitting her name, Peplau had left for her cross-country summer workshop tour and so was away from Rutgers during the meetings of the committee. Moreover, although Hilda did not know it, Provost Schlatter and Rutgers President Mason Gross had consulted with Dean Stonsby about the search for a new dean. They knew that Stonsby was physically ill, but were respectful of the fact that she was the founding dean of the college and that her early years as dean had been quite productive and innovative.[2] They also knew that it was Stonsby who had persuaded Peplau to come to Rutgers, thus ensuring the development of graduate education simultaneously with the development of the undergraduate program.

As she often noted herself, Hilda Peplau was not at all "political." She was too straightforward and too intolerant of irrationality in the professional setting to play the political game well. Her first mistake was to assume that a long and thoughtful letter to the search committee would be taken on its merits. In this letter she spelled out the tasks and challenges facing the college as she saw them and proposed several possible scenarios and agendas for meeting them. It was a strong and positive statement, one that left plenty of room for faculty involvement and choice. It provided alternative visions and practical and realistic choices for the immediate future. She concluded her letter by suggesting that the deans of the 10 leading colleges of nursing across the country be contacted as references and listed them by name. She also suggested contacting Marion Johnson, the dean of the Graduate School in New Brunswick; Dr. William McGlothlin, president of the University of Louisville; and Dr. Henry Davidson, medical director of Overbrook Hospital.[3] From any other candidate, this letter would have been regarded as a remarkable document. For any other search committee, it would have ensured that Peplau was a peerless candidate.

Hilda then wrote to her references herself, informing them that she had given their names to the search committee and alerting them that they would hear from the Rutgers search committee.[4] The chair of the search committee wrote to Hilda in July advising her that "the Committee has submitted your name to President Gross for consideration for the position of Dean of the College of Nursing."[5]

During the course of the summer, each referee responded enthusiastically to the news that Peplau would accept this challenge, but some expressed concern that in accepting the deanship she would effectively be leaving the field of psychiatric nursing.[6] Some expressed puzzlement that they had not heard from Rutgers. A sampling of these letters establishes unambiguously that Peplau would have been enthusiastically welcomed into the circle of deans, and had that happened, the reputation of the Rutgers College of Nursing would have been substantially enhanced:

You know well . . . of my belief that you are one of the most forward thinkers in nursing and that your contributions have been of an order not achieved by many . . . I will consider it a pleasure to write a letter strongly supporting you. (Emily Holmquist, Dean, University of Indiana)

I shall do so with great pleasure and complete conviction that you will make a distinguished Dean for Rutgers. (Mary Kelly Mullane, Dean, University of Illinois)

. . . I'll be tempted to write a discouraging account, however, because we need your leadership so desperately in psychiatric nursing. (Elizabeth Kemble, Dean, University of North Carolina)

You are unquestionably the person for this Deanship—but I will save all the reasons why for the Committee. (Florence Wald, Dean, Yale University)

I am not sure I want you to be Dean. Why should psychiatric nursing lose its most distinguished educator to the never-never land of administrative bureaucracy? (Henry Davidson, MD)[7]

To Hilda's embarrassment, none of the persons she suggested be contacted as references on behalf of her candidacy ever heard from Rutgers. She was never interviewed by the search committee.[8] Over the course of the summer, the search committee interviewed only one candidate, and—presumably to head off Peplau's candidacy—the committee immediately forwarded that candidate's name to President Gross and then met with him, urging him to make the appointment straightaway. For reasons unknown, the president agreed to this very unorthodox strategy. The university's senior officials never learned of the high regard in which Peplau was held by leaders in nursing education from across the country.

Returning from her cross-country summer workshop tour in September, full of stories of adventure and new case material for clinical research papers, Hilda was eager for classes to begin and was fully engaged in her writing and her national committee and organizational work. She was happy and optimistic, and looked forward to her meetings with the search committee and university officials. She was stunned to discover, the day that classes began, that the college already had a new dean, Bernice Chapman.[9] Hilda Peplau had not been given even the courtesy of a meeting with the search committee. In nursing circles nationally it had been assumed that Peplau would be the next dean at Rutgers. This snub would lead to a rift within the faculty that would endure beyond her retirement in 1974.

FINDING A NATIONAL FORUM

At the time, Hilda tried to put her disappointment behind her, going about her business and interacting with the new dean of the College of

Nursing and nonpsychiatric nursing faculty only when necessary. The fall of 1963 marked another turning point in Hilda's life. After spending the summer working in Ghana with the Experiment in International Living, Tish entered Bennington College, following in her mother's footsteps. Letitia Anne Peplau was not Hilda, however, and in contrast to Hilda's own growing-up years, Tish's childhood and school years had been rich in books, ideas, and challenging experiences. In her first term at Bennington Tish especially enjoyed an English writing course taught by Hilda's former instructor, Catherine Foster Osgood, and in light of her advanced work in French language studies, she was placed in the senior seminar for French majors. Bennington had changed considerably since Hilda's time there in the 1930s, however, and Tish soon became impatient with the Bennington attitude of nonconformity for its own sake. In fall 1964, after 1 year at Bennington, she transferred to Pembroke College, the women's college of Brown University in Providence, Rhode Island. She would graduate summa cum laude from Pembroke in 1967 with a degree in psychology, a Phi Beta Kappa key, a National Science Foundation Fellowship, and a Danforth Teaching Fellowship for the graduate school of her choice. With Tish away at school for most of the academic year, Hilda was free after 1963 to step up her already whirlwind conference and speaking schedule. For the next 10 years, Hilda would spend little time physically on the Newark campus.

Peplau's outside commitments had become a problem to the former dean, Ella Stonsby, as early as the late 1950s. This seems understandable when one reviews Peplau's consulting, speaking and workshop schedule toward the end of Stonsby's tenure as dean. During the first semester of the academic year 1959–1960, for example, she consulted at Veterans Administration hospitals in Indiana, Wisconsin, Virginia, Massachusetts, North Carolina, Ohio, Iowa, and Illinois. In January, she conducted workshops for the Wisconsin League for Nursing and at Adelphi University on Long Island and at the University in Ohio; in February she was in North Carolina and Wisconsin; and in March she was in Iowa and Indiana. In May she presented a paper on "Modern Psychiatric Nursing Workshops" at the American Psychological Association meetings in Chicago,[10] and by this time, she had also begun to accept invitations to give college graduation speeches before taking off on her cross-country summer workshop tours. In May 1960 she gave four commencement speeches. For Hilda Peplau, there would be no empty blocks on her calendar.

These workshops and speaking engagements were overlaid on top of her already extensive work with national and international committees, including those of the American Nurses Association (ANA) and the American Psychiatric Association (APA). Even during Stonsby's tenure Peplau served as a consultant to the National Institute of Mental Health (NIMH) as well as the U.S. Public Health Service (USPHS) training committees which set policies for the expenditure of NIMH funds for the four major mental health professions (psychiatry, psychology, social work, and nursing). She also served as consultant to the Mental Health Council of the Southern Regional Education board, as the nurse consultant to the Veterans Administration, and as the nurse member of the World Health Organization expert advisory panel.

During this period, Dean Stonsby became more and more insistent that Peplau spend more time on campus. Hilda made it a point to never miss a class, but this often meant trips up and down the east coast touching down in Newark to teach while on her perpetual circuit between New York and Washington, D.C. To Stonsby Hilda must have seemed a whirling dervish, zooming in and out with dozens of commitments pressing on her each time she appeared on campus.

After being passed over for the deanship, and with Tish away at college, Hilda rapidly increased the scope and the pace of her outreach. She seemed constitutionally unable to say no. For all of the next decade, if the request had anything to do with helping to reform nursing care for the mentally ill, or with reforming and upgrading the profession as whole, and if her schedule permitted, she just said yes. She was a one-person band, constantly banging her drum—do more, do it better, study, research, write, focus on the clinical—do it for nursing, do it for the ill, do it to help yourself as a professional—look at the clinical substance of what you do, analyze it, document it, and inform the world. While Peplau never neglected her graduate students, she was nonetheless increasingly focused on her mission to professionalize nursing. Most of her life in the years between 1963 and 1974 were remembered by her in the context of what nursing meeting she was rushing to or from at the time.

She began to add speaking engagements and workshops on the west coast to her regular schedule, which meant she often flew across country in the morning and red-eyed it back to Newark in the evening. In addition to her nearly endless national and increasingly international committee meetings, Peplau almost never turned down invitations to speak to Sigma Theta Tau, the National Honor Society for Nursing. No matter how tired she became in the last decade of her career, no matter how stretched out she was from over-commitment, she seldom declined a request from Sigma Theta Tau. In addition, she always responded to students who wrote to her after these talks. Typically, a student would write a one-paragraph query and Peplau would respond with three pages of handwritten single-spaced exposition, always beginning with the comment, "the question you raise is important." She never tired from urging nurses on to greater heights, always urging more education, or more thought and publication, or more reading and professional involvement.[11] Her recurring themes were graduate education for nurses, research by nurses, and professionalization of the field of nursing.

By 1964 Peplau had expanded her work with the VA hospital network, having been appointed to the Veterans Administration Advisory Council on Nursing, as well as to the Nursing Studies and Special Projects Division of the VA.[12] Here her suggestions for research by nurses in VA hospitals were met with encouragement, allowing her a transitory note of optimism concerning the future of nursing: "It enlarges my confidence that nursing will become a profession, and that it will develop a nursing science and achieve colleague status for nurses based upon merit."[13] For her work, she received many letters of appreciation from VA Nursing Directors.[14]

In February 1964 Hilda attended the "First National Conference for Professional Nurses and Physicians" in Williamsburg, Virginia. As usual, she took copious notes while there and then wrote deans and colleagues with suggestions of how to follow up.[15] Few did. In October, 1965, she attended the second national conference organized by the ANA and AMA to discuss "Nurse-Physician Collaboration Toward Improved Patient Care." With the exception of Peplau, who truly understood the nature of collaboration and had thought seriously about how to foster it, the nurse-participants seemed suspicious and unimaginative.[16] The physicians would soon give up on this effort.

At a large conference organized at the University of Pittsburgh on "Graduate Education in Psychiatric Mental Health Nursing," held in November 1964, Peplau presented a long paper on "Identification of Knowledge Necessary to Function in Community Mental Health Services." Her presentation was the only one with references and footnotes, and the only one seeking to establish what nursing could do in the context of national developments.[17] A month later Peplau directed the first Annual Workshop Conference of the Southern Regional Education Board in Atlanta entitled "Mental Health and Psychiatric Nursing." As usual, always looking for new material, she kept verbatim notes of the presentations, demonstrating again that it was not only the meetings themselves that ate up her life, since whenever she served on a committee, she almost always ended up taking responsibility for writing the reports. From what seemed to be the unending cycle of conferences she attended there were notes, notes, notes, and papers, papers, and papers, and many reels of verbatim tapes.[18] Because she considered the reports from these meetings to be important, she put enormous time and energy into them.[19] They were always detailed and exhaustive, leaving the author drained.

In 1964 Hilda was asked by Dr. Robert Felix, the longtime director of the National Institute of Mental Health, to serve a 4-year term as a member of the National Clearinghouse for Mental Health Information, a group that developed policies regarding a computerized retrieval system.[20] Later in 1964 Felix retired from the Public Health Service after serving for 31 years as the first director of the NIMH. Hilda was momentarily bereft at his retirement. Dr. Felix had been a stable, able, gigantic, and effective advocate for the mentally ill for so long. Under his tutelage and through serving on so many NIMH committees, Peplau had learned a great deal about grantsmanship and how to operate effectively in Washington, D.C. She would be forever grateful to Felix, not only for the doors opened to her but for all he did for the mentally ill in this country. Nonetheless, her final commitment to Felix, through service on the National Clearing house, as well as her increasing work within the American Nurses Association, had the added effect of taking her out of New Jersey on multiple assignments for a good part of each year.

Somehow—and it is hard to imagine how it could be so—the momentum of her involvement in national committees and advisory boards continued to build after 1964. From 1965 on she also served 4-year terms as consultant to the Research and Study Section, Division of Nursing of the Public Health Service, and as a member of the Nurse Scientist Graduate Training Committee of the Nursing Division of the Department of Health, Education, and Welfare, charged with promoting the development of nurse-scientist programs and reviewing grant applications. From 1965 to 1972, Peplau was National Nurse Consultant to the Surgeon General of the United States, working to expand the role of nurses in the armed services.[21]

Her calendar was incredibly dense. Her schedule for September and October in the fall of 1965 looked like this: visits and presentations to Air Force nurses in Texas, Labrador (Canada), and Alabama; Sigma Theta Tau lectures in New Jersey, New York, Pennsylvania, and Virginia; workshops for the Ohio League for Nursing, the Southern California Nurses Association, the Indiana and Ohio State Nurses Associations; scholarly presentations on acute patients group work in Mendocino, California, and on hallucinations at a Nurse Scientist conference in Minneapolis, Minnesota; as well as the presentation of two papers on the Integration of Mental Health Aspects of Care at nursing conferences in Denver and Atlanta, and two additional papers submitted for publication.[22] After this, she was off to Europe visiting air bases in November. In late December, she visited VA hospitals in Arkansas, Virginia, Louisiana, Alabama, and North Carolina.

By the mid-1960s, Hilda Peplau had become a towering figure in nursing. Her achievements, though, were not appreciated at Rutgers, where most of her colleagues on the faculty of nursing felt left behind, left out, ignored, and embittered. Seeming to forget the nationally visible and highly embarrassing snub they had dealt her in 1963, they were resentful of the fact that Peplau was so active nationally, so seldom on campus, and, they felt, "did very little for the College of Nursing."[23] Their inability to discredit Peplau and her growing national reputation irked College of Nursing faculty and administrators to no end. During the remaining years of Peplau's tenure at Rutgers they would do all in their very limited power to make her days as difficult as possible. Peplau was cordial, but tried to stay out of Dean Chapman's way.

By 1964 Peplau's own Graduate Program in Psychiatric Nursing was solidly grounded in the Graduate School in New Brunswick, and her students took their classes on that campus, effectively removing Hilda from the vortex of the administrative circles of the College of Nursing in Newark. She continued to be as intensely involved in her students' education as ever, making long and painstakingly detailed notes on all student work. As always, student papers were thoroughly dissected and commented upon, and her evaluations of each student were full and frank. Often, the notes of the instructor were as long or longer than the student's paper itself.[24]

Peplau also was criticized in her home state of New Jersey, allegedly for doing so little for the State Nurses Association (SNA) while doing so much on the national scene.[25] Here too, however, the written record suggests Peplau was repeatedly stymied when trying to operate within her own state. In 1965 she expressed some of this frustration to her old friend and colleague since her days at Teachers College, psychiatrist Joe Geller: "Sometimes the situation is most discouraging . . . In the [SNA] task force I have met only overt resistance to any definitive ideas by nurses and there's little interest in the nature of education we offer."[26] She went on to explain that when opposition to her work was particularly intense, she retreated so as not to provoke restrictions on the work her students were doing, but that when she met someone more encouraging she ventured to present more of herself and the work being done at Rutgers.[27] She wrote Geller a few weeks later that

> The situation, of course, is not helped by the lack of nurse leadership within the State. The previous Dean made my position in this regard difficult to say the least. In fact, only now is the State Nurses Association beginning to even treat me with courtesy, let alone to listen to anything I might have to say.[28]

Under the new dean, as well, she did not feel much better about her colleagues at the College of Nursing. She confided to Geller that

> Under the present regime, the College of Nursing sits on its hands while the entire university is developing, strengthening, expanding, and moving with the trends in higher education. I think I am making considerable impact on the profession at large—through papers, speeches, clinical workshops in summer, and such. Clinical interest and capability in working directly with psychiatric patients is evolving in many other nursing centers. Eventually, maybe the news will reach New Jersey.[29]

Hilda's frustration, sharp wit, and barbed tongue cannot have helped the situation. In her defense, Joe Geller, who was now director of a large psychiatric clinic in New Jersey, was indefatigable in sending letters to the New Jersey State Bureau of Community Health Services, the Division of Mental Health Hospitals, and the Department of Institutions and Agencies trying to clarify, explain, and promote Peplau and her work. Finally, after 2 years of effort, Geller was able to give Hilda some good news about New Jersey. In 1967 he informed her that the State Community Mental Health Advisory Council had approved a resolution permitting nurse clinical specialists from the Rutgers Psychiatric Nursing Program to work in community mental health centers as therapists, thus recognizing nurses as professional therapists for the first time.[30] This major coup marked a turning point. Now, Peplau could begin to feel she'd succeeded in making a contribution on her home ground.

SEEING THE WORLD

By the mid-1960s Peplau's international work was picking up. In 1965 when she accepted the Surgeon General's appointment as the National Nurse Consultant to the Air Force, she took on the responsibility for visiting Air Force bases not only around the country but internationally. (Her service in this position occasioned a rare letter of recognition from Rutgers President Mason Gross.)[31] Between October 23 and November 19 of 1965 she visited nurses in Air Force hospital facilities in England, Germany, Greece, and France. This European tour, happily, allowed her to spend a weekend in Paris with Tish who was taking a junior year abroad on a program sponsored by Hamilton College. The two took a bus tour to Versailles and the French countryside, and Tish was treated to meals in Paris restaurants that she could not have afforded as a student. Upon her return, Hilda wrote a long, detailed report for the Air Force, as well as long letters of information, suggestions, and thank you notes to the majors and colonels she met along the way.[32] Thus began an international correspondence with nursing administrators from around the world, and the beginning of many invitations to return—many of which she honored.[33]

During the spring and summer of 1966, she attended 15 different Air Force "case conferences" where she offered suggestions and recommendations and followed up with thoughtful critiques. For her efforts, she received many kudos from the military brass. For the next 3 years she would crisscross the United States visiting Air Force hospitals, giving talks, graduation addresses, attending special exercises, and talking to nurses in flight school evacuation classes. She became a one-person consulting firm on the need for mental health concepts in flight nurse training programs.

Wherever she went, she made notes on everything she saw, and sent back observations to her sponsors. In 1968, in addition to bases in the contiguous United States, she added Alaska and a second trip to Labrador to her itinerary. A list of command nurses from around the world compiled in 1969 indicates that she had met fully half of them.[34]

Hilda's international travels offered her another opportunity to fulfill her promise to Tish that Tish would "see the world." During Tish's high school years this promise had been met with their summer cross-country trips together. During Tish's college and graduate school years their travels together during Christmas and summer vacations were increasingly international. In the summer of 1966 Hilda traveled to Latin America to lead seminars and workshops sponsored by the Kellogg and Rockefeller foundations. Tish, returning from her junior year in France, accompanied her to Panama, Peru, and Colombia before Hilda went on to Puerto Rico for yet another workshop before getting on with her U.S. summer workshop schedule. As always, the two managed sightseeing along the way. The next summer Tish traveled with Hilda again, to Europe, Kenya, Mexico, and Alaska. For Christmas 1967, during Tish's winter break from her senior year at Pembroke, Hilda and Tish took a trip to Israel. This was not the usual work-related trip, however. "Israel is strictly vacation—personally paid for," she wrote, "The first such vacation trip I have taken in twenty or more years. I feel entitled! . . . We are celebrating Tisha's upcoming graduation with a B.A. in June 1968."[35] Tish entered Harvard Graduate School in the fall of 1968 and that year Hilda and Tish celebrated the holidays in Hawaii. In the summer of 1969 Tish again joined Hilda on the summer workshop circuit. Hilda was concluding a family therapy workshop with Bill Field and Shirley Smoyak in Albuquerque when terrible news reached them. Hilda's beloved brother Walter had suffered a heart attack while sitting in a living room chair after mowing the lawn at Walter and Anne's home in Poughkeepsie. He was pronounced dead on arrival at the hospital on August 7, 1969, at the age of 56. Hilda and Walter and his wife Anne had been close throughout their adult lives. It was Walter who had helped Hilda conceal the circumstances of Tish's birth by assuming the putative role of Tish's adoptive father, thus allowing Hilda, for professional reasons, to present Tish as the "niece" she was raising. Hilda and Tish both were devastated by the loss of Walter, who had held such a central place in their hearts. They rushed home from Albuquerque to attend the funeral and grieve with other members of the family.

In 1967 Hilda accepted the challenge of offering a seminar and workshop experience to nurses in West Africa at the University of Ibadan in Nigeria.[36] The nursing program at Ibadan was an intercountry project jointly sponsored by the Government of Nigeria, the World Health Organization (WHO), UNICEF, and the Rockefeller Foundation. The Department of Nursing at Ibadan was under the faculty of medicine, but unlike in the

United States, where nurse faculty were often wary of medicine's domination, the relationship in Nigeria worked beautifully. The physicians were exceedingly supportive of professional nursing. This would be the first nursing program leading to a university degree in Africa. The first faculty members were international nurse educators funded by the WHO. (A former Peplau student from Rutgers, Mary Abbott, had served as a WHO representative in Nigeria helping in the development of the nursing program.) African counterparts would be sponsored for graduate study abroad, to return and replace the international nurses.[37] Hilda was excited about the unlimited opportunities here for nursing research in relation to local needs and by the enthusiasm of the students for designing and conducting such research. She was "absolutely delighted" and "thrilled" with all she found in Ibadan. She was particularly intrigued and impressed with the work of Dr. Adeoyo Lambo, Dean of the Medical School and Chair of the Department of Psychiatry, whose hospital in the Aro Community Center at Abeokuta in the Western Region of Nigeria combined Western and African traditional ways of working with the mentally ill.[38]

Harry Stack Sullivan, Peplau's intellectual inspiration since those early years at Chestnut Lodge, was again, near the end of her professional career, relevant. Here, in Nigeria, Sullivan's emphasis on interpersonal relations, which had altered psychiatry's traditional concern with the individual, was being adapted by Adeoyo Lambo to focus on the interpersonal phenomena in the traditional African village setting. The emphasis was on the relationship among people as members of an extended family system and the social context of their behavior. Lambo had built a therapeutic community where milieu therapy was on display. Peplau could see in practice the interpersonal theory that she had intuitively believed. She was encouraged because—in this African setting— all her early training, so challenged by American nursing, seemed vindicated. She was discouraged, though, because she was aware changes developing in the healthcare system in the United States meant that therapeutic communities such as these would never be given a chance there. One of the best things about Nigeria was that she and Lambo immediately recognized the kindred soul, one of the other, and became long and fast friends.

After the humid heat of tropical Nigeria, Peplau was not quite prepared for the moonscape of Iceland, where she went to give one of her last workshops for the WHO in 1968. Perhaps because it is so otherworldly, Iceland leaves a curious impression on the mind. Although Hildegard's weeklong workshop was held in the spotlessly clean and very humane mental hospital in Reykjavik, the days spent there seemed, as she later described them, as an interlude from life, a sojourn in some other, nether, twilight zone of the mind.[39] She had been warned a bit about the peculiarities of the place—no beer and no TV on Thursdays, for example—but she was not prepared for no trees and no fresh vegetables. More than 80% of Iceland consists of nothing but ice fields, barren mountains, lava, and tundra so lunar that NASA astronauts trained there. Iceland is a duck-shaped island with 8 million puffins and considerably less than a million people.

The most striking thing, to Hilda, about Reykjavik was its extraordinary stillness. The overwhelming impression on the tiny, empty streets, was of silence. Peplau was like an Alice-in-Wonderland, in a quaint and quiet place, as silent as a photograph. Rows of tiny, clean, white boxes set out in geometric grids, with roofs of red, blue, and green, as in a storybook. Iceland is famous for having no mansions and no slums, in much the same way that its language has no accents and no dialects. With a population smaller than that of Colorado Springs, uniformity is not hard to achieve, and because nearly all the houses are geothermally heated, the city shines silent in the unpolluted air. For once she had no real idea of what to do to help the silent souls, chronically mentally disturbed, who were the patients in Reykjavik's hospital. Iceland was unforgettable, a stabilizer after the energy of Nigeria, but it was to Nigeria she would return in the years to come.

In the summer of 1968 Peplau returned to Latin America, going to Chile to consult with the Pan American Health Organization, before her return to Nigeria. She sent off her usual long and thorough report before heading off on her cross-country workshop odyssey. That her efforts in Nigeria were appreciated is evident in this note from Dr. Lambo:

> Thank you for your letter . . . kind of you to write so soon . . . a great honour for this University to be able to have a nurse educator of your international stature and repute . . . Your recommendations will go to the Faculty of Medicine . . . but at this juncture, I should like to thank you most sincerely for writing at length and so thoughtfully. It is most stimulating to read some of your most penetrating comments and practical suggestions. We are very grateful.[40]

Following her 1966 workshops in Latin America the Kellogg Foundation had written to say that they had "received your report and what a magnificent report it is."[41] Similarly, the Rockefeller Foundation thanked her for a great seminar in Cali, Colombia, and hoped she would return in January 1968 for another workshop.[42] Never one to turn down such an invitation, Hilda jetted down to Colombia on a Thursday for a Friday presentation before flying back up to Cherokee, Iowa for a Saturday morning workshop.[43]

The spring and summer of 1969 found her on the road again, going to Chile once again in April, then to Nigeria in July, and on to Indiana, Wisconsin, North Carolina, and Texas during the summer. As 1969 moved toward 1970, during which time she was also serving as the executive director of the ANA, the pace became even more frantic. That winter she accepted invitations to give keynote addresses to state nurses association meetings in North Carolina, Tennessee, Texas, and Wisconsin. As she explained to her good friend, Bill Field: "If we can just keep plugging away, this sagging profession may yet be saved."[44]

THE CHAPMAN YEARS

As had Dean Stonsby before her, Dean Chapman soon began to question the time Hilda spent away from Rutgers and to request detailed information on Hilda's travel plans. In October 1968, when the ANA wrote to Dean Chapman to inform her of the honor Dr. Peplau had received having been designated by the ANA as its liaison representative to the National Advisory Mental Health Council, Chapman responded with a two-sentence note to Hilda: "This sounds like you are adding some more work. Will you please keep me informed as to when you will be away for meetings of this Council."[45] Normally, such an honor to a member of the faculty would be met with a note of congratulations from the dean.

Peplau's Program in Psychiatric Nursing, however, located as it was under the wing of the Graduate School in New Brunswick, at some distance from the College of Nursing in Newark, maintained its relative autonomy and continued to grow stronger. From 1967 through 1969, the Rutgers students in New Brunswick were joined by New York University doctoral students who came to Rutgers to do their practice teaching under Peplau. As always, Hilda took her responsibilities seriously, and prepared long, elaborate plans for the NYU students.[46] These students too joined the "Peplau Circle."

By this time, Peplau had assured considerable financial assistance for the Psychiatric Nursing Program, having secured NIMH-funded positions for four additional instructors and for the NYU students, who were in residence, to help with instruction and clinical supervision. Since all of the appointees had trained with her, Peplau felt the program well in hand. In 1968 Dr. Irwin W. Pollack assumed the Chair in Psychiatry at the Rutgers Medical School. An innovative and creative man, Dr. Pollack, far from being suspicious of Peplau's work, was impressed with what she was doing. In 1968, with Pollack's encouragement, the Program in Psychiatric Nursing was given space at the new medical school in New Brunswick, and the program's faculty spent more and more time in the offices allotted to them there. Pollack welcomed Peplau's students into the Community Mental Health Center located on the Medical School campus. In Pollack, Peplau had finally met an academic physician who understood and encouraged the work her students were doing to the point of inviting her to share his turf.[47] She knew she had passed a significant milestone when, early in 1969, the Dean of the Medical School wrote her a note: "Let's get together soon for a really hard discussion of the Mental Health Center planning with Harold Logan and Dr. Pollack."[48] Subsequently, the psychiatric nursing faculty were given adjunct appointments in the Department of Psychiatry and were treated as full members of the staff in the mental health center.[49] This was an extraordinary recognition of Peplau's work and such appointments were probably unique in the United States at that time.

For the first time, Peplau would have had colleagues with whom to work, discuss, and share her work had she not at this time accepted an appointment that ultimately led her to the presidency of the American Nurses Association and duties that would consume her time and energies for the next 4 years. In 1968, at the time of the move to the Medical School campus, Hilda was serving as a member of the ANA committee named to seek a new executive director for the association. The search came to an end when the committee unanimously chose to ask Peplau herself to assume the position, at least on an interim basis. Never able to say no, she reluctantly agreed to accept the responsibility, taking a partial leave from Rutgers.[50] The partial leave would require her to teach two courses as well as to continue to exercise overall responsibility for the Psychiatric Graduate Program in order to assure the continuity of the NIMH grants supporting it.[51] The university routinely granted leaves of absence for such professional work in other disciplines—but it was not to be so in the College of Nursing. By the terms of her agreement with the College of Nursing, Peplau was required to carry virtually full-time responsibility at Rutgers while also directing the affairs of the American Nurses Association, one of the nation's largest professional associations.

Fortunately, Peplau's former student, friend, and professional colleague Shirley Smoyak, who had just received her own PhD, was named acting director of the program and in Hilda's absence began to assume more and more responsibility. With the Medical School affiliation afforded by Dr. Pollack, many of the things Peplau had worked so hard to achieve in her graduate program were now coming to fruition, but for all practical purposes, she would not be present to enjoy its success.

The affiliation of the psychiatric nursing faculty with the Mental Health Center and the Medical School, together with the fact that all the graduate courses in psychiatric nursing were offered on the New Brunswick campus, made it all the more obvious that the program was an anomaly in the College of Nursing. Shirley Smoyak pressed this point more aggressively, arguing that the Psychiatric Nursing Program should be a freestanding program on the New Brunswick campus, independent of the College of Nursing in every way. In June, Provost Schlatter agreed in principle and appointed a committee to design a master plan for health education in the university, including nursing. Dean Chapman was most definitely not pleased with this turn of events and spent most of 1969 try-ing both to stop the master planning process and to reverse the decision to move graduate psychiatric nursing to New Brunswick.[52] Schlatter held firm, however, and it was announced that the Program in Psychiatric Nursing would officially move to the New Brunswick campus in Septem-ber 1970.[53] Since the faculty and staff were already physically on the New Brunswick campus, this decision really meant that the program's staff would be freed from the administrative oversight of the dean of the College of Nursing. After this, the tension between Chapman and Peplau became more acute, and once again Hilda found herself in a constant bat-tle to defend her program, even though she was, for all practical purposes, not even on the scene.

In 1969, in addition to her full-time position at the ANA, Hilda contin-ued to work on the national and international scenes. In May 1969 she had planned to leave for Chile immediately after her last class in order to conduct a workshop under the auspices of the Rockefeller Foundation. Peplau formally petitioned her dean to be excused from the university graduation that spring, pointing out that nowhere in the university's offi-cial regulations was it stated that attendance at graduation was *required.* The dean responded thus:

> I guess attendance at Commencement is not compulsory . . . since it has been discontinued as compulsory for students, there has been more leniency in granting the faculty members' requests to be excused. Since you will be out of the country again at that time and have made previ-ous commitments, I see no way of handling it but to excuse you.[54]

The exchange of memos from this period preserved in the university's personnel file reflect a growing gulf between Peplau and her dean and colleagues in the College of Nursing. As well, in the university at large, she was still perceived by those who did not know her personally as an eminent but difficult "troublemaker."[55]

COLLAPSE OF A DEANSHIP

By 1970, Dean Chapman was increasingly overwhelmed by the adminis-trative pressures on deans at Rutgers. A new State Department of Higher Education (DHE) in Trenton began monitoring state higher education institutions, and in the process developed new accounting and account-ability formulas. DHE formulas had to be used in generating a university budget, and this put increasingly complex demands on deans to develop the required data. Dean Chapman simply could not produce the informa-tion required for the College of Nursing.[56] In her frustration she blamed

Peplau for her problems—primarily because Hilda did not have the time (nor the inclination) to help her out of them. Letters from outside the university praising Peplau's work on the national level simply increased Dean Chapman's frustration that her most distinguished faculty member wasn't around to help her with the increasing burden of the deanship.[57]

In 1970, Peplau was elected President of the American Nurses Association, and the terms of her partial leave were revised so that her teaching load would be reduced, but she was still expected to be on campus on Mondays. Her ANA responsibilities, however, required extensive traveling. The travel schedule submitted to Dean Chapman for the fall semester 1970 indicates that Peplau expected to be out of the state of New Jersey for part of every single week of the semester. Having to check in at Rutgers each Monday while attending to the affairs of the ANA, and traveling throughout the country and the world was to prove totally exhausting. In addition, in 1970 Peplau was a passenger in a serious automobile accident, sustaining injuries from which she never truly recovered.[58]

Thus it was that Peplau's last years at Rutgers were characterized by fatigue and physical exhaustion. She kept up her travel schedule, but her time back in New Jersey was full of physical pain, as well as the tension of the situation at Rutgers. On the one hand, her graduate program was flourishing. The move to New Brunswick had stimulated both faculty and students. Demand for the program was higher than ever, the number of students accepted (28) was the largest ever, and finally the program was gaining respect in larger university circles. Finally too, Peplau had students about whom she was truly excited, students whom she was sure would make a difference in the professionalization of the field through their clinical work and publications. On the other hand, her relationship, such as it was, with Dean Chapman had clearly deteriorated.

Soon faculty members were once again petitioning the university's administrators for a change in the deanship. Chapman's difficulties with administering the college were obvious. As before, upper-level university administrators did not want to deal with "the nursing problem." Peplau's diary of this time records a litany of faculty discontent, but dwells mostly on her nearly continuous back, neck, and head pain incurred as a result of the automobile accident.[59] She noted she was too busy to go to the doctor, and thus suffered on without medical treatment. While the diaries note the difficulties at Rutgers, it is clear that any energy Peplau could muster was expended on her ANA work, its required travel, and dealing with nearly constant pain. At Rutgers, she lent her name to the efforts of the younger faculty to once again remove the dean, but she was not an organizer of this effort nor did she play a central role in it. Nonetheless, university administrators chose to see the difficulties in the college as the result of a "personality clash" between Peplau and Chapman and their respective followers.[60]

On May 8, 1971, Provost Schlatter became the acting president of Rutgers when President Mason Gross resigned due to an illness that would take his life before the year was out. One of Schlatter's first acts was to appoint a Committee to Plan for Nursing Education at Rutgers, to be chaired by Shirley Smoyak. Aware of Peplau's considerable national stature, and of the fact that the Chapman deanship was problematic, he asked Hilda to serve as a member of the committee. She reluctantly agreed, stating that her travel would preclude her full participation. In fact, she attended only one meeting of this committee and noted in her diary that she simply no longer had the stamina to cope with the situation. In just 4 months' time, Rutgers had a new president, Edward J. Bloustein. The nursing committee was so fraught with internal differences that it never issued a report. Once again, at the upper levels of the administration, Peplau would be somehow held responsible for not saving it, reinforcing the opinion that once again "the nurses just couldn't get it together."[61]

In September 1972, after the nursing committee dismissed itself, declaring its differences irreconcilable, Shirley Smoyak led a group of faculty members to see the new acting provost, Horace DePodwin, on the Newark campus.[62] The meeting did not go well. Instead of summarizing their concerns, the nurses had a list of 22 complaints against the dean. Not a patient man, DePodwin was annoyed. He interrupted in the middle of the litany. "Come off it," he said, "it's a personality difficulty—that's the root of all the difficulty."[63] In October, several of the senior faculty caught up with Peplau when she was in town and tried to make the case that she ought to "do something about the College of Nursing . . ."[64] Hilda was privately infuriated, since several of those calling on her now had been on the search committee that chose Chapman in the first place—and without even giving Peplau the courtesy of an interview. So, she told them that it was their responsibility to do something about Chapman, and no, she would not help. It was simply too late. She was ready to retire.[65] What she didn't tell them was that she was too physically and mentally exhausted to even think about the issues.

In November 1972 Dean Chapman bowed to the inevitable and resigned, effective June 30, 1973. In December 1972 there was yet another crisis. The 5-year accreditation visit from the National League for Nursing was coming up, and as was the case a decade earlier with Dean Stonsby, Dean Chapman had not been able to put together the self-study report required for such a visit. She, as had Stonsby, called upon Peplau at the last minute, at first asserting it was Peplau's fault that there was no report because she had not been around to work on it. Chapman called repeatedly the weekend before the visit, clearly in a panic and asking for advice. Peplau, however, was simply too sick and exhausted to respond. She literally could not do it. As Hilda noted, "She phoned three times on

Saturday and three times on Sunday. She really doesn't know what she's doing, but I can't do it for her; I did respond to questions and gave suggestions. I am too exhausted, too dizzy, in too much pain, to do more."[66]

This was the Hilda Peplau that the new president, Edward Bloustein, asked to chair a search committee for a new dean. While in years past Hilda would have jumped at the opportunity and scoured the nation to find the best possible candidates, this time she very reluctantly agreed to serve on the committee, but adamantly refused to chair it.[67] She simply had neither the energy nor the heart for this effort in 1973. Peplau was more annoyed than flattered when several of her colleagues, including some of the members of the 1963 search committee, tried to convince her she "owed" it to the college to "save it" by being a candidate herself. Peplau leaves no doubt concerning her feelings about the matter:

> There's so much to do and I have no energy. I am too exhausted. They had their chance six years ago. Now I am NOT interested. Now I am weary . . . I just couldn't take it on. Now, with six years of deterioration in the school—no! I am weary of the people, the work, and the noise. I am not up to fighting, and so little thought goes into anything in nursing.[68]

The president had appointed her to the committee despite her reluctance in order to ensure that good candidates would be found, but Peplau had virtually no support within the committee. The majority of its members were not comfortable with the candidates she encouraged and did all they could to ensure that they would not be considered. Hilda had reason to be worried. In February, the committee finally agreed on a preliminary list of three candidates, one of whom was strongly recommended by Peplau over the other two. When, at a faculty meeting on February 28, it was announced that only two of three candidates recommended by the search committee would be invited to campus, Hilda was livid. The third candidate was the only one Hilda had endorsed.

Confronted again with what she considered to be the perfidy of the system, Hilda Peplau in the summer of 1973 distanced herself as much as possible from the ongoing search for a dean of the College of Nursing at Rutgers. In the end, neither of the two candidates brought in by the search committee was appointed by the university president, and therefore the process dragged on through the summer and into the next fall. As the process wore on, Hilda commented that she was "weary of fighting the destructiveness of nurses of nursing. So, Shirley Smoyak, with a stronger stomach than mine, will try for nineteen more years, no doubt."[69] In November the search committee was tied in a vote taken on the only two new candidates they could agree upon. In the end, one candidate withdrew so the final candidate became the committee's only recommendation. Peplau thought the final candidate might be all right, but she

expressed "an undefinable nagging doubt,"[70] a doubt she did not publicly express, but which would be validated 4 years later when Rutgers
would again be searching for a new dean of nursing.[71]

It should be noted that the "dean problem," as it was experienced at
the Rutgers College of Nursing, was not limited to Rutgers. While
Rutgers may have had more than its share of troubled deanships in the
College of Nursing, the problem was by no means unique to that university. Rather, many schools of nursing from the 1960s through the 1980s
went through similar traumas. While the problem was not unique to
Rutgers, the nature of the problem does seem unique to nursing. Perhaps
this is because until very recently nursing deans lacked the academic standing and background held by deans in most other academic disciplines.
Thus, this insecurity played out in faculty politics. The nursing dean could
complain to those above her about how very difficult her faculty, and thus
her life, was, and her problem would be shifted back downstairs for solution. The subsequent interplay worked to make the incumbent dean
increasingly unstable, both personally and in terms of her command of her
position. The situation would deteriorate, eventually leading to a "coup."
As at Rutgers, in many colleges the weaker or more threatened faculty
members, likely representing a majority on the faculty, controlled the
searches for deans. A new dean would be sought who inevitably was not
the best candidate for the position, and the cycle would start again.

At Rutgers, January 1974 began with a new dean in place, and with
Peplau counting the days to retirement at the end of the semester. In her
diary she noted "I will be glad to be done with the charade called nursing
education at Rutgers."[72] She would retire in just a few months time, on
July 1, 1974, tired and disillusioned.

Bone weary though she was, Hilda's description of nursing education
at Rutgers as a "charade" took a far too narrow view. Her own program,
resented as it was by a nursing faculty that she had long since left behind,
was flourishing. Because Peplau's impact was so great on so many, she
was often accused by envious colleagues of developing "disciples." There
could not be a more unfair characterization. Hilda always had the deep-
est respect for individual ability, and was constantly challenging those
with whom she had contact to aspire to their personal best and thereby to
make solid contributions to their profession. Her passion was for her
work, and it was this passion for linking theory to practice in order to
make a difference in patient care that translated to distinctive careers for
many of her students. The charge of "discipleship" arose, perhaps, around
this untiring effort to maximize the leadership potential of each student
coupled with her insistence on limiting the numbers of students admitted
to her program. It should be no surprise that graduates of the Program in
Psychiatric Nursing quickly became nationally visible. They were told
from the very beginning that they would be leaders, and they were.[73]

In her 20 years at Rutgers, Peplau's program produced only 128 advanced clinical specialists, but these 128 nurses had an enormous impact on their profession. Her legacy from the Rutgers years was not so much to the College of Nursing, but to the profession at large, as her Rutgers students fanned out across the country making major contributions in a wide variety of settings. They defined themselves as clinical nurse specialists and were very clear that they wanted to work directly with patients. They assumed leadership roles across the country as clinical practitioners, administrators, consultants, educators, and researchers. They worked in community, VA, state, and county hospitals; community mental health centers; colleges and universities; federal and state policy planning and regulatory offices; national and state nurses associations; publishing companies; and in private and group psychotherapy practices in 30 different states. Twenty-one of them continued their education, earning their doctorates and assuming posts in universities across the land. Thus, although small in number, their impact was widespread. They became leaders within the health and education institutions where they practiced, and carried Peplau's influence to institutions and organizations across the country.

ENDNOTES

1. Letter from Hilda Peplau to Elizabeth Fenlason, May 22, 1963, Rutgers Personnel Files.
2. Interview, Richard Schlatter, June 12, 1992.
3. Letter from Hildegard Peplau to Elizabeth Fenlason, May 22, 1963.
4. These materials may be found in Box 17, #582, at the Schlesinger Library. The 10 deans were Dean Helen Nahm, University of California Medical Center at San Francisco; Dean Elizabeth Kemble, University of North Carolina at Chapel Hill; Dean Rozella Schlotfeldt, Case Western Reserve; Dean Katharine Hoffman, University of Washington; Dean Emily Holmquist, University of Indiana; Dean Helen Bunge, University of Wisconsin; Dean Mary Maher, University of Massachusetts; Dean Mary Mullane, University of Illinois; Dean Edna Fritz, University of Minnesota; and Dean Florence Wald, Yale University. Letters to these deans from Dr. Peplau and all their responses are in this collection. In addition to the Deans, Hilda suggested the committee contact Dr. Marion Johnson, Dean of the Graduate School at Rutgers; Dr. William McGlothlin, President of the University of Louisville; and Dr. Henry Davidson, Medical Director of the Essex Country Overbrook Hospital.
5. Letter from Elizabeth M. Fenlason to Hildegard Peplau, July 5, 1963.
6. See materials in Box 17, #586.
7. Letters from Holmquist, Kemble, Wald, and Davidson in Box 17, #582.
8. Interview, Hildegard Peplau, January 22, 1992.
9. Bernice Chapman had initiated but not completed work on a doctorate from TC several years before. She came to Rutgers after having served as the founding dean of the Brigham Young University College of Nursing in Utah.
10. Correspondence about many of these activities may be found in Box 22, #742–764.

11. Many of these letters to and from students may be found in Box 38, #1399.
12. Materials on Peplau's work with the Veterans Administration may be found in Box 39, #1411–1412.
13. Letter from Hilda Peplau to Mrs. Gertrude Abraham, Chief, Nursing Studies, Veterans Administration, March 9, 1964, in Box 39, #1412.
14. Examples of such letters may be found in Box 39, #1412.
15. Peplau's notes and letters to colleagues about this conference may be found in Box 23, #805 and #806.
16. See materials in Box 24, #827.
17. This paper may be found in Box 23, #816. Many of her papers given at workshops or at conferences would later appear in volumes of proceedings. Inevitably, her paper would be the only one with footnotes, for she always read the literature before writing, and made enormous efforts to always be up to date.
18. Papers, notes, and tapes may be found in Box 23, #806–820.
19. Several examples of such reports may be found in Box 22, #754, in the Schlesinger Library.
20. Letter from Hilda Peplau to R. H. Felix, September 17, 1964, accepting the appointment was found in her Rutgers Personnel File.
21. See letters of appointment to various committees and posts in Box 20, #693, Schlesinger Library.
22. Materials related to all of this, along with many of the papers and transcripts of the workshops, may be found in Box 23, #792–820.
23. This was a comment often made by former faculty members at the College of Nursing, 10 of whom were interviewed for this book. Because they are all still living and feelings are still very strong, I've chosen not to quote them directly or by name.
24. Much of this material, with sample student papers and long evaluation notes, may be found in the Schlesinger Library in Box 17, #583–597. Elaborate course outlines and study guides, together with reams of materials for students may be found in #596.
25. Interview, Lucille Joel, November 18, 1992.
26. Letter from Hilda Peplau to Joseph J. Geller, MD, February 10, 1965, in Box 16, #580.
27. Ibid. By this time, it was clear that what many of her students were doing was practicing psychotherapy—and in 1965 this would have been severely criticized in many quarters were it more widely known.
28. Letter from Hilda Peplau to Joseph J. Geller, MD, March 1, 1965, in Box 16, #580.
29. Letter from Hilda Peplau to Joe Geller, March 22, 1965, also found in Box 16, #580.
30. Letter from Joseph J. Geller, MD to Hilda Peplau, April 11, 1967, Box 16, #580.
31. Letter from Mason Gross to Hildegard Peplau, October 14, 1965, Box 24, #827.
32. This report, along with letters and notes, may be found in Box 24, #882.
33. See programs, letters, correspondence, copies of talks and addresses, courses devised and given, protocols observed, etc., on these Air Force forays in Boxes 38 and 39, #1400–1410.
34. Ibid.
35. Hildegard Peplau, Christmas Letter to Friends, 1967, Box 4, #121.
36. For details of the arrangements and notes taken during the Nigerian trips, see Box 25, #894.
37. Unfortunately this program was interrupted by the Nigerian civil war in 1967. While the nursing program continued, it never developed the graduate programs and programs of nursing research envisioned in 1966. See letters from Mary Abbott and Evelyn Zimmerman to Hildegard Peplau in Box 25, #895; and interview, Evelyn Zimmerman, April 28, 1993.

38. Papers, correspondence, and materials related to these experiences may be found in Box 25, #894, #909, #930, and #931.
39. Interview, Hildegard Peplau, February 5, 1992, and descriptions and comments on the trip to Iceland found in Box 25, #917.
40. Letter from T. S. Lambo to Hilda Peplau, September 13, 1969, Box 25, #908.
41. Letter from M. G. Candau, MD to Hilda Peplau, January 29, 1966, in Box 39, #1421.
42. Letter from Robert Caldwell to Hildegard Peplau, May 20, 1967.
43. Correspondence and itineraries in Box 24, #882.
44. Letter from Hilda Peplau to Bill Field, February 14, 1968, Box 25, #908.
45. Letter from L. Bernice Chapman to Hilda E. Peplau, November 7, 1968, Rutgers Personnel File.
46. These notes and plans may be found in Box 17, #589.
47. Interviews, Hildegard Peplau and Irwin W. Pollack, March 12, 1992. The Community Mental Health Center had been built with state and federal funds and had its own staff, but was affiliated with the Department of Psychiatry in the Medical School. Dr. Pollack served as both the Chair of the Department and as Director of the CMHC. According to Peplau, he was the first psychiatrist to treat her students as colleagues and to give them access to acutely ill rather than only chronically ill patients.
48. Dean James W. MacKenzie to Hilda Peplau, February 11, 1969, Box 25, #921. In 1970, the Rutgers Medical School in New Brunswick was severed from Rutgers by the New Jersey legislature and joined to a freestanding medical school based in Newark, the College of Medicine and Dentistry of New Jersey.
49. See agreements in Box 15, #529.
50. For details see note from Hilda E. Peplau to L. Bernice Chapman, May 22, 1969, confirming arrangements for the leave, Rutgers Personnel File.
51. These details are contained in a letter from Hilda Peplau to Esther Garrison, May 26, 1969, found in the Rutgers Personnel File. This letter also carries the signature of Dean Chapman, and was intended to confirm the mutual understandings between NIMH and Rutgers in regard to Peplau's grants as well as the terms of the conditions of Peplau's leave. In a further letter to Provost Schlatter, dated June 20, 1969, Dean Chapman assured the Provost that Peplau would not only teach her two classes on Monday mornings, but would supervise theses work on Monday afternoons and Saturdays, as well as maintain overall responsibility for the program and the clinical assignments of students.
52. Interview, Evelyn Wilson, Director of Program Development and Planning, October 15, 1996, in New Brunswick, NJ. See Box 15, #532 for a collection of memos from Chapman to Smoyak and Peplau, challenging them in every conceivable way in regard to the running of the program. As time passed, Peplau's responses get shorter and snappier. Clearly relationships had deteriorated.
53. Materials concerning the move to New Brunswick may be found in Box 15, #529. While the graduate program itself had been under the aegis of the New Brunswick graduate school for some time, the faculty members were still members of the College of Nursing faculty and had their faculty offices in Newark. Thus, classes and students were in New Brunswick, but the faculty itself was resident in Newark until the fall of 1970.
54. Bernice Chapman to Hilda Peplau, May 15, 1969, Box 25, #921.
55. Interviews, former Provosts Horace J. DePodwin, October 10, 1995, in Newark, New Jersey, and James E. Young, July 5, 1997, in Vermont.
56. Interviews, Elinor Gersman, former Academic Planning Officer in the Office of the Vice President for Budgeting at Rutgers University, May 10, 1994, by telephone from Tokyo, Japan; and Evelyn Wilson, Associate Vice President for Budgeting and Program Development, October 15, 1996, in Kennett Square, Pennsylvania.

57. A letter from Leonard D. Finniger, MD, Director of the Bureau of Health Professions Education at the Department of Health, Education, and Welfare, praising Peplau for her work on the Nurse Scientist Graduate Training Committee moved Dean Chapman to refer to Hilda as "that irresponsible power grabber." Letter from Leonard Finniger to L. Bernice Chapman, August 20, 1969, Rutgers Archives, and interview, Leonard Finniger, March 22, 1993.

58. This accident and its consequences will be discussed more fully in chapter 13.

59. In 1972, the last year of her ANA presidency, Peplau kept a fairly detailed diary. This diary may be found in Box 8 of the Schlesinger collection.

60. Interview, Horace DePodwin, October 10, 1995, in Newark, New Jersey.

61. Interview, Evelyn Wilson, October 15, 1996.

62. One of President Bloustien's first acts was to announce a reorganization of the university, giving the two branch campuses in Newark and Camden greater autonomy. In Newark, the Dean of the Graduate School of Management, Horace DePodwin, was named Acting Provost while a search was conducted for the position.

63. Interviews, Shirley Smoyak, September 9, 1997, and Horace DePodwin, October 10, 1995, and recorded in Peplau's diary on September 16, 1972. The diary is in Box 8, Schlesinger Library.

64. Diary entry, October 22, 1972.

65. Ibid.

66. Diary entry, December 10, 1972.

67. Interview, Hildegard Peplau, January 29, 1992, and diary entry, November 24, 1972.

68. Diary entry, January 7, 1973.

69. Diary entry, August 24, 1973.

70. Diary entry, November 10, 1973.

71. In fact, the Rutgers College of Nursing was to continue to suffer from weak leadership and an under-credentialed faculty for several more years. It was not until well into the 1980s and several deans later that the college began to find its stride—and to reach back to claim Hilda Peplau as a revered and treasured former colleague.

72. Diary entries, January–March, 1974.

73. For a report on Rutgers graduates and their affiliations across the country see "Brief Summary of Accomplishments of Graduates of the Rutgers Graduate Psychiatric Nursing Program, 1957–1974" in Box 17, #603. For a detailed list of graduates, showing year of graduation and current positions in 1978, see a report prepared by Shirley A. Smoyak, also in Box 17, #604.

Vision of a Profession   12

We had nothing like hard scientific knowledge to take to colleagues in other professions—there was no intellectual dialogue in nursing, thus we had nothing to offer other professions . . . If we could train nurses as clinical specialists, and do it right, then we'd have something to contribute in dialogue with other professions.

—Hildegard Peplau
February 10, 1992

Peplau's career was multifaceted and played out on several different local and national stages. While her impact on psychiatric nursing care in public mental hospitals was major and profound, and the impact of her graduate program at Rutgers was certainly national in scope, a third focus of her long career was much more problematic. As the years went by, her increasing involvement in nursing's professional associations was to be a source of growing frustration and disillusionment. By 1955, when she went to Rutgers, Hilda knew she would

> . . . have to do something about nursing. Until then we had nothing like hard scientific knowledge to take to colleagues in other professions— there was no intellectual dialogue in nursing, thus we had nothing to offer other professions . . . This is why I decided to go to Rutgers and go after the grants. If we could train nurses as clinical specialists, and do it right, then we'd have something to contribute in dialogue with other professions.[1]

Hilda believed this lack of a definitive clinical focus in nursing profoundly limited nursing's ability to develop as a profession. While today Peplau is widely recognized and honored as "the mother of psychiatric nursing," her efforts to move all of nursing in the direction taken by other health care professions are much less widely acknowledged and generally not yet understood. Yet, for more than half a century, she either initiated or was active in every major effort to professionalize nursing. Through her work in nursing's two major professional organizations, the National League for Nursing (NLN) and the American Nurses Association (ANA), Peplau sought to bring together her efforts in education and practice to advance nursing's professional image.

Hilda Peplau's own career path diverged greatly from that taken by most hospital-trained nurses of her generation. That path was determined from the earliest years by a deeply personal sense that nursing, as a profession, could and must make its own distinct contribution to the science and practice of health care. She had set herself upon that path as early as the 1930s when, as camp nurse at the New York University summer camp, she worked with instructors from Smith, Barnard, Vassar, and Mount Holyoke colleges, and New York and Columbia Universities. They accepted her as a professional and began to socialize her into thinking of herself as such, rather than as "just a nurse." Then, while she was a nurse and a student at Bennington College, both Wilmoth Osborne and Joseph Chassell regarded her as a professional equal, assuming she had the appropriate education and experience to make independent judgments in her own domain. During long winter breaks, her Bennington field experiences (8 weeks in New York working with Dr. David M. Levy on a research project the first year, 8 weeks at Bellevue Hospital the second, and then 12 weeks at Chestnut Lodge the third year) added to her perceptions of what constituted a profession. During World War II, while at the 312th Station Hospital, she deepened her understanding of psychiatric theory while interacting with men who later came to be among the ranks of America's leading psychiatrists. It was then that Peplau began to think analytically about nursing in relation to medicine, and the complementary roles of each in health care. Increasingly she visualized the nursing and medical professions as sharing some common ground, but with different and separate contributions to make to the health needs of people.

During the early years at Teachers College (TC), when she taught in the summer session, she had many discussions with sociologist C. Everett Hughes about his own field, the sociology of professions. At this time she began to think conceptually about the scope of professional practice in nursing. At Highland Hospital in North Carolina, she had begun to develop an integrated nursing education and practice program when the hospital fire caused her to reconsider her direction. She returned to New York and Teachers College to earn a doctoral degree and to pursue her ideas for the advancement of nursing through academic channels. Finally, before joining the faculty at Rutgers in 1954 she developed a private practice in Manhattan (a practice she continued after moving to New Jersey) where she began to visualize therapeutic roles for nurse clinical specialists holding graduate degrees.

From the mid-1950s on, Hilda Peplau's career had a two-track trajectory. Within her specialty of psychiatric nursing she constantly pushed the boundaries of practice, while in her involvement with national and international nursing associations she argued for the professionalization of the entire field of nursing. Peplau merged her experiences outside the traditional nursing framework with a deep involvement in the substance and practice of her own specialty. In the process she formulated a clear concept of what a profession is and does, and thus a vision of what nursing, if practiced as a true profession, could and should be doing. Essentially, she believed that nursing must be able to delineate the scope of nursing practice; it must define and certify clinical competence; it must have clear minimum requirements for licensure; and, finally, it must have processes of certification for advanced or specialized practice. This model of a profession guided her work in nursing's associations. Her unrelenting efforts caused continuous controversy around her. It is not surprising that *this* thrust of her career remained largely misunderstood and unacknowledged even as nursing's highest honors were later bestowed upon her.

EDUCATIONAL REFORM: A VISION

Peplau saw that the necessary first step in the professionalization of nursing was to move nursing education from hospital-based nursing schools to colleges. In the 1950s, the national consensus was that the profession of medicine, practiced by doctors, required graduate academic and clinical training leading to the MD degree. Specialization was a further option, requiring additional training and certification. In contrast, the educational background of nurses could range from a 2-year hospital-based program under the tutelage of physicians on through, in very few cases, to a PhD or somewhat more commonly to an EdD in nursing education. For nursing to qualify itself as a profession, as Hilda saw it, nursing education had to be controlled by nurses, and minimal educational standards had to be established, including a shift from hospital-based to college-based education. Nurse leaders needed to identify the ways in which the work of nurses was distinct from that of other health care professionals. Nurse theorists needed to develop concepts and models to guide nursing practice, and nurse researchers needed to provide an empirical basis to support those models. It was a grand vision, but resistance was deep.

The roots of resistance to Peplau's vision are not hard to find, beginning with Hilda's own reputation within the nursing community. One of professional nursing's fundamental problems is a strong undercurrent of class consciousness. Because Peplau possessed an earned doctorate, many rank-and-file nurses did not realize that she, like they, had graduated from a small hospital school and came from a working-class rather than a middle-class background. It was erroneously assumed that she had "never practiced." In fact, from working in the emergency room at Pottstown

Hospital through working in the field hospital during the war, and in her drive to reform nursing care in public mental health hospitals, Peplau was as concerned with nursing practice as any other nursing leader. She was perceived first as an educator, however, and so also, by definition, an elitist. No characterization could have been less apt, but the perception remained, creating a practical gap between Peplau and the "sisterhood" of working nurses whose status she hoped to elevate.

In the 1950s, when Peplau was formulating her vision for a profession of nursing nearly 40% of all RNs were practicing private-duty nursing, and the leading magazine for private-duty nurses was *The Trained Nurse*.[2] Its 1950s editorials emphasized "character"—not professionalism—and continued to define the good nurse by the 19th-century "Nightingale" model, which emphasized innate womanly characteristics and devotion to service, self-sacrifice, and a higher moral good. *The Trained Nurse*, which was distributed through state nurses associations, had, at its peak, a circulation of some 200,000. Consistently, the journal attacked efforts to raise entry-level educational requirements for nursing, and editorialized that education was no substitute for discipline and devotion to the service of others. The journal portrayed professional nursing's concern with education as irrelevant to the needs of the working nurse.[3]

Historically, while a small subset of nursing leaders was concerned with raising educational requirements, nurses in practice—those reached by *The Trained Nurse*—were concerned primarily with conditions of work and opposed to any reform that might raise educational requirements for them. These rank-and-file nurses, an overwhelming majority of whom were graduates of hospital schools, resisted any effort to move nursing education into institutions of higher learning. Too, hospital administrators fought hard to retain the schools and their students, who provided, at so little cost, so much of a hospital's daily workforce. The notion of clinical nurse specialists, holding graduate degrees, was simply beyond the imagination and expectations of most nurses, and beyond financial feasibility in the minds of hospital administrators. Physicians, who certainly understood the professional issues involved, offered little or no support. By and large, they wanted nurses to perform as well-trained subordinates. And the general public was certainly not interested in the concept of a "professional nurse." Since nursing itself had not differentiated between a hospital-trained nurse, a college-educated nurse, or a clinical specialist with a graduate degree, similarly members of the public seldom made a distinction between a nurse's aide and a registered nurse (RN).

In her own work consulting and conducting workshops in hospitals across the country Peplau experienced repeated examples of the ambiguity that nurses themselves felt over their place in the hospital hierarchy. For example, in late 1963 she had been invited to talk to nurses at the Montefiore Hospital in New York City about the nurse-patient interpersonal relationship and issues and trends in nursing. When she arrived she found an undercurrent of discontent. The nurses were angry and the doctors were puzzled. The physicians were taken aback that "their" nurses, whom they genuinely liked, seemed angry at *them*. The director of nursing asked Hilda if she would try to analyze the increasing tension between the doctors and the nurses at Montefiore. The nurses had complained cryptically to the director that the doctors were treating them badly, but they didn't want to talk about it. Peplau agreed to talk with the nurses, and then with the doctors. She began by trying to get the nurses to pinpoint what had angered them. "We are angry about the docs" is all she could get from them. Gradually, the story emerged.

The precipitating event occurred on the day of President John F. Kennedy's assassination. Television sets had been on in the children's unit as the nurses were preparing the children for naps when news of the shooting came over the airways. A few children were mesmerized by the commotion on the screens, and soon all the children were crying. The nurses organized immediately, talking to and comforting the children. Two nurses, students of Peplau, began taking notes, getting down as much of the verbatim material as they could. The next morning, when the chief pediatrician came on his rounds with an entourage, he asked as he was leaving, "Anything new?" "Well, yes," replied one of the nurses, "The President of the United States was assassinated yesterday." She went on to explain the children's distress and mentioned that she and her colleague had taken notes on children's reactions. The pediatrician then said he'd like to see the notes. He took the notebooks and simply walked off, followed by the entourage. Shortly thereafter, on the morning news, the nurses saw that very doctor with several of his entourage appearing on television. He had called a national news conference to talk about how *they* had dealt with the children. No nurses had been invited, consulted, or credited. That was what the nurses were angry about. The physicians remained puzzled. After all, they *had* used the nurses' notes! The doctors had so thoroughly incorporated "their" nurses into their personas that they were truly surprised the nurses felt that their data had been appropriated.

Never one to miss an opportunity when she saw it, Peplau suggested that physicians and nurses at Montefiore work on a joint grant proposal to seek funding for studies of nurse-doctor collaboration. Dr. Harold Laufman, professor of clinical surgery, liked the idea. Peplau then spent an enormous amount of time helping the Montefiore nurses develop a proposal to the Department of Health, Education and Welfare (HEW) to establish a special nurse-doctor surgical center. She was deeply disappointed when it was not funded. She later learned that it was the nurse consultant at HEW, not the physicians, who had shelved the proposal. The consultant felt that it threatened the established status-quo relationship between doctors and nurses.[4] In Peplau's vision for educational reform, such collaboration between professional equals in clinical research would be a given.

NURSING'S DILEMMA

In the 1960s, as Peplau labored to instill concepts of professionalism, nursing's primary professional association, the American Nurses Association, concerned itself more and more intensively with union-like activities directed to economic issues rather than with the development of educational thresholds and clinical expertise. In this period, the majority of hospital nurses were working long hours and split shifts for low pay under authoritarian supervision and rigid rules. For this reason, many of these nurses began to leave hospital work altogether for private-duty nursing, taking care of individual private patients on a one-to-one basis. It is therefore not surprising that the American Nurses Association—which defined itself as an organization representing the interests of individual nurses rather than of the nursing profession—spent much of its organizational energy in supporting calls for better hours, better pay, in-house education, and better pensions.[5] Accordingly, the largest section of the ANA was the division concerned with "Economic and General Welfare." This emphasis was reflected in the fact that, unlike medical professional meetings where the focus was on clinical sessions and research presentations, professional organizational meetings in nursing focused largely on economic issues.

Moreover, as hospitals became larger and more complex, there was a reordering of the division of labor. The fact that many nurses moved in and out of hospital work and private duty meant that there was often high turnover in hospital nursing services, thus giving nursing supervisors both more responsibility and more power. As nursing services became ever more central to hospital care, their directors were paid accordingly. Within the ANA, these directors became a powerful force in opposition to professional upgrading and reform. Well paid and well ensconced in hospitals, they had a vested interest in fostering the union mentality rather than instilling a professional mentality in the legion of rank-and-file nurses. Certainly the ANA reinforced this tendency in nursing, to the frustration and disappointment of Hilda Peplau and a few other nursing leaders.

PREACHING THE MESSAGE

Hilda Peplau was not naive in her assessment of the forces arrayed in support of the status quo, but her vision was clear. For nearly 2 decades, she was indefatigable in her efforts to carry her message of the need to professionalize both to nursing's leadership and to nurses in the field. Through the 1960s and into the 1970s she traveled constantly, at great cost to her own health and well-being. She spoke widely, published extensively, served on almost innumerable national and international committees and commissions, and toward the end of her career generously spent the last of her depleted energies in an effort to move the ANA itself forward on behalf of the profession. Wherever Peplau went in support of the professionalization of nursing, she not only shared her considerable expertise in psychiatric nursing but also her pride and optimism about the future of nursing as a whole. She seemed to think that if she talked to enough nurses in enough settings, if she explained, presented, and met with enough members of the profession, she could rally them to the reforms necessary to move ahead. For nearly 15 years, she never sat still. She seemed driven as she dashed from state to state, meeting to meeting, venue to venue—talking, explaining, cajoling, always making the extra effort to convince nurses of the need to raise educational standards, to specialize in clinical areas, and to increase their professional image.

In government agencies, in endless committee work, in professional associations, and in hospital-school and university graduation speeches, Peplau constantly reiterated the theme that if nursing could move its educational base into colleges and universities, and develop graduate programs offering clinical specialty tracks, nursing could make significant contributions to health care while at the same time raising its own professional status. Peplau believed that just as nurses with graduate degrees in psychiatric nursing could help patients by establishing one-on-one therapeutic relationships with them, so could nurses working in public health agencies or in hospitals, emergency rooms, and intensive care units, make unique and substantive contributions to the health of their patients.

Peplau tried to inspire nursing to learn from other professions that were also dealing with professional issues related to practice, particularly psychology and social work. It was hard going. Her constant efforts to infuse science and scientific methods into nursing education made others uncomfortable. Her efforts to professionalize nursing were seen as violating the very "soul" of nursing. She was perceived as being "uncaring," and her approach to nursing was labeled too "mechanistic."[6] This effort also ran into opposition from physicians and hospital administrators, including the administrators of nursing services, who measured good nursing according to how "efficient," that is, how cheap, it was. Precisely because these groups *did* equate nursing with "women's work" and "caring," they devalued it.

The class issues that underlay the hostility toward reform efforts, particularly the effort to move nursing education from hospitals and community colleges to 4-year colleges and universities, could not be overcome. Rather than address the issue head on, nursing's leadership kept trying to bring about reform incrementally, and without a major confrontation. Thus, both the American Nurses Association and the National League for Nursing encouraged collegiate education while seeking at the same time to upgrade the standards in the hospital schools and community colleges. Because the majority of nurses worked in hospitals where administrators and supervisors were suspicious of, if not hostile to, the college graduates, however, reform was never seriously addressed at the grassroots level. For their part, college graduates were not as willing to accept hospital routines without question as were the diploma graduates, but their energies, too, were directed primarily toward demands for higher salaries. As the health care system moved to contain costs, the salary issue became critical. By not setting basic educational requirements as a gateway into the profession, nursing may have lost its opportunity ever to do so. Peplau saw this coming 30 years before managed care was on the horizon, but in spite of heroic efforts, she was not able to rally nursing to reform itself.

AN EDUCATOR FIRST

Peplau was first and foremost an educator, and it was in thinking about her field of psychiatric nursing that she also began to formulate her positions concerning the advancement of professionalization in nursing. Through her work to develop graduate education in psychiatric nursing, she began to see a paradigm for nursing as a whole. Psychiatric nursing was also her entree into professional nursing associations. When she was not in the classroom, she was either serving on national committees concerned with the development of graduate education in her field or on the road explaining the significance of what was happening in psychiatric nursing education to others, both inside and outside of nursing. Because her role as an educator framed all she did, it is important to put this contribution into a wider professional context.

By the time she came to Rutgers in 1954, Peplau was a major grants woman, securing funds for faculty salaries, travel, equipment, and for tuition stipends for graduates to pursue graduate education in other fields. By the time her program was up and running in 1956, Peplau had served on the planning committee for an NLN-sponsored national conference on "Trends in Psychiatric Nursing" and then played the central role in the conference itself held in Washington, D.C., in April 1956. After this, she was inundated with invitations to consult in hospitals, clinics, colleges, and with state departments of health. Nurses from around the country began to write to her, and she spent an inordinate amount of time sending long, detailed, and thoughtful, responses to their requests.[7] In the early years at Rutgers, she was in full academic swing: publishing, giving papers at professional meetings, serving on national panels, and accepting countless invitations to speak. These speeches were always long, dense, serious, and thoughtful, and always raised issues of nursing's image as a profession.[8] Through all of this, her influence continued to expand.

Her first book, *Interpersonal Relations in Nursing,* quickly became a classic. It is remarkable that 50 years after its first publication, *Interpersonal Relations* was still considered relevant and was reissued without revisions in 1996. This work has helped to frame nearly every subsequent text in psychiatric nursing.[9] Although accepted as common sense today, Peplau's conceptualization of the process of the nurse-patient interaction and its possibilities stands as one of the first major delineations of what is (or could be) distinctive about nursing. Her paradigm for psychiatric nursing stressed that both nurse and patient participate in and contribute to the nurse-patient relationship, and that the relationship itself could and should be therapeutic. In psychiatric nursing, the emphasis should be on understanding the problematic, psychosocial behavioral problems of patients rather than upon diagnostic categories of mental illness, which was domain of the psychiatrist. In this way, each professional contribution could be delineated and applied. By developing a focus and body of knowledge of its own, Peplau argued, psychiatric nursing would professionalize itself. Other fields in nursing could and should follow the same model, she asserted. Rather than attempt to develop grand theory themselves, Peplau urged that nurses adapt appropriate theories, wherever they be found, to the practice of nursing care. Her call was for theoretical pluralism, in which nurses choose an appropriate theory for a specific situation and apply it appropriately in practice. The critical question nursing students should be taught to ask was, Does this theory or explanation of this patient's problem enable me to identify interventions that will help this patient move toward recovery or health?[10] Always she reiterated the refrain: Examine the phenomenon, observe it, describe it, analyze it, extract the themes, and apply them to the next situation as appropriate for effective nursing intervention.

Peplau was famous for using clinical settings up and down the eastern seaboard for her teaching and for getting her students involved in interdisciplinary health care meetings taking place within a radius of several hundred miles of Rutgers. By 1958, to demonstrate what graduate nurses could do, she had her students conducting "ward studies" in all the hospitals in which they worked. She dreamed of being able to use these studies to demonstrate the difference that nursing could make in patient improvement in the hospital. She constantly urged upon nursing the benefits of specialization in nursing practice, believing that specialists' concerns could push the whole profession forward. Thus, her consultation and teaching took her out of the classroom into diverse clinical settings across the country to share what she had developed and learned in her own specialty of psychiatric nursing.

Peplau's Program in Psychiatric Nursing at Rutgers was noted for its rigor and emphasis on research into and application of psychiatric concepts. As time went by and the 1950s moved into the 1960s, other programs developed that explicitly rejected this approach and found the Peplau example objectionable—as "not really nursing." While she strove mightily to interest nurses in the intellectual work of nursing, most nurse educators did not understand her. A few program leaders who did understand her point were nonetheless temperamentally, if not ideologically, opposed to Peplau's emphases on psychiatric concepts and their clinical application in nursing. To them, nursing was fundamentally about caring.[11]

One such program was directed by June Mellow at Boston University. Mellow was the first to use the term "therapy" to describe what psychiatric nurses were doing when talking to patients in a "one-to-one relationship," but her conception of the nurse-patient relationship was diametrically opposed to Peplau's. In April 1968 a symposium featuring Mellow and Peplau was held at Yale University to explore these alternative approaches.[12] The 200-page transcript reveals the deep differences between the two. Mellow argued that therapy was "more artistic than scientific" and could work only when the therapist became emotionally involved with the patient, stressing that therapy was essentially a "professional form of love." She asserted that women made particularly good therapists because they identified with the patient more easily than did male therapists and were not afraid of feeling the emotion inevitable in a therapeutic relationship. As different cases were presented, Peplau and Mellow outlined the approaches each would take. The audience clearly identified with Mellow and found Peplau unfeeling and "too objective." After much heated discussion, someone asked, "Wouldn't you both get results?" This excerpt from Peplau's response provides a good summary of her thinking on this point:

> Yes, but my concern is for the enduring nature of the results and my claim is that if the therapist builds in these interpersonal competencies, they will endure over time and be usable in other situations . . . I am of the general opinion that there is a structure to mental illness, and that there are scientific aspects to it that we can develop—that there are reliable explanatory theories in this field as there are in other fields. We can study the phenomena of disturbed behavior in an individual . . . there is a logical approach. This doesn't mean that feeling and intuition and inference don't matter—of course they do—but there will also be a

substantive scientific core that will be useful to recognize. And that core will be dealing with universals—things you see in all people. The uniqueness comes not in terms of the patterns, but in terms of the variance of the pattern . . .

Now you can go on loving until you are blue in the face, but if you don't know what the pathology is that you're working with, then you can't remedy it. If you don't understand what the problem is then you can't solve it . . . Therapy is a one-to-one relationship that minimizes the burden on the patient and yet in a gradual way evokes and develops the needed intellectual and personal competencies . . . You have to help the patient name the problem. This is terribly important. If the patient is anxious, you have to help the patient name it.[13]

The audience reacted negatively to this statement, asserting that Peplau was not talking about nursing, that nursing was about *caring*. Hilda exclaimed plaintively at one point, "I would hate for you to think I'm an uncaring person. I think of myself otherwise!"[14] She might have thought of herself otherwise, but it is clear from the transcript that the audience did not share that perception.

As is clear from her remarks at the Yale conference, Peplau did not believe that there were rigid models of nursing care that students could be taught, but rather that there are "reliable explanatory theories" that could assist nurses in therapeutic relationships with the patients. The use of terms like *model* or *theory* to define her own work, however, concerned her because she believed that such terms were either too simple or produced distortions of her work. Peplau used the theories of *others* to visualize a distinctive role for nursing in the care of patients. She urged that observations and explanatory concepts be used to make clinical judgments to determine a nursing intervention. She believed that the word *model* was an oversimplification of this process of inquiry. As she stated it, "I cannot see the vast complexities of a nursing science, or of a service and the people it serves, somehow being fitted into a model."[15] She added, "A careful reading of everything I've ever published will show that I have not used the words *model* or *theory*. Others have attributed the terms to my work, or foisted them upon me."[16]

In the late 1950s, Peplau began to accept invitations to speak to physicians about the new direction of psychiatric nursing, particularly in the public mental hospitals. The talks were long, closely written, full of facts and figures and details, and perhaps overly cautious so as not to engender a negative reaction.[17] Those who listened were impressed. Her trouble would not come from physicians. In these talks, Peplau gave examples of how a "well-trained" nurse could function therapeutically in order to make a difference on the wards, to intervene when patients were undergoing severe anxiety or panic. She described a progression of nursing roles, from "customary mothering functions" such as bathing, feeding, and dressing the patients, to "therapeutic roles" in which nurses communicate with patients "in order to prepare that patient for therapy with the doctor." This last remark was made somewhat facetiously, since both Hilda and the physicians knew that the chance of a patient in a public mental hospital actually being seen therapeutically by a physician was very remote. The physicians who heard her, however, were more inclined to be supportive than were members of the nursing profession itself. So long as she was talking about working with patients in mental hospitals, Peplau would receive no opposition from psychiatrists. Opposition would come when she began openly to use graduate education to prepare nurses for private practice, and then, again, not so much from the medical profession as from nursing itself, and from social workers and psychologists, who saw nursing as encroaching on their territory.[18]

While Peplau was successful in explaining her goals to psychiatrists serving state mental hospitals, she would be considerably less successful in her efforts to effect change in the entrenched attitudes of nurses toward physicians and vice versa. The transcripts of the jointly sponsored AMA-ANA 1964 and 1965 conferences dealing with the nurse-doctor relationship make it clear that both nurses and physicians had a way to go before professional relationships between the two could become a reality.[19] The physicians referred to the nurses as "the girls," and the nurses referred to the physicians as "the docs." Peplau sought to get the nurses to understand that words matter, and to acknowledge that it was hard to be colleagues when there were such marked differences in education, income, status, and gender. In the end, the nurse participants did agree, in principle, that there was a "definite need for basic standards in nursing education of the kind that would roughly approximate the uniformity of standards in medical education."[20]

By 1968 physicians were writing Peplau from all over the country requesting her suggestions for revising manuals of care, for consultations on the role of nursing in psychiatric clinics, for her advice on psychiatric nursing services, and for participation in discussions concerning the physician-nurse relationship. It was not always smooth sailing. Dr. Charles Gardner, Jr., the director of the Yale Psychiatric Institute, made the mistake of inviting Hilda to participate in a case conference and sending her the "protocol of the patient" to be the subject of the conference. Gardner would learn his lesson, as had many before him. Peplau took the case apart, sentence by sentence.[21] In Peplau's mind, the nurse-physician relationship was one of equals.[22] By this point in her career, she was confident that she did indeed have something to offer, even if most others in her field did not.

On the appointed day, she drove up to Yale. An eminent European psychiatrist had also been invited and was clearly regarded as the honored guest. Dr. Gardner had apparently expected Peplau to be deferential and not to take a substantive role in the discussion. After making grand rounds, the conferees convened in an elegant wood-paneled room complete with an imposing conference table, crystal chandeliers, and a silver coffee service. The subject of the conference, a 13- to 14-year-old boy suffering from depression, was brought in. Peplau was appalled. First of all, the young man must have been intimidated by the room itself, and second, this group of terribly serious adults could not have been reassuring. Then, the questions started. They were all of a strictly Freudian nature. After the patient left, the "great one" was asked to speak. He held forth for an hour with his Freudian theories, based on a deeply flawed case write-up, at least in Peplau's view, and 15 terribly artificial minutes with the boy. He diagnosed the boy as homoerotic with repressed sexual drives. Peplau had always harbored great reservations about psychoanalysis. She felt the interview with the boy was too brief to jump to a diagnosis and that the "diagnosis" itself was full of canned psychoanalytic interpretations. After the eminent guest's Freudian analysis, the group broke for lunch, Peplau going off with the residents while the physicians took the honored guest for a tête-à-tête.

When they reconvened after lunch for a wrap-up session, Peplau was asked if she had anything to add. She did. She asked that the boy be brought back in, much to the discomfort of the assembled group. When the boy reappeared, she spoke with him reassuringly, asking him about himself, and then honing in on the period when he had been sent away to school while his parents were out of the country. She asked him about his friends, his relationship to them, his feelings about the school, and his feelings when his parents returned. It soon became clear the boy did have problems and fears about abandonment, but they were not sexual in nature. Rather than being homoerotic, the boy was simply lonely. After the patient left the room, using a developmental rather than a Freudian interpretation, Peplau pointed out gaps in the data, made suggestions on its meaning, and suggested the directions *she* would pursue. By this time, the tension in the room was so high she was afraid to breathe.[23] The physicians were defensive and upset. A mere nurse had seen something they missed, and this group was highly offended, perhaps because of the presence of their distinguished guest.

CLINICAL SPECIALISTS

As early as 1956 Peplau realized that not only educational reform but also a new vision of nursing practice was essential to advance professionalization. She envisioned nurse clinical specialists holding master's degrees, working in hospitals, nursing homes, or in the private practice of their specialties.[24] In this vision, nurses would function much as physicians did, setting their own schedules, defining their own protocols, and offering clinical expertise in specified areas of nursing practice. The prototype, of course, was psychiatric nursing. She traveled the country presenting her ideas on university-based nursing education and practice. In her vision, undergraduate education would focus on the needs of institutions (such as hospitals and clinics), and prepare nurses to assume staffing and leadership roles in them. Master's level programs would produce clinical specialists in areas such as medical/surgical nursing, intensive care nursing, pediatric, and psychiatric nursing. Doctoral programs would be developed to generate nursing research on clinical and health care issues, and would produce graduates to assume faculty roles in colleges of nursing. By the late 1950s, Peplau was utterly convinced nursing would not advance until it began to make distinctions among nurses based on educational requirements and certification. In her view, not only should the hospital schools be phased out, but differentiations in college and university education should be clear. In short, Peplau had decided to confront head on the prevailing ideology that "a nurse is a nurse is a nurse."

In pursuit of this proposal, she traveled continuously, speaking wherever she was invited. Her relentless travel and speaking schedule generated voluminous correspondence from nurses across the country—much of it quibbling with one point or another she had made, while studiously avoiding the issue itself.[25] As is often typical of faculty members in other disciplines, the nurses picked apart the specifics of the proposal instead of endorsing the principle and then working on the details. Peplau took all of the critiques seriously, attempting to answer them thoughtfully and intelligently. She also wrote long treatises for psychiatrists and hospital and nursing service directors trying to explain what a clinical specialist could do for them and trying to enlist their support.

In response to seemingly endless letters from nurses uncomfortable with the term clinical specialist, Hilda wrote a 3-page summary of "The Nurse Clinical Specialist Role," trying to clarify what a clinical specialist could do that other nurses could not. She sent the paper out for comment, but what she got back was more quibbling about definitions, descriptions, classifications, etc.[26] Some did get the point, but had difficulty conceiving how in practice a clinical specialist would work in their setting. Peplau was frustrated by the confusion caused by a word she considered self-explanatory. Ever concrete, however, she took the confusion seriously and developed an instrument to conduct a national survey to determine the understanding of the word "specialist" in order to develop a definition clear to all. She sought in vain to secure funding for such a study. During 1957 and 1958, she had her graduate students at Rutgers writing papers and designing research projects on the "functions of the clinical specialist."[27]

All of this was to no avail. Hilda Peplau was a voice in the wilderness. Most graduate education in nursing consisted of 1-year master's level programs that produced nurses qualified to teach, direct nursing services, or to practice. Clinical expertise was not a focus, and often not even an option.

Peplau believed that if she could convince a significant core of nursing's leadership that educational restructuring would change nursing's opportunities, they would take action. In her work with the Southern Regional Education Board (SREB), as with all her government work, she constantly urged deans and directors to take advantage of federal programs to get nursing moving—to apply for funding, train and then hire good faculty, develop graduate programs, and develop strong clinical foci—just get started.[28] Suspicion, petty jealousies, and insecurities, however, would continue to bedevil nursing throughout Hilda's active career.

In 1960 Peplau began to push for wider acceptance of psychiatric nursing in the broader therapeutic community. She proposed to the American Group Psychotherapy Association that membership be extended to psychiatric nurses. The president, Maurice E. Linden, MD, responded that the association was "not prepared this year to admit them."[29] A year later, Jay Fidler, MD, chairman of the program committee for the association's annual meeting, wrote to ask Hilda to make a presentation on the uses of group psychotherapy by nurses. She agreed.[30] She worked diligently on her presentation, for she did not want to offend. In January 1962 she drove to Atlantic City for the panel. Her presentation went well, but the occupational therapists and social workers in the audience were hostile. Once again, it was the psychiatrists who understood what Hilda was doing and rose to her defense. One, Dr. David Alman, took the time to write:

> I was very much impressed by the whole concept of nurse-counseling; beyond that I was quite moved by the intensity of your style, the firmness with which you shunned the platitudes in which much of all therapeutic rhetoric is engulfed, and with what I can only call your unrelenting orientation to patients. You know better than I do how rare it is to find both original thinking and militant teaching in the same person in any profession, and when it occurs it ought to be—but isn't— trumpeted in style.[31]

Later that year, in addition to writing a contribution for the *American Handbook of Psychiatry*, she was asked to write (and did) a piece on "Principles of Psychiatric Nursing" for the *Handbook of Psychology*.[32]

THE NURSE PRACTITIONER MOVEMENT

In the early 1960s, the federal government provided funding to give "nurse practitioners" the skills needed to conduct basic physical assessments.

When nurse practitioner programs were established to provide this training, Peplau initially endorsed them. While continuing to urge the development of graduate clinical specialist programs in nursing, she realized that the shorter practitioner programs would be more attractive to the large majority of nurses who did not wish to pursue graduate degrees and would present an opportunity for them to upgrade their skills. She soon realized that the nurse practitioner movement was giving rise to a concept of "advanced practice" in nursing without any agreement on educational prerequisites. She sought agreement that the concept of advanced practice implied the master's degree as the basic educational requirement. Such a consensus could not be reached, as nurses without college degrees, let alone graduate work, took advantage of the nurse practitioner programs to enter "advanced practice." Because they lacked the essential educational credentials themselves, they would not support resolutions that required the master's degree for "advanced practice." Over time, the master's degree became the norm for nurse practitioners, but in the early days of this specialty this was not the case.

In 1966 Peplau succeeded in getting funding for 5 years for a nationwide series of 10-day "general practitioner" workshops to be given in university settings or through university continuing education programs. These workshops would introduce basic psychiatric nursing concepts and physical assessment skills to nurses in order that they might work in the newly established community mental health centers. Because of her consulting role with government agencies, she was keenly aware of new initiatives to move patients out of the public mental hospitals into communities to be served by community mental health centers. Hilda envisioned practitioner programs as a short-term, stopgap phenomenon, not as an alternative to overall educational reform. Although in the best of worlds psychiatric nurses would pursue graduate degrees, she recognized that in the short run this was not an attainable goal. For the same reason, she had embarked upon the summer workshops as a way of reaching frontline nurses and improving their skills, if not their academic preparation. Thus, as she explained to Helen Tibbits, the executive secretary to the Nursing Study Section of the National Institutes of Health,

> I seem to be getting an increasing number of letters from nurses about where to get some short course help with specialist training and research . . . Of course, I think a PhD program is the only sound approach, but, as with the clinical specialists in psych nursing, I believe short courses might help plow up the field and get some seeds planted—either to find more applications for PhD study or to light fires to aid and abet nursing research.[33]

Thus, she began adding short courses on nursing research methods to her repertoire and traveling schedule.

BACK TO BASICS

Beginning in 1915 a few of nursing's leaders in the ANA struggled to move nursing education into the country's colleges and universities.[34] Through the years many meetings and many committees sought to define professional standards and to delineate education requirements necessary to meet them. Nearly every ANA president in this century has dealt with the issue, either supporting collegiate education as basic to professional nursing, or establishing committees to study the issue. In 1960, the ANA Long-Term Planning Committee finally recommended that baccalaureate education be required for nurse licensure, but not until 1964 did the ANA House of Delegates recommend that the ANA "work toward baccalaureate education as the educational foundation for professional nursing."[35] Ten years later, however, even this small step was undercut. In 1973, the House of Delegates voted "to examine the contemporary relevance of the terms 'professional' and 'technical' and to distinguish the basic preparation for nursing practice, and to recognize all registered nurses as professionals."[36] The inability of nursing to take this basic step opened the door for ancillary health care workers to erode the boundaries of nursing practice, until, in the 1990s, hospitals began to substitute less expensive aides and "practical" nurses for the more highly paid "professional" nurses (nurses who had passed the state boards for registered nurses).

The scenario of nurses fighting within their own ranks for the dubious privilege of retaining the lowest educational entry requirement among all health professions was profoundly discouraging to Peplau as she approached the end of her career. Even at the graduate level, instead of going in the direction of clinical specialist training, as she had advocated, graduate nursing curriculums seemed to be moving in the opposite direction.

At the beginning of the 21st century, nurses still had not resolved the problem of a common education requirement for entry into the profession. A nurse can still earn the same RN license through a hospital school, a community college, or a university. In fact, the majority of RNs still do not hold a baccalaureate degree, although the numbers of RNs with a baccalaureate degree or higher has grown significantly since Peplau's era (43%).[37] Peplau never gave up, however. In 1968 she wrote the newly elected governor of New Jersey suggesting that he appoint a commission to decide the "fastest, most economical way of closing the state's thirty-five hospital-operated nursing schools."[38] Because the move was so controversial and divisive, she was asked to give radio and television commentary on the issue, which she did willingly and with great frequency. New Jersey entered the 21st century with this issue remaining unresolved. Hilda's failure in this regard was offset by one small victory: In

1965, when serving as nurse consultant to the Air Force, she strongly recommended that the armed forces begin to recruit only college-educated
nurses.[39] This soon became Air Force official policy.

REFORMER IN NURSING ASSOCIATIONS

Never one to give up, Peplau in the 1950s and 1960s redoubled her efforts
to work within nursing's established associations, first in the National
League for Nursing, and then in the American Nurses Association. The
ANA, in contrast to the NLN, always defined itself an organization for
"nurses," not for "nursing," much to Peplau's frustration. In this work,
Peplau sat through endless meetings for over 2 decades, trying to contain
her frustration as nurses evaded the issues and muddled on obsessively
trying to find consensus on what it was they were about.[40] Although
often frustrated with her nursing colleagues, Peplau did manage to keep
a sense of humor in regard to the endless, often useless committee meetings. As she wrote to a friend and colleague, Helen Arnold, in 1965 following one of these meetings,

> Unfortunately, we had such a chairman that we drifted around and
> never got to one item on the agenda—and little else too. Before the
> meeting was over, I managed to fix that. We spent a bit of time on vot-
> ing in a new chairman.[41]

Her concern about this emphasis in the ANA was well-placed, for both
its members and its leadership continued to target economic issues as
their top priority. Although there was great debate in the organization
about whether collective bargaining was consistent with the ANA image
as a professional organization, over time the association nonetheless
encouraged nurses to engage in collective bargaining to gain better pay
and better working conditions. Nurses wanted it both ways. They supported collective bargaining to assure economic security, and they wanted
their professional organization, rather than a union, to do the bargaining.
Because the ANA was nursing's only professional organization, however,
Hilda felt she had no choice but to work for reform within its ranks to
move the organization away from its trade-union mentality. She wanted
it clear that nurses were, or could be, independent practitioners, not
assembly-line workers.[42]

In one area, however, Peplau found some fulfillment. Her participation in ANA efforts to purge state nurses associations of racial barriers
was successful. In 1958, she was asked to serve as a member of the ANA's
Intergroup Relations Committee and then, in 1959, to chair it. The Intergroup Relations program had been established in 1950 to "open opportunities to all racial and religious groups in the ANA."[43] That year the ANA

had agreed to absorb the National Association of Colored Graduate Nurses (NACGN). The Intergroup Relations Program was established to facilitate their integration into the association. At that time, 15 southern states barred colored nurses from membership in their state nurses associations (SNAs), thus precluding their membership in the ANA, which was a constituent rather than a direct membership organization. To deal with this issue, the ANA Board extended the category of individual membership, originally created for those serving in the armed forces during the war, to nurses barred from membership in their SNAs because of their race.

In 1959 ANA President Matilda Scheuer called Peplau at Rutgers to discuss the ANA principle of nondiscrimination adopted by the ANA Board in 1948, shortly after the end of the Second World War.[44] They agreed that the Committee on Intergroup Relations would prepare a resolution to be introduced at the ANA meetings in Miami in May 1960 barring SNAs that continued to discriminate on the basis of race from participation in the association. Peplau wrote the resolution and persuaded the committee to vote to recommend it as a part of its report to the House of Delegates. As word about the resolution circulated among the delegates in Miami, tensions rose. By the time Peplau was called upon to give the report, the entire ANA Board was seated on the platform, along with the ANA lawyer, the parliamentarian, and Dr. Robert Merton, the sociologist hired as a consultant to the board. It was a very stormy meeting, with endless motions, counter-motions, points of order, and parliamentary challenges, but in the end, the resolution passed.[45] The state of Georgia was the only holdout. Georgia was then given 2 years to be in compliance with the ANA policy.[46] The category of individual membership was eliminated, and all nurses became members of the ANA through their state associations.

In the summer of 1963 Peplau attended a meeting of the Public Health Nurses of Alabama in Birmingham where she gave a series of lectures. On the third day, as she walked into the meeting room she sensed enormous tension. Several African American nurses were in the audience. Peplau immediately greeted them personally and in her opening remarks stressed that nursing was one community, and that *all* were a part of it. During the lecture, several security guards entered the room and stood at the back. Peplau ignored them and tried to stimulate discussion of her lecture. None was forthcoming. When the session broke for lunch southern hospitality failed: No one invited Hilda to join them. As she stood alone wondering what to do, one of the security guards approached her. He was an "observer" sent by Governor George Wallace, a strident segregationist who preached White supremacy as the engine that drove Alabama politics.[47] The governor's observer invited Hilda to his office for lunch, which was sent in. The observer spent the time talking about how misunderstood the governor was and offering an apologia for segregation in Alabama. When Peplau informed him that Tish, her "niece," was in Ghana with the Experiment for International Living, lunch was quickly concluded.[48]

NATIONAL COMMITTEE WOMAN

From the time she entered Columbia's Teachers College as a student in 1945, and for the rest of her career, Peplau was active on federal government advisory committees on nursing. These included multiple appointments to committees and consultancies for the National Institute of Mental Health; the Veterans Administration; the U.S. Public Health Service; the Department of Health, Education and Welfare; and the World Health Organization. In addition, Peplau devoted a lot of time in the 1950s to the Nurse Advisory Panel to the Southern Regional Education Board. The SREB was set up in 1949 by the governors of the nine southern states to coordinate educational developments in the region. Peplau, along with Esther Garrison, represented nursing education on the advisory panel.[49] She loved working with this group of serious and dedicated educators who thought seriously about the nature of education and the challenges faced by the South which lagged behind much of the rest of the country. In her work with the SREB, Peplau urged an ever broadening perception of nursing education and laid out an agenda of baccalaureate and graduate education. As a result, in the South, at least, new nursing programs would be college- or university-based from the 1950s on.[50]

After each session of the SREB there were many, many letters of thanks and appreciation for her hard work and substantive contributions to the work of the council. As Virginia Crenshaw, then dean of nursing at Vanderbilt University wrote: ". . . we owe you a debt of immense gratitude for all you have done."[51] William J. McGlothlin, president of the University of Louisville, sent a note thanking her for her "substantial" contributions and stating that it was "a rare pleasure to work with someone so constructive."[52] Peplau herself constantly sent memos and reports from the SREB to all deans of colleges of nursing and presidents of state nurses associations about the work of the council, urging them too to work to develop models of professional nursing education.

In her work with the Public Health Service (PHS) Peplau was concerned with assuring that there was funding for nursing research, and that there would be nurses who could do research qualified for the funding. The PHS grants were given in three categories: to specific projects, in lump sums to schools of nursing to fund faculty research, and as faculty research development grants to designated programs.[53] When not in committee meetings, Hilda was out on the speaking circuit urging colleges to apply for grants in the relevant categories. Her goal was to encourage colleges of nursing to develop graduate programs and to assure them federal funding if they did. She advocated and consulted ceaselessly, absolutely convinced that if enough nurses pursued enough education, the overall professionalism of nursing was bound to rise.

By 1964, Peplau was well known throughout nursing, not just in psychiatric nursing. As Earl Shephard, an editor at John Wiley and Sons wrote,

> After meeting so many of your friends and admirers at the various nursing schools which I have visited recently, I was indeed delighted to meet you last week at Rutgers and truly moved by our open and frank discussion . . . You have caused a radical change in my thinking about how we should go about starting a new series of nursing books here.[54]

He then proposed that Peplau edit such a series, but for once she realized this was more than she could take on.

That year Hilda published her second book, *Basic Principles of Patient Counseling*. It received rave reviews.[55] In it she again reiterated her thesis that nurses needed to relate to patients as individuals, not as objects or subjects being treated exclusively by doctors. The focus on the relationship between nurses and patients, independent from the physician's relationship to the patient, represented a major paradigm shift in nursing and had an enormous impact on the way in which "nursing process" courses were taught in the college-based programs. Peplau stressed that the relationship of each nurse to an individual patient makes a substantial difference in what that patient will learn through the experience of illness. She hypothesized that the behavior of nurses in relation to patients with different kinds of health problems provided a rich focus for research into practice, and that from this a science of nursing could evolve.

By 1968 Hilda Peplau had become a nonstop whirlwind, presenting papers at colleges, at the American Psychiatric Association, the American Nurses Association, the American Public Health Association, to staff nurses, at graduations, for Sigma Theta Tau, for Air Force base graduation classes, at VA hospitals, to community health conferences, to SNAs, and to college of nursing alumni associations. Her themes seldom changed. She continued to urge nurses to become interested in clinical problems. By this time, she was literally begging nurses to break out of the supervisor, teacher, hospital bedside track, and work directly with patients in clinical settings or on clinical problems. She urged psychiatric nurses in particular to give direct care to a selected caseload of patients, and then to report on their practice through publications.

While Peplau received numerous expressions of appreciation for her workshops, and high praise for her books, her innovative scholarly papers and policy recommendations were not so enthusiastically received. She did not, however, lack for supporters. One who invariably expressed appreciation for Hilda's "always invaluable work," was Dr. Helen Nahm, who was dean of the College of Nursing at the University of California, San Francisco (UCSF), in the mid-1960s.[56] Peplau first met Helen Nahm in 1947 at a workshop at Duke University just before she accepted the position of instructor at TC. Nahm and Peplau then worked together on the NLN "Structure Study" of 1950.[57] Nahm was a great supporter of the summer workshops, and, as dean at UCSF, assured the workshops in California by securing an NIMH grant for them. During these years, she and Peplau also served on various Western Council of Higher Education Network committees as the consultants. Helen Nahm, Emily Holmquist, Esther Garrison, and Helen Arnold were among only a handful of nurse friends who were not former students, who truly seemed to understand what she was trying to do, and who were supportive in every way they could be.

Nor did her efforts go unrecognized in other quarters. As early as 1952 Dr. Jay Hoffman, who had been the chief medical officer at the 312th Station Hospital and later served with the Veterans Administration, wrote,

Dear Pep:

Thank you for the copies of your two papers . . . In recent weeks I have been particularly impressed by the fact that you by yourself are still a small band, and that the great majority of your sisters prefer to be the passive partners in the traditional marriage of doctor and nurse . . . Nursing will never quite establish itself as a separate profession until it has produced a considerable number of its own, of sufficient capacity and stature as to erect a foundation for the profession.[58]

Toward the end of her career at Rutgers, Hilda had begun to concede that this was a cause she could not advance by willpower and hard work alone. Once in a while, she saw a ray of hope, some indication that her work was understood and appreciated as a whole. Thus, in 1969, she was both surprised and pleased when Columbia's Teachers College awarded her its Nursing Practice Award, for "documented excellence and innovation as a clinician, making a significant, unique contribution to nursing practice, and engaging in scholarly activities related to nursing practice and disseminates those efforts through publications, presentations, and consultations to advance the profession of nursing." She was even more surprised later that same year to be awarded, of all things, the R. Louise McManus Medal, "In recognition of long standing contributions, of a distinguished nature, to the nursing profession."[59]

ENDNOTES

1. Interview, Hildegard Peplau, February 10, 1992, in Sherman Oaks, California.

2. See Susan Reverby, *Ordered to Care: The Dilemma of American Nursing, 1850–1945* (Cambridge: Cambridge University Press, 1987), 137.

3. Reverby, 137–142.

4. This grant proposal may be found in Box 24, #876; her feelings about it were discussed with Hildegard Peplau in a discussion on June 14, 1996, in Washington, D.C.

5. See Beatrice J. Kalish and Philip A. Kalish, *The Advance of America Nursing* (Boston, Little Brown, 1986), 493.

6. See a 200-page typescript of an emotional panel discussion between Peplau and June Mellow, April 17, 1968, on the general issue of "caring" vs. a scientific approach to nursing practice found in Box 25, #904.

7. A collection of this material may be found in Box 21, #699–703.

8. A collection of speeches and papers given during 1954–1956 may be found in Box 20, #675–679.

9. See for example Grayce Sills, "Psychiatric Nursing Theory and Practice, Milieu— 1946–1974," in *Psychiatric Nursing 1946–1974: A Report on the State of the Art* (New York: The American Journal of Nursing Company, 1975); Shirley Burd and Margaret Marshall, *Some Clinical Approaches to Psychiatric Nursing* (New York: Macmillan, 1963); Shirley Smoyak, ed., *The Psychiatric Nurse as a Family Therapist* (New York: Wiley and Sons, 1975); and Joanne Hall and Barbara Weaver, eds., *Nursing of Families in Crisis* (Philadelphia: J. B. Lippincott Company, 1974).

10. Interview, Hildegard Peplau, March 18, 1992.

11. The emphasis on "caring" in the nursing literature of the 1990s caused Peplau dismay. She referred to them (interview, April 23, 1992) as "nursing mystics who wish to focus on caring as a non-spiritual event" and quite the opposite from the rigorous form of inquiry she began nearly a half-century ago. For an overview of the "caring literature," see J. Watson, *Nursing: Human Science and Human Care* (Norwalk: Appleton Century Crofts, 1985); "Watson's Philosophy and Theory of Human Caring in Nursing," in J. Riehl-Sisca, *Conceptual Models for Nursing Practice*, 3rd ed. (Norwalk: Appleton and Lange, 1989); C. Kirby and O. Slevin, "A New Curriculum for Care," in O. Slevin and M. Buckenham eds., *Project 2000—Innovations in the Nursing Curriculum* (Edinburgh: Campion Press, 1992); and recent articles (1994–1998) in the nursing journal *Revolution*.

12. Transcripts of this meeting may be found in Box 24, #904.

13. Ibid, 153.

14. Ibid, 178.

15. Paraphrased from Phil Barker, "The Peplau Legacy," in *Nursing Times 89* (1993), 48–51.

16. Interview, Hildegard Peplau, March 18, 1992. See, for example, H. Simpson, *Peplau's Model in Action* (London: MacMillan, 1991) and A. R. Pede, "The Evolution of an Intervention—the Use of Peplau's Process of Practice-based Theory Development," in *Journal of Psychiatric and Mental Health Nursing* (May, 1998), 173–178.

17. A collection of these talks may be found in Box 21, #727.

18. Two nursing leaders who objected to Peplau's encouragement of nurses entering private practice as clinical specialists were Dorothy Mereness, herself a psychiatric nurse and dean of the College of Nursing at the University of Pittsburgh and ironically, Jane Schmahl—the same Jane Schmahl who had entered the William Alanson White Institute with Hilda in the late 1940s. In 1962 Schmahl wrote, "Because psychotherapy is an autonomous specialty, as is nursing, I believe it is impossible for the psychiatric nurse to become a practicing psychotherapist and at the same time retain her identity as a nurse," and in 1964 Mereness wrote that "Even though there is a serious shortage of therapists, it is logical that the concept of a professional person who is a psychiatric nurse may vanish if nurses continue to expand

their role by preparing and assuming responsibility for therapeutic activities that are recognized as part of the work role of other professional groups." Jane Schmahl, "The Psychiatric Nurse and Psychotherapy," *Nursing Outlook 10* (July, 1962): 460–465; Dorothy Mereness, "The Psychiatric Nurse Specialist and Her Professional Identity," *Perspectives in Psychiatric Care 1* (March–April, 1963): 18–19.

19. Materials from these conferences may be found in Box 39, #1410.
20. Ibid.
21. The letter from Charles Gardner, MD, the case protocol, and related materials, together with Peplau's detailed notes may be found in Box 25, #916; and interview, Hildegard Peplau, April 21, 1992.
22. See Box 25, #912 and #913, and Box 26, for correspondence with physicians on a wide range of subjects. The professional respect evidenced on both sides is clear.
23. Interview, Hildegard Peplau, April 23, 1992.
24. See Hildegard Peplau, "Present Day Trends in Psychiatric Nursing," *Neuropsychiatry* (1956): 190–204.
25. Much of this correspondence may be found in Box 21, #708, along with a collection of speeches and writings on this subject.
26. Ibid.
27. See material in Box 21.
28. Interview, Hildegard Peplau, February 6, 1992.
29. Letter from Maurice E. Linden, MD, to Hilda Peplau, October 17, 1960, in Box 21, #739, Schlesinger Library.
30. See letter from Jay Fidler, MD, to Hilda Peplau, March 20, 1961, and letter from Hilda Peplau to Jay Fidler, April 13, 1961, both in Box 21, #379, Schlesinger Library. Peplau's recollection of this session are recorded in an interview with Lee Spray, November 4, 1995, at the Inn at Honeyrun, Pennsylvania.
31. Letter from David Alman, MD, to Hilda Peplau, July 22, 1962, found in Box 41, #1495.
32. The galleys for these pieces may be found in Box 22, #742.
33. Letter, Hilda E. Peplau to Helen Tibbits, September, 1967, in Box 24, #853.
34. Annie Goodrich was president of the ANA from 1915–1919 and made it her goal to move nursing education into institutions of higher learning. Annie Goodrich then became the first dean of the Army School of Nursing, and in 1923 the founding dean of the Yale University School of Nursing. See Lydia Flanagan, compiler, *One Strong Voice* (Kansas City: The Lowell Press, 1976), 407.
35. Flanagan, 185.
36. Flanagan, 249.
37. According to the findings of the preliminary 2001 national survey of nurses, 22% of RNs are hospital diploma program graduates, while 34% hold associate degrees. Hence, 66% of registered nurses still do not have a baccalaureate degree. See "The Registered Nurse Population: National Sample Survey of Registered Nurses— Preliminary Findings, February 2001," Division of Nursing, Bureau of Health Professions, Health Resources and Services Administration, U.S. Department of Health and Human Services.
38. Letter from Hildegard Peplau to Robert Meyner, December 11, 1968, in Box 21, #726.
39. See letters of appointment from the Surgeon General of the United States to Hilda Peplau for the years between 1955 and 1960, and correspondence and related materials in Box 20, #693.
40. In 1951 the National League of Nursing held its second conference on Advanced Programs in Psychiatric and Mental Health Nursing in Cincinnati, Ohio. Teacher's College sent Hilda Peplau to this meeting. The conference discussion centered around an effort to differentiate between what content should define graduate and

undergraduate programs in psychiatric nursing. No agreement was reached. Interview, Dorothy E. Gregg, October 12, 1994, in Denver, Colorado.

41. Letter from Hilda Peplau to Helen Arnold, April 15, 1965, Box 38, #1398.

42. The contradiction came into sharp focus in 1968, when the California State Nurses Association began labor negotiations with the Veteran's Administration on behalf of nurses working in the VA system in California. As a member of the VA Nurse Advisory Committee and as Executive Director of the ANA, Peplau asked that the ANA Board meet with the VA Advisory committee to discuss difficulties that were arising as a consequence of nursing's professional organizations functioning as labor unions. The concern was that President Kennedy had issued an Executive Order prohibiting nurses employed by the Veteran's Administration from joining unions or of serving as officers in organizations, such as the ANA, that functioned as unions. In a contentious meeting in January, 1969, presided over by the ever cautious, tactful, and thoughtful Rozella Schlotfeldt, Peplau pressed her concern that "professional employees of the federal government were being represented in union negotiations by their *professional* association," which in effect disenfranchised the VA nurses within the ANA. In spite of Schlotfeldt's diplomacy and Peplau's advocacy that the ANA function as a professional association and not as a union, the ANA Board held firm in its position that the state nurses associations had the right, indeed the responsibility, to negotiate on behalf of their members.

43. ANA Archives, Mugar Library, Boston University, Box 179.

44. ANA Archives, Box 179.

45. A verbatim transcript of this meeting may be found in the ANA Archives, Box 87.

46. ANA Archives, Box 179.

47. Stephen Lesher, *George Wallace: American Populist* (New York: Addison-Wesley Publishing Company, 1994).

48. Interview, Hildegard Peplau, March 9, 1992. Anne (Tish) Peplau later took part in the 1965 civil rights march from Selma to Montgomery; she was then completing her sophomore year at Pembroke. Although she traveled to Selma on a bus with fellow students, Hilda sent her daughter a plane ticket to return to Madison. Tish continued her study of race relations as a graduate student in social psychology at Harvard.

49. It was this Board Ella Stonsby had suggested to Hilda Peplau that she resign from, since it took her away from the College of Nursing several times during the academic year. The request enraged Peplau, and certainly contributed to her disillusionment with the Dean.

50. Peplau's major contribution here was the report she presented to the Southern Governor's Conference in Boca Raton, Florida, in November 1954, entitled "Mental Health Training and Research in the Southern States," which laid out an agenda of baccalaureate and graduate education. This report may be found in Box 20, #679. Other materials on the SREB and Peplau's work in and with it are found in Box 20, #679–684.

51. Letter from Virginia Crenshaw to Hilda Peplau, April 28, 1954, Box 20, #683.

52. Letter from William J. McGlothlin to Hilda E. Peplau, May 6, 1955, Box 20, #684.

53. Interviews, Gwen Tudor Will, October 8, 1994, in Denver, Colorado, and Hildegard Peplau, March 22, 1994, in Sherman Oaks, California.

54. Letter from Earl Shephard to Hilda Peplau, March 10, 1964, Box 39, #1446.

55. Hilda E. Peplau, *Basic Principles of Patient Counseling* (New York: Smith, Kline and French, 1964). Many comments and reviews may be found in Box 39, scattered throughout the file folders.

56. See letter from Helen Nahm to Hilda Peplau, September 14, 1964, in Box 23, #814.

57. In regard to this study, Helen Nahm funded a study of psychiatric nursing functions that Peplau designed, Dr. Emma Spaney "blueprinted," and Claire Mintzer

Fagin administered (eventually published as "Desirable Functions and Qualifications of Psychiatric Nurses"). As a result of the work of this committee, the NLN established the "Interdivisional Council" of Psychiatric Nursing. Helen Nahm sponsored a resolution that was adopted by the NLN Board stating that all undergraduate nursing programs should offer a clinical course in psychiatric nursing as a part of the curriculum. Later still, at Peplau's urging, it was Helen Nahm who applied for and got the 5-year grant for clinical workshops at NAPA and Moffitt, the UCSF Teaching Hospital in San Francisco that would keep Peplau on her cross-country migrations during the latter 1960s.

58. Letter from Jay Hoffman, MD, to Hildegard Peplau, March 8, 1952, Box 39, #1436.
59. "Criteria for NEAA Alumni Achievement Awards, 1969," TC Archives, Columbia University.

ANA: The Professional Challenge

13

Do I arise early because of depression, or am I depressed because of lack of sleep—the latter resulting from rumination about the seemingly unsolvable problems . . . This is a time to face up to hard realities and face them squarely and try to rebuild.

—*Hildegard Peplau*
January 1970

In 1969 Hilda Peplau's intense loyalty to her profession led her to accept an assignment for which she was desperately needed, but not ideally suited—that of interim executive director of the American Nurses Association. The fall of 1969 had been an difficult time. In August her beloved brother Walter, who had been of such enormous support in the years immediately following the Second World War, died suddenly of a heart attack. In September, Tish went off for her second year at Harvard graduate school. Tish was now settling into her own adult life—supporting herself, making her own decisions, fashioning her own career. She had a Volkswagen, an apartment shared with a classmate, and fellowships to cover her tuition and living expenses herself.[1] After more than 15 years at Rutgers, Hilda was beginning to look forward to handing the graduate program over to a successor and phasing herself out of the faculty and its myriad problems. She could retire in 1974, and had begun to think seriously about doing so. Hilda was ready for a change. The period from September 1969 through the summer of 1970 brought change, but challenged all of her skills and left her exhausted mentally, physically, and spiritually.

By 1969, the ANA leadership knew that the organization was in trouble. Financial reports were not good, and worse, such accounting as there was made no sense. The organization's executive director was clearly in

343

over her head, and the staff seemed unable to serve the board. After years of benign neglect of the mounting problems, the ANA Board of Directors finally took the decision to relieve the longtime executive director of her responsibilities and conduct a national search for a replacement. Hilda Peplau was one of those asked to serve on the search committee.[2]

The committee had a difficult time. Either there was disagreement among committee members as to who had the skills necessary to undertake the responsibility for the ANA, or prospective appointees declined to serve. Either way, by the end of May 1969 no candidate's name remained on the table. Because it was scheduled on the same day as Rutgers graduation ceremonies and because graduation was such an important day for her students, Hilda found it necessary to miss a meeting of the committee. This was unusual for her since, as a point of honor, she never accepted a responsibility that she did not intend to fulfill completely. Missing this particular meeting would have important consequences. In her absence, the committee decided that Hilda Peplau should be asked to assume the responsibilities of the executive director on an interim basis while the search for a permanent appointee continued. Emily Holmquist, the dean at Indiana University, in particular, urged that Peplau be persuaded to take a leave from Rutgers in order to help the ANA put its house in order.[3] Although taken by surprise and somewhat apprehensive, Peplau did not resist the challenge. She immediately assessed the interim appointment as an opportunity to push the ANA to move nursing forward as a profession.

The appointment would turn out, however, to be a near total mismatch between person and organization. Totally dedicated as she was to the professionalization of nursing, Peplau simply would not or could not accept the fact that the ANA had already turned the corner and opted for trade-unionism and a working-class ethos over advancement of professional standing for nurses. She believed that by force of reason and will, she could make a difference in ANA attitudes and priorities. She accepted the position full of optimism about its potential and negotiated a partial leave of absence from Rutgers, that essentially committed her to teach on Mondays and be at ANA headquarters in Manhattan the other 4 days of the work week.[4] Initially she even wished she were younger and therefore a viable candidate for the permanent position.[5] She was 61 years old.

On Friday, September 5, 1969, Peplau arrived at the ANA headquarters offices to assume her role as interim executive director of the organization. On this day she was feted at a large reception, complete with case after case of good wine and a steady flow of trays heaped with fancy hors d'oeuvres. Walter's funeral had been on Monday, and thus it was the end of a rather sad week, but on this day it did seem as though a new chapter was beginning. The champagne was flowing, the table arrangements were beautiful, and everyone was very gracious. There were masses of floral arrangements sent by Rutgers and other well-wishers, photographers snapped photos, and nursing's leadership gave warm welcome speeches.[6] Hilda Peplau stood tall, her light blue suit setting off the clear blue in her eyes, and it seemed for the moment, at least, that her profession was ready to accept her leadership, ready to make a start toward the changes she knew were needed. It seemed to Hilda that anything might be possible. She was wrong, however. The festive reception scene was deceptive: It disguised deep, nearly fatal, problems at the American Nurses Association.

THE AMERICAN NURSES ASSOCIATION

The American Nurses Association (ANA) traces its origins to the first general meeting of nurses in the United States held in conjunction with the International Congress of Charities, Correction, and Philanthropy meeting at the Chicago's World Fair in June 1893. At this meeting, Isabel Hampton Robb, principal of the nurse-training school at the Johns Hopkins Hospital in Baltimore, was designated as chairman of a subsection on nursing.[7] Under Robb's leadership, the group in Chicago recommended that two nursing professional associations be established: one for the superintendents of training schools and one for the alumnae. Later in 1893 the superintendents established the American Society of Superintendents of Training Schools for Nurses. This group would evolve into the National League for Nursing Education (NLNE, later just NLN). Five years later the Nurses Associated Alumnae of the United States and Canada was established, and Robb was elected president. This organization would evolve into the ANA.

Robb was an early advocate of setting national educational standards for nurse instruction in the hospital training schools.[8] As the first president of what would become the ANA, she stressed that nursing could not attain the dignity of a profession until it established and controlled nationally recognized educational standards. Under her leadership, State Nurses Associations (SNAs) were organized to work for the passage of nurse practice acts in their respective states. In 1911, the Nurses Associated Alumnae changed its name to the American Nurses Association. Strictly speaking, the ANA is not a membership organization. Rather, it is an organization of constituent associations. Individual nurses participate in the ANA through their membership in a SNA or other constituent organization such at the U.S. military.

Soon a problem became evident. The nurse members of the SNAs brought with them educational backgrounds ranging from 8th-grade certificates and hospital diplomas to university degrees. Obviously, nursing would have a hard time becoming recognized as a profession with this wide variation in professional preparation. This was a problem that would not be solved. In 1918 the Rockefeller Foundation sponsored the work of a 23-person committee to study nursing education. In 1923 this committee produced the Winslow-Goldmark Report on nursing education that recommended that university programs for nurses be developed and strengthened and that hospital nurse-training programs be phased out.

From the time of the Goldmark report onward, the ANA tried, without success, to deal with nursing's inability to establish professional bona fides. Over the years, nursing spent an enormous amount of energy in defining its relationship to hospitals, to patients, to physicians, and to allied health professions, as well as trying to document "what nurses do" through"time and efficiency" studies. Seemingly, in the end these studies always advocated salary enhancements rather than educational reform. By 1970, nursing was preoccupied with distinguishing between nurse practitioners, nurse clinicians, nurse specialists, registered nurses (RNs), and practical nurses in terms of what each was qualified to do, but with no agreement on basic educational differentiation. Failing to reach closure in this debate, the ANA increasingly focused on"promoting the interests of nurses." Its most important division, the Division on Economic and General Welfare, increasingly came to play the role of a labor union for nurses.

Initially, Hilda thought that her greatest challenge during the year she would be interim executive director would be to move the ANA Board of Directors to a focus on issues of professionalization and the closely related issues of education, and away from a focus on collective bargaining and concern with terms and conditions of nursing "labor." The emphasis at ANA conventions was not on professional goals, but rather on authority and responsibility, on wages and salary. When Hilda traveled the country, she spoke of nursing's clinical and professional interests; but the ANA was moving to support the economic interests of *nurses* as opposed to the enhancement of *nursing* as a profession coequal with other health care professions. The board was making major moves to accommodate more and more of the collective bargaining activities of the SNAs, believing that would attract more members at the state level.

Peplau jumped at the opportunity of leading the ANA because she saw it as a last opportunity to advance her vision of the ANA as a professional association that would advance the cause of professionalization in nursing. In this she had clear goals for American nursing and hoped through hard work and thorough preparation to lead the board to adopt them as its own. In her vision, the ANA would take the lead in encouraging nursing to

- become an autonomous profession,
- carve out its own territory for nursing practice and research,
- be self-governing and create its own standards,

- move toward high educational standards and practice,
- work as equal colleagues with physicians and other health professionals,
- foster the development of professional nursing around the world, and
- assure that nursing research added to scientific knowledge about human responses to illness.[9]

No one person could assure that nursing reached all these goals, but Peplau tried to set change in motion and had developed a two-pronged approach. Her first, and continuing approach, was to work directly with several generations of nursing students and through workshops with nurses in practice to encourage them to become the leaders and researchers who would advance her own goals for the profession. Her second was to work within nursing's organizations to adopt policies and programs that would advance this agenda. Given this, serving as interim executive director was an irresistible challenge.

DISMAL DISCOVERIES

Upon accepting the appointment as ANA interim executive director, Hilda had secured an apartment, sight unseen, within walking distance of the ANA headquarters. She had arranged to sublet the apartment from an ANA staff member who would be on leave, and the opportunity to secure a place in such a convenient location seemed promising as it would enable her to leave her car in New Jersey. Hilda was looking forward to becoming reacquainted with New York, the city she had left in 1954. On the day before her welcoming reception, Hilda and Tish drove from Madison into the city. They located the apartment in the Lincoln Towers behind Lincoln Center, and Hilda was soon dismayed. Hilda was neat and a minimalist. Her home in Madison was comfortable, but sparingly furnished. The apartment she entered that dark September day in 1969 was full of overstuffed furniture and every window was heavily draped, letting in little light. Even worse, everywhere she stepped, she hit another hanging mobile, and every surface was covered with knickknacks teetering in unlikely positions, some on the edges of tables and others swinging from lights or from curtain rods. Tish, ever the no-nonsense child, took one look and headed out to find boxes. They designated one closet for storage and set about boxing up the knickknacks, artificial flowers, mobiles, and personal mementos. By midnight, they had cleared space, taken down the dark drapes, and made the bed. Tish left to go back to Madison to pack for Harvard, and Hilda went to sleep.

On Saturday, Hilda returned to Madison to be with Tish before she left for Cambridge, and to get her own linen and towels to take back to the apartment. On Sunday, they drove back to New York with Tish's Volkswagen full of their personal things. Together they cleaned the dreary apartment, moved lamps and furniture, and Tish made curtains while Hilda scoured the kitchen and bathroom. On Sunday Tish left for Cambridge, leaving Hilda feeling slightly depressed: she knew that on Monday morning the real work would begin, and she knew it would not be easy. From serving on ANA committees, she was well aware that staff work was often inadequate and that there never seemed to be enough money to support the work of those committees.

She spent the first hour that Monday morning with the outgoing executive director, who Peplau found to be"totally dedicated to ANA, but very disorganized" and "scattered"[10] The ANA president, Dorothy Cornelius of Ohio, was also in town and the morning was spent in staff briefings, that Peplau also found to be "very disorganized," as was seemingly everything else at the ANA. The three of them went to lunch and Hilda sat quietly while the other two discussed ANA business, a discussion that left Hilda to inquire in her diary that night, "Will I ever be clued in?"[11] Later that afternoon, she observed a meeting of an ANA "Congress on Clinical Specialists," called to set guidelines for certification. This, she wryly observed in her diary, "is going nowhere." Seven options for deciding what to do about certification for clinical specialties were on the table, but "sharing diverse opinion takes courage and involves risks of ostracism, so the work grinds on and on as all the unverbalized private thought and opinion stymies discussion and decision-making."[12] Before going back to her apartment that night, Peplau was briefed on ANA negotiations with unions, about which she observed, "The decision-making process leaves much to be desired."[13]

On her second day at the ANA Peplau met with a young man from Arthur Young, the accounting firm the ANA had hired to audit its books. She had been told there were disagreements around the conduct of an audit. Given the lavish character of the reception on Friday, it had not occurred to Hilda that the fiscal problems of which she had been warned were as critical as she later found them to be. She readily agreed to the auditor's suggestion that she and he actually visit the accounting department rather than just look at the books. Over the strenuous objections of the outgoing executive director and her deputies, Hilda and the Arthur Young auditor went in together. They found an office in total disarray. They learned that ANA's bank, Chase Manhattan, was threatening to take the organization to bankruptcy court for overdrafts on their accounts and the telephone and electricity companies were threatening to discontinue services due to nonpayment of bills. Peplau immediately asked the auditors to send over a team so that the situation could be assessed as quickly as possible, which the firm did the very next day.[14]

On Wednesday, leaving the Arthur Young accountants to do their work, Peplau began meeting with the senior staff, asking for clarification on procedures and lines of responsibility and authority that pertained among the ANA Board, the executive director, and the staff. Staff members she interviewed were not responsive to her queries, appeared anxious, and professed to feeling overworked. To make the gap in communication worse, the staff at that time was frantically trying to prepare for a meeting of the board of directors the next week. Peplau found it impossible to get systematic information on any subject. By the end of the week, the picture darkened even further. The Arthur Young auditors gave her their preliminary report: The ANA was in debt to the tune of $1,258,000. For some time, the ANA business manager had been inappropriately moving money from the pension fund to pay current expenses. Even so, there remained an overdraft of at least $200,000 on the Chase Manhattan account.[15]

By the time the board met at the end of the month, Hilda described herself as "in shock."[16] Because she was so new, and because she did not yet feel she had a handle on what was really going on, she was "a silent observer" at that board meeting.[17] The board heard the report from the Arthur Young consultants and tensely directed Peplau to handle the crisis.[18] Then they adjourned for the final good-bye party for the outgoing executive director, whom they had effectively fired. As she noted in her diary, "I've never seen anything like it . . . I've never seen so much kissing and hugging. Presents. Flowers. You would never guess the true occasion."[19] Finally, after the director's departure, Hilda was able to close the doors and begin to go through the files, in which she found nothing but "utter chaos and disorganization."[20] She began making lists of things to do, prioritizing, trying to make sense of what had happened and what was happening and what options there might be.

By October, it was clear that Peplau's relations with the staff would be difficult. The staff rapidly went from being solicitous to exhibiting distant formality. Peplau had come to the conclusion that the business manager was at the fulcrum of the disorder. It was on his watch that the financial crises had developed and grown. He had joined the ANA staff in 1950, and in his 20-year career there had assiduously created classic mutual dependencies between himself and the rest of the staff.

By November Hilda knew the ANA was sinking; she took full responsibility for putting the ship in order before a permanent executive director was appointed. She understood intuitively the board had hired her to make the hard decisions for the organization that it could not or would not make itself. Her first major act would be to replace the business manager. The Arthur Young accountants had found boxes of unpaid bills stacked up in his office—unpaid because there were no funds from which to pay them. He had made documented, but unauthorized withdrawals, from the pension funds and had made no payments on the $200,000 overdraft at the Chase Manhattan Bank. On November 9, Peplau ordered him out of the building, giving him the choice of either signing a letter of resignation dated November 9, 1969, or of accepting a summary dismissal signed by Hildegard E. Peplau. Under protest, and not without unduly upsetting a good portion of the staff, he signed the letter of resignation giving 2 weeks notice.[21] He left that day, but remained on the payroll until November 19, 1969. Now the work could begin.

After the business manager's departure, Peplau herself went into his office to sort out the disarray. Boxes of files, loose pieces of paper, unpaid bills, un-deposited checks, and random notes were everywhere. She began putting the files back together, and with the help of the deputy director, Margaret Carroll, began to restore order in the business office. With the help of the auditors, Peplau established that the board-approved budget for that year had already been overspent by $500,000. She discovered a report to the board presented by consultants in 1968 citing serious deficiencies in billing and accounting procedures. When she was asked to accept the position of interim executive director, Peplau had not been told of any of this, nor had the report been shared with her.[22] Had the board been more forthcoming, the trauma to come that year might have been mitigated.

By December it had become abundantly clear to Hilda that drastic action had to be taken to set things on course, to establish appropriate procedures and responsible bookkeeping, and to professionalize the way the organization was run. The waste and personal indulgences of the immediate past years had to stop. Although still somewhat shy or reserved on a personal level, Hilda had by the late 1960s attained professional poise and considerable self-confidence. Certainly she was secure in her understanding of what had to be done. Hence, in the months remaining in her interim term, she acted decisively, and virtually alone, to deal with the crises she had inherited. Her personality was such that she would be resisted and challenged every step of the way. Put simply, and to quote Rutgers Provost Richard Schlatter, Hildegard Peplau was a "formidable woman." She spoke with the authority of a powerful intellect and with incisive clarity about issues and problems. Clearly, her straightforward approach to dealing with the problems at the ANA was not only unsettling, but threatening to staff.[23] In later years, most of these staff members simply could not or would not discuss their experience of this period.[24]

Certainly the day-to-day atmosphere at ANA headquarters was increasingly tense. Because of the financial crisis, one of Peplau's first acts had been to collect all the staff credit cards and decree that there would be no advances for staff travel without her approval. Early in December, the associate director informed Peplau she would be attending a professional meeting the following week and would take four staff members with her. Hilda refused to approve the trip as there were no funds to send a delegation. The associate director defied her and attended the meeting along with other staff. When she returned, Peplau gave her a letter demoting her and informing her that "there will be a salary adjustment which will be communicated to you within the week."[25] By this action, Peplau had made an enemy for life. As a champion of ANA's preoccupation with the "economic welfare" of nurses, the associate director was very popular. The next day, December 5, 1969, the associate director resigned, after handing Peplau a letter in which she stated: ". . . I can only conclude that the intent of your remarks and this demotion constitute summary dismissal . . . and accordingly, I shall leave immediately."[26] There was an equally immediate outcry across the country at the "summary dismissal" of such a faithful staff member who had "given" 18 years to the ANA. As Hilda remarked in her diary recording these events, "I did not fire her summarily, I only demoted her. She quit summarily."[27] A new associate director was soon appointed by the board.

What had started so full of possibility in September had turned into a nightmare by December. After this incident, Hilda announced that *all* expenditures by staff must be authorized by her and that staff travel, including official visits, was, for the foreseeable future, to be canceled. Further, she announced, most major programs and projects were to be drastically reduced or suspended, and meetings of commissions and committees were to be streamlined or canceled. It had become clear that the financial crisis had developed between 1966 and 1969 as the ANA had greatly increased its staff and program activities to accommodate recommendations made by the board. Antiquated and outright incompetent financial control had then contributed to what had become an out-of-control budget disaster.[28] Knowing that an even deeper staff cut would have to come, Peplau released 29 "nonessential" staff on December 18, 1969, most of whom were short-term employees hired in response to increased programming at the ANA. This was incredibly hard for Hilda. She agonized about how painful this was for employees, and all the more so to have it occur at Christmas. On the other hand, carrying these short-term employees into the new year would simply be financially irresponsible. By the end of December morale at ANA headquarters was very glum indeed. As 1969 drew to a close, Hilda resolved to do her best, to put the ANA house in order, and to expect no reward for her efforts. Her own agenda would be put in abeyance.

The promise and potential of the ANA as an organization seemed far removed from the reality of incompetence and financial disarray. Hilda knew that she was already tired at this stage in her life. This was the job that needed doing, though; she had accepted it, and thus she resolved to find the energy to do what needed to be done.[29] Her actions had not made her popular at the ANA. She knew she would have to go it alone.

By this time the required Mondays spent teaching at Rutgers provided a break. Throughout the fall Hilda had usually returned to Madison on Friday evenings and spent Saturday attending to household chores, answering accumulated mail, paying the bills, reading student papers and Rutgers mail she'd had sent out to Madison during the week, and preparing for class on Monday. Sundays she reserved for catching up on ANA reading. On Monday mornings she met with faculty and students at Rutgers, and by Monday afternoons she was back in New York at the ANA. Occasionally she stayed in the city on Friday nights, but generally she allowed herself no free time, no distance from the pressure of day-to-day events. She did find a compatible friend in Phillip Day, the managing director of the *American Journal of Nursing* Company. Occasionally she'd have dinner with him, and found in him a man seemingly interested in the bigger issues in nursing and the vexing question of how to validate a distinction between nursing and medicine. These meetings provided one of the few opportunities for intellectual discussions she would have that year.[30]

THE CRISIS DEEPENS

After Christmas, it became obvious that 1970 was going to be an even more difficult year. When she returned to ANA headquarters on January 3, 1970, Peplau found that the editor of the *American Journal of Nursing* (AJN), nursing's journal of record, had effectively rejected a manuscript she had submitted.[31] Rarely were Peplau's manuscripts rejected, and she certainly did not expect it at this stage in her career. The editor, however, was a close friend of the departed associate director, who had left the ANA in a huff after Peplau had demoted her.[32]

That first week in January, Peplau faced another major frustration when Bernice Chapman, dean of the College of Nursing at Rutgers, refused to sign the application for a new nursing building. Hilda did not have time to fight this battle however, and, perhaps, as a consequence, Rutgers would not get a building dedicated to nursing.[33] January 1970 quickly degenerated into a waking nightmare. Hilda found herself spending 15-hour days at the ANA. As the severity of the crisis became ever more apparent, the staff became more confused, angry, and hostile. Peplau alerted the board, and began taking the additional steps she thought necessary to rectify the situation.

She urged Dorothy Cornelius, the ANA President, to make an appeal to the membership for emergency financial help. She began to discuss the possibility of a loan from the AJN company to the ANA to cover immediate operating expenses, and upset Phil Day by suggesting that the AJN solicit advertising or sell stock to increase its revenue.[34] With the help of the new comptroller, Gerald Dorfman, Hilda began to set up new financial protocols and update the accounting system (which had remained unchanged for 75 years). She also recruited a group of college of nursing deans (Eleanor Lambertson, Dorothy White, Lulu Hassenplug, and Rozella Schlotfeldt) to write grants seeking foundation support to underwrite some of ANA's activities.[35] Increasingly the evidence indicated that both the former executive director and the former business manager had known for some time that the organization was in deepening financial trouble and had directed their efforts not toward solving the problem but toward covering up the enormity of it. Hilda discovered that the ANA Financial Committee had kept no minutes after 1964. She noted in her diary that the information given the committee was "too confusing—no one could have understood it," and that as a result the committee had simply ceased to present a report.[36] At that time, also, the budget format had been changed, thus further mystifying the budget. In later years Peplau would reflect that she was not sure the former executive director ever truly understood either the nature or the extent of the problem.[37]

January 1970 would be one of the most difficult months in Hilda's long life. The board had promoted a staff member about whom she had grave doubts to the Associate Director position. Her January 1970 diary conveys something of the stress and emotional toll of those days and decisions:

> *January 8:* February 13 has been set as the date for an emergency board meeting to officially state the facts [i.e., for the record] about ANA finances . . . The board's Finance Committee wants ANA to just go on as though nothing has happened and hope the money turns up! It was precisely this kind of thinking that got them into this situation. This is a time to face up to hard realities and face them squarely and try to rebuild.

> *January 9:* [the former associate director] keeps coming in to visit with staff. If looks could kill, I'd be dead. I feel as though I am sitting on a volcano . . . The effect of the stress and trauma is hate, revenge, and derogation—the way those most affected seek to mobilize in order to cope. It's unbearable to watch.

> *January 10:* In again at 5:00 a.m. Do I arise early because of depression, or am I depressed because of lack of sleep—the latter resulting from rumination about the seemingly unsolvable problems? . . . You really cannot imagine the troubled guilt, concern, alarm, and general avoidance of the task. They want to leave all hard decisions for the executive council and board to decide . . . I am becoming more of a social hermit every day.

> *January 20:* The board is more puzzled than angry . . . How could this have happened? They are in a state of shock. Everyone has a rather standoffish attitude toward me.

January 21: I felt some of the hostility toward me is melting, but it is there. I am not sure why. Have found out [the new associate director] is in great disagreement with me over the staff cutbacks, she refuses to believe they are necessary. Why hasn't she spoken to me? She just can't handle reality.

January 23: Several of the board are clearly aggrieved at me . . . [doubt the necessity for] the staff layoffs . . . I am too open. I stand on sub-stance and am not good at rituals . . . It leaves me with ominous feel-ings, but I'll leave in August and have a good vacation.

Undoubtedly, the worst day that winter was Wednesday, January 27, when an additional 41 of the ANA's remaining 124 staff members were given notice that they would be terminated on February 27, with the reluctant concurrence of the board. As Hilda recorded that day,

January 27: The staff lay-offs were announced. There's shock rather than grief. I had the staff heads tell their people. I just couldn't do it . . . There's anger and hostility. People don't answer when I speak to them. Whispers on the elevator. My fatigue today is total—I know I have to stay and clean up the mess. It seems hopeless at times.

Hilda's fatigue was indeed total, but so was the personal distress she felt over the layoffs. While she had supervisors meet first with the indi-viduals to be terminated, she then met with the staff as a whole to explain the layoffs. The decision to lay off staff was not one that she had come to easily nor was it made without great empathy for the personal pain that could result from a job loss. She was at that time still grieving deeply the loss the previous August of her brother Walter, and she vividly recalled, and emotionally relived in this meeting, the experience, some years earli-er, when Walter had unexpectedly been laid off a job he held after his retirement from the military. Walter found another position, but the memo-ry of the shock of the lay-off and Walter's feeling of devastation remained in Hilda's mind.[38] In the circumstances in which she found herself at the ANA, Hilda knew that she had no choice but to reduce staff. The survival of the organization was at stake. In announcing the layoffs, though, Hilda remembered Walter and began to cry uncontrollably. This was the first time and only time she broke down in tears in public.

The stress heaped on Peplau and the climate of tension in the ANA offices remained unabated into February. Hilda found out at the begin-ning of the month that the former associate director had found a new position—she would become the executive director of the International Council of Nurses based in Geneva. As Hilda noted with some resigna-tion in her diary at the time: "Ah well—she'll spread her word about me far and wide." In her February 1970 diary, Hilda recorded that the day-to-day dollars and cents existence was difficult for all and that not surprisingly the looming staff terminations cast a pall over everything.

Added to this was the necessity to plan and make arrangements for the biennial ANA convention scheduled to take place in Miami in May. The convention exhibit contracts and agreements had been found among the tangle of papers left behind by the business manager in November. Thus, in the midst of the fiscal and morale problems that had descended in January and February, Peplau worked to reactivate planning for the Miami convention. In this period she used income coming in for the exhibits to pay for day-to-day ANA operations. Here she had some much needed help from Margaret Carroll, who "worked day and night to straighten it out." Later she noted, "M. Carroll has a helleva situation under control. She's cleaning up the unanswered mail—has reduced the 30 form letters to 3. I am so lucky to have her."[39] Hilda's only solace during the dreary month of January was that the new comptroller she had hired, Gerald Dorfman, was proving to be a godsend. She respected his judgement and he in turn became a constant source of support for Hilda. In the wake of the layoffs, he took charge of consolidating the remaining staff on the 23rd and 25th floors of the building, inventorying space and equipment, and securing renters for the vacated space and buyers for the surplus equipment.[40] Although he would later rescind it and agree to remain with ANA until Hilda's term as the interim executive director expired in August, in early February he brought her a letter of resignation. As she recorded it in her diary,

February 9. Another day. It's endless. Jerry quit. He says he has no confidence in [the new associate director], and can't grasp what ANA is all about. Staff is not top quality, panic disables everyone, etc. Staff meetings have deteriorated again. More scattering . . . Feeling the problems of being a lame duck. [The interim appointment was for 1 year, and there had been no discussion of extending Peplau's contract beyond that.] Unable to get decisions on restructuring.[41]

As February moved into March, as long-term employees left in pain and anger, as the remaining staff obstructed rather than facilitated the salvage efforts, Hilda began to give in to a depression of her own. Nothing seemed to be going right. The archives give evidence of the enormous sense of personal responsibility Peplau assumed for the financial fate of the ANA and its psychic cost to her. There are over 20 files on the ANA financial crises with many, many worksheets generated in January and February of 1970 in an attempt to decode an underlying "system." No such system was to be found. As early as January it had become apparent that a large influx of cash was essential if the ANA was to avoid bankruptcy.

At Hilda's urging, the board reluctantly agreed to investigate the possibility of soliciting the membership directly for financial contributions.

Peplau prepared a letter, approved by Dorothy Cornelius, which was test-mailed on January 9 to 240 representatives of the ANA member organizations. The letter went to SNA presidents and executive directors, members of commissions, and ANA officers and committee members. They were asked to respond with checks and opinions in regard to the letter. The response to the appeal was immediate and positive. Eighty-five percent of the recipients sent checks and endorsed the letter. Thus, on February 24, a second letter written by Peplau and signed jointly by Peplau and Cornelius was mailed directly to the individual members of the ANA's constituent organizations. This letter was unprecedented in the sense that it was sent directly to individuals rather than through the parent organizations, which constituted the actual "membership" of the ANA. It explained the immediate crisis and appealed for contributions to an emergency fund to "Save the ANA."[42]

Nurses responded. By the middle of March, responses were pouring into the ANA by the thousands. Checks came by mail, telegraph, and courier, singly and in bulk, from individuals and from groups. The checks came by regular mail, airmail, certified mail, and special delivery. New stamps, no stamps, and a large number of uncancelled stamps were on the envelopes that came from all over the world, from nurses and non-nurses alike. Many checks came from groups—hospital school alumni associations, Sigma Theta Tau chapters, district and state nurses associations, professional groups—as well as from active and retired nurses.[43] Some nurses sent checks with prayer cards, sympathy cards, or get-well cards. Others wrote letters offering advice, and still others were angry—the latter usually from friends of laid-off staff members. Some cited problems related to the central membership and billing services. Peplau insisted that each and every letter be answered. More form letters were designed, but she wanted to read all the correspondence herself.[44]

Tish recalls staying with Hilda over her spring break and observing the deep sense of responsibility that Hilda felt to use wisely and carefully the hard-earned money sent in by individual nurses from throughout the country. Hilda knew that some of the nurses who sent contributions could barely afford to do so, that it was a sacrifice on their part for their professional organization. The contrast between the previous high-living style of ANA officers and staff members and the generosity of nurses on meager incomes was enormous.[45] It would be clear throughout Peplau's tenure with the ANA that she would be far more successful in her efforts to connect with rank-and-file nurses than she would be with the highly politicized ANA leadership and headquarters staff.

As Peplau began to sink under the sheer volume of the response to the fund appeal letter, Claire Fagin, a former student at Teacher's College who was then chair of the department of nursing at CUNY-Lehman, sent two doctoral students to help.[46] They were joined by two faculty members,

one from Adelphi and one from Columbia Presbyterian, and by other former Peplau students. The group would usually assemble around 5:00 in
the afternoon, and the daily sorting, counting, stamping, and recording
would begin, continuing until around 11:00 at night. It was a massive and
exhausting undertaking. While the days working with an increasingly
hostile staff were pure agony, the easy comradeship of the evenings provided relief for Hilda from what was otherwise very lonely and discouraging work. At the end, she could report to the board that expenditures
had been curbed to equal anticipated income, bankruptcy had been
averted, and the slow climb to financial health had begun. In addition,
while Hilda appealed to the membership for money, sorted donations,
and responded to donors, Dorfman developed new and more appropriate accounting guidelines and financial controls.

Peplau had accomplished a near superhuman feat. She had, indeed,
saved the ANA from bankruptcy, but the work had taken its toll. The hours
had been long, the pressure unremitting, and the appreciation sparse. Once
the immediate emergency had been dealt with, those hurt in the process
prevailed upon their friends who had survived the crisis for sympathy.
Antipathy toward the woman who had managed it pervaded the staff. In
late April the AJN published a letter from the former executive director
defending her directorship and implying that the financial crisis had
been manufactured by Peplau in order to reduce staff. Hilda was stunned
that the AJN would publish such a letter and infuriated that it would be
published without her being offered the courtesy of a rebuttal. Realizing
that she was losing ground with the staff, Peplau began to withdraw, to
keep her thoughts to herself, to be less willing than before to share her
opinions with others. As April turned into May, the days seemed endless
and tiring. She felt the increasing hostility, and she did not know how to
cope with it.[47]

During this time, the Executive Committee of the ANA Board was
meeting monthly to deal with the ongoing crises at headquarters. The
ups and downs of these days are revealed in the following excerpts from
the February diary:

> *February 12:* Dorothy Cornelius came to town to try to convince the
> comptroller to stay on. [He] said no—nurses won't take a position and
> stick with it, incompetence of the staff, lack of a sense of mission. Not a
> profession. The bypassing of authority, no sense of order or discipline.
> The files, the horrible workload, the long hours, unable to get home to
> his family. Made it clear I was in the same predicament. He'd hoped I'd
> be there two more years. I pleaded again for Jerry to stay until August
> 1 [1970]. He'll think about it over the weekend.[48]

The next day the Executive Committee convened for its meeting, at which
the full extent of the financial crisis and the actions needed to resolve it

would be formally presented. Peplau hoped this meeting would bring the beginning of closure on this sad chapter. Even so, the atmosphere offered little relief to the embattled executive director. Hilda noted in her diary that

> . . . all the whining, wheedling, manipulating, preaching, distrust, grudging recognition of achievement or judgment or ability of the other. Refusal or inability to deal with reality or focus head-on on an issue, inability to hold confidential information. All there plain to see at the board meeting, as Dorfman does every day. And I am very depressed about that . . . I've known for a long time that nursing taken as a group lacks intelligence, competent leadership, but I have always thought that under stress it would rise to the crisis. This is not to indict the whole board.[49]

Evidently the ANA Board was more supportive of her efforts than Hilda realized. After the February meeting, President Dorothy Cornelius called with the news that the Ohio State Nurses Association would like to nominate Peplau for the presidency of the ANA.[50] Taken aback, Hilda invited Phil Day to cocktails and dinner for a"long overdue talk." Day accepted her dinner invitation, the two had the long overdue conversation, and Hilda decided to make herself available for the nomination to the ANA presidency.[51] Earlier that day, Dorfman had informed her that he would agree to stay on until August. So, for a moment, there appeared to be light at the end of the tunnel. She wrote in her diary that, "We seem to be over the hump and everything is going for us at least." She continued in this vein the next day:

> I've been "in charge" at the ANA for six months. We've gone from pleasant though anxiety-laden rituals, to high anxiety and fear, to utter helplessness as staff had to be let go not due to their own performance, to peeling out the seriousness of the problems, to utter chaos and despair, and now the beginning of optimism and readiness to rebuild . . . Things are looking up.[52]

Such optimism was to be short-lived. By March 1, Peplau was again discouraged. It had become clear that the board would designate the newly appointed associate director as her successor as executive director, and it was becoming alarmingly obvious that the transition would not go well. During the first week of March, Hilda recorded that

> . . . all is for naught. I wonder about the worth of the investment. I find myself growing apprehensive about ANA and feel terribly helpless. My work is an exercise in futility . . . Why do I even think about being ANA president? It can only increase the headaches. Well, at least I'll get the

debts paid before I leave ANA . . . [the associate director] complaining of staff shortage. Well, of course we're short. We cut 2/3 of the staff. Her voice whines and her hands wring and her face shows contempt. [She is] trying to get it said that the debts mounted "since September." She's still denying the crisis . . .[53] The ANA is becoming a society of hand-wringing, whining martyrs who haven't practiced nursing in years.[54]

By the end of March, all hope of a successful and upbeat conclusion to her months of hard work and heartbreak at the ANA had vanished. Even Dorothy Cornelius now seemed distant when she came into the ANA headquarters. Hilda was puzzled and truly did not understand the dynamic at play. As it became clear that she would earn only grudging respect for "saving" the ANA—and gain no friends from the experience—she became even more disillusioned. Undoubtedly, she was depressed, but in spite of being a psychiatric nurse, it never occurred to her to seek help for herself. She would simply keep her head down, do what had to be done, and move on—to the presidency were she to be elected or to a final few years at Rutgers if not.

The sheer volume of other work did not diminish. The archives contain hundreds of pages of Hilda's notes and drafts of reports written in this period as she prepared for the April board meeting.[55] That meeting, held from April 28 to May 1, immediately prior to the convention in Miami, would be her last as executive director. While Peplau presented her long and detailed financial report to the full board, her designated successor sat shuffling papers and sighing. In the report Peplau laid out her analysis of the origin of the crisis and detailed the steps taken to deal with it.[56] She pledged that she would continue to work to establish new procedures to ensure that future boards would be better prepared to oversee fiscal accountability and integrity. At the conclusion of the report, Peplau recommended that the board set priorities and bring in a consultant to help reorganize the personnel and administrative functions to support these priorities. She urged board members to put in place a process for long-range planning, the setting of clear goals, and the development of an overarching vision. The board listened politely, then the treasurer moved that further discussion and decisionmaking be postponed until June. The board members stalled, electing to "see where we are in May."[57] In effect, Hilda's exhausting, debilitating 9 months in the ANA's chief staff position had ended with the immediate crisis averted, but with the future of the ANA as a professional organization unresolved.

The ANA had been brought back from the brink of disaster. Near certain bankruptcy had been averted, but the personal cost had been high. Seventy staff members had lost their jobs, operations had been scaled back, and progressive new procedures had been introduced. An exhausted and disillusioned Hilda Peplau watched with considerable reservation while her supporters rallied to put on a campaign to elect her president of this organization. As she thought back over her career, she longed for the days of doing "the real work of nursing," working in hospitals and clinics, teaching students who would make a difference in the lives of the mentally ill, debating the intellectual component of nursing. Yet, she also felt the irresistible pull of one last challenge. Perhaps as the leader of the national organization, as nursing's chief spokesperson, she could rally the profession to move ahead, to finally take its place as an equal in the health professions. She had to try.[58]

Thus it was with very mixed feelings that Hilda Peplau prepared to go to Miami for a campaign and a convention that could elect her to nursing's highest office. She had officially asked Rutgers for permission to seek the office, and Vice President Henry Winkler had responded that her election "would be an honor for the university."[59] At the ANA headquarters she watched with disappointment as the staff reverted to its former disorganization. She pensively recorded her thoughts about the circumstances:

> The campaign is going well . . . but why I'd even want the presidency in view of all the problems is an enigma . . . I really think it will be difficult to work with [the new executive director] knowing what I already know . . . staff seems to be waiting for me just to go away so the martyrs and hand wringers can return to "normal" we-against-the-board work.[60]

She had analyzed it right, but seemed unable to accept the meaning of the analysis: if she became president, the board would be manipulated by the staff. The fact that she knew the staff, and anticipated what would happen, would be of no help. The board had placed her in an impossible situation when they asked her to assume the interim executive directorship. They had in effect given her a task, save the ANA, but as a group would not share the responsibility for what had to be done. Hilda was in a very real sense operating alone. She quickly understood that her assignment was to reorganize, introduce new procedures, increase productivity, hold people accountable, reduce expenses, let people go, reduce the budget, and to do it all within the year. She set about "downsizing" before the concept was an understood or accepted term.

In the short run, Hilda was an impressively successful executive director. She straightened out the chaotic finances and put the ANA back on sound footing. This success earned her the enmity of the staff, however, and the board compounded the situation by appointing as her successor the associate director who had long been a member of this staff. As she headed to Miami, this did not bode well.

ENDNOTES

1. Hildegard Peplau, 1969 Christmas Letter, Box 5, #196, in the Peplau collection, Schlesinger Library.
2. Materials in regard to the Search Committee may be found in Box 33, #1221, Schlesinger Library.
3. Interview, Emily Holmquist, June 16, 1996, in Washington, D.C. According to Hilda Peplau, a member of the search committee called her on a Sunday morning to inform her that the search committee had decided that she should be appointed to the position. See Grayce Sills, "Peplau and Professionalism: The Emergence of a Paradigm of Professionalization," *Journal of Psychiatric and Mental Health Nursing* V (June 1998): 170.
4. See letters in Peplau's Personnel File at Rutgers, specifically letter dated August 3, 1969, from Richard Schlatter to Hilda Peplau.
5. Hilda Peplau, 1969 Christmas letter, Box 5, #196.
6. Diary entry, September 5, 1969, found in Box 8, #242.
7. For a succinct history of the ANA, see Lydia Flanagan, compiler, *One Strong Voice: The Story of the American Nurses' Association* (Kansas City: American Nurses' Association, 1976).
8. See Lavinia Dock, "The Relation of Training Schools to Hospitals," in Isabel Hampton, ed., *Nursing the Sick* (New York: McGraw Hill Book Company, 1949), 17.
9. This list represents the author's summation of hundreds of Peplau's speeches and papers on this subject.
10. Diary entry, September 8, 1969.
11. Ibid.
12. Ibid.
13. Diary entry, September 10, 1969.
14. Ibid.
15. For the full report on ANA's financial situation, see Arthur Young Company to the American Nurses Association, November 30, 1969, "A Statement of Financial Condition," in the ANA Archives, the Mugar Library, Box 72.
16. Diary entry, September 25, 1969.
17. Ibid.
18. Board minutes, September 25, 1969, ANA Archives, Mugar Library, Box 73.
19. Diary entry, September 26, 1969.
20. Ibid.
21. Letter to Hilda Peplau, November 9, 1969, in Box 33, #1218.
22. Interview, Hildegard Peplau, February 10, 1992.
23. Insights related by Grayce Sills in an interview, February 13, 1999.
24. Hilda Peplau provided the author with the names, addresses, and phone numbers of dozens of former nurse colleagues and ANA staff members involved in the many events described in this chapter. With few exceptions, they would not speak. Either they claimed not to have been a part of events that documentary evidence established; or they claimed to have forgotten the details, no matter how traumatic; or they refused to speak about them on the grounds that "such information does not belong in a biography." As was the case in regard to events at TC in 1953, nursing's leadership suffers from collective amnesia when events are traumatic.
25. Letter from Hilda Peplau to Associate Director, December 4, 1969, in Box 32, #1273.
26. Letter from Associate Director to Hilda Peplau, December 5, 1969, ibid.
27. Handwritten observations in Box 32, #1273.
28. For a documentation of the development of the financial crisis see *Report of ANA's*

Financial Situation (American Nurses Association, April 1970) in Box 33, #1219 at the Schlesinger Library and *Book of Reports* 1968–1970, Exhibit A, "Statement of Financial Condition," December 31, 1969, page XII, in the ANA Archives in the Mugar Library, Box 72. The Arthur Young report submitted to the Board in September, 1969, noted that annual costs had increased 184% between 1964 and 1968. This report may be found in Box 33, #1237 in the Schlesinger Library collection.

29. Interview, Hildegard Peplau, April 23, 1992.
30. Ibid.
31. Letter from AJN editor to Hilda Peplau, January 2, 1969, Box 40, #1455: "I am returning to you your paper on 'The Generation Gap,' since I was unable to sell it as it stands and you indicated, when we last talked about it, that you were unwilling to revise it." Notations by Peplau indicate that the revisions suggested would have made for a completely different paper, which she did not have time to write given the emergencies erupting at ANA.
32. 1970 Diary, entry for January 5, 1970.
33. Peplau had worked hard to ready this grant for submission over the Christmas break, only to be met by resistance from a Dean under attack from her faculty. Chapman always believed that Peplau was fomenting the unrest, when in fact Peplau was more than fully engaged in the traumas of the ANA and not at all tuned into the faculty turmoil at Rutgers. Most publicly supported colleges of nursing in the country secured federal funds for new buildings during these years, as did many private institutions. Seton Hall, a private university just 5 miles from the Rutgers campus in Newark, won such funds, for example. For Peplau's notes on these events, see Box 40, #1455.
34. The AJN is considered nursing's journal of record, but it is a freestanding fiduciary company. The ANA has a representative on the AJN Board—usually the organization's outgoing president—but there is no other legal connection between the two and the journal is considered to be a freestanding and independent organization in its own right.
35. See notes, correspondence, and other material in Box 8, #242 in the Schlesinger Library.
36. Diary entry, January 15, 1970.
37. Interview, Hildegard Peplau, April 23, 1992.
38. Letter from Anne Peplau to Barbara Callaway, January 11, 1999.
39. Diary entry, January 15, 1970. The various form letters developed during this time may be found in Box 33, #1219.
40. See *Financial Situation* report in Box 33, #1219.
41. Diary entry, February 9, 1970.
42. See Gerald Dorfman and Hilda Peplau, *Report of ANA's Financial Situation* (Washington: American Nurses Association, 1970), Box 33, #1219, for the final text of this letter together with a summary of events leading to its issue. There are also literally hundreds of pages of notes, drafts, and various versions of the letters and the final report.
43. Altogether, slightly over 15,000 of the 160,000 individual members of the SNAs to whom the letter was sent responded to the appeal.
44. The form letter developed to help respond to this outpouring of support may be found in Box 33, #1219.
45. Letter from Anne Peplau to Barbara Callaway, January 6, 1999. At this point in time, Hilda Peplau was very ill, but she continued to elaborate on her thoughts and observations to the author through her daughter.
46. Interview, Claire Fagin, October 29, 1992, St. Louis, Missouri.
47. See entries for March and April, Diary #2 for 1970, in Box 8, #243. Also, letter from Hilda Peplau to Anne Warner, Director of Public Relations, ANA, April 24, 1970, in Box 32, #1273.

48. Diary entry, February 12, 1970.
49. Ibid.
50. This would be a nomination from the floor as the Nominating Committee had already presented a slate of candidates. Letter from Grayce Sills to Barbara Callaway, February 13, 1999.
51. In addition to the heart-to-heart talk, Peplau also informed Day that without a $500,000 line of credit collateralized through the AJN Company, the ANA literally could not continue to function through the present crisis. Day was supportive of Hilda's efforts, but gave no assurances in regard to AJN financial help for the ANA.
52. See entry for January 17–18, 1970 Diary, in Box 8, #242.
53. Diary entry, March 9, 1970.
54. Diary entry, March 10, 1970.
55. This material may be found in Box 32, Files #1239–1241, and Box 33, Files #1224–1235.
56. See *Report of ANA's Financial Situation* by Hilda Peplau and Gerald Dorfman, April, 1970, in Box 33, #1219. In essence, her analysis was that the ANA House of Delegates had set too many priorities for the staff without providing appropriate dues increases to fund these escalating priorities. As late as 1968, when a crisis was already visible, additional space had been leased, renovations made, furniture bought, and new staff members added without any concomitant increase in incoming funds. An antiquated accounting system made matters worse. Essentially, the former business manager used a cash system of accounting, wherein income was recorded as received and expenditures noted only when actually paid. There was no system at all for tracking bills on hand for goods and services not yet paid, even for such essentials as rent, insurance, leases, etc. No priorities had been set, and as programs and expenses mounted, the board had rightly become alarmed at the lack of comprehensible financial reports. Finally, upon the recommendation of Arthur Young and Company, a new controller was authorized to establish a modern accounting and control system. It was under this directive that Peplau hired Gerald Dorfman in November, 1969, and began to address the problem. At this date, the ANA was in debt to the tune of $1,200,000. In addition, $112,000 had been diverted from the pension fund; $213,000 had been taken as an unauthorized loan from the membership account, there was a $200,000 bank overdraft, and there was $375,000 in unpaid bills. On December 18, 1969, 29 part-time and temporary staff members had been terminated, and on January 27, 1970, 41 full-time staff had reluctantly been notified they would be let go by the end of February, 1970. Thus, by February 1, 1970, a staff of 153 had been reduced to 70. What then became extra space was leased out, leased equipment was returned, publications were suspended, consultancies were terminated, and scheduled salary increases were not paid.
57. Board minutes, February 12, 1970, ANA archives, Mugar Library, Box 75.
58. Diary entries, April, 1970.
59. Letter from Henry R. Winkler to Hilda E. Peplau, April 17, 1970, in the Peplau Personnel File in the Rutgers University Personnel Archives.
60. Diary #2 for 1970, entry for April 21, 1970.

ANA: The Professional Nightmare

14

*I've worked terribly hard to change ANA and the members' percep-
tion of it, and just possibly all I've done is to raise hopes [that won't]
be realized and thus made the situation worse than ever.*

—Hildegard Peplau
May 1971

The May 1970 American Nurses Association convention in Miami
did not begin well. On May 4, the evening of the opening ceremonies, Hilda Peplau and outgoing ANA President Dorothy
Cornelius set out from the hotel for the convention hall in one of two
small Renault cars provided the executive director and the president for
the duration of the convention. Hilda had loaned the Renault designated
for her use to Gerald Dorfman for the evening, explaining that she would
travel with Cornelius. Cornelius was driving, and her longtime associate
and friend Elaine Martyn was in the passenger seat. Hilda rode in back
with Captain Joanne Kennedy of the U. S. Air Force. Suddenly, a Lincoln
Continental roared up the wrong side of the road directly at them. The
Lincoln hit the Renault head on. The small, French-made car, which was
not equipped with seat belts, was no match for the heavy Lincoln. Hilda
was bounced from seat to ceiling to floor, then to the ceiling again. She
was knocked unconscious. She came to, dizzy, dazed, disoriented, and in
great pain. She was aware of faces staring in through the car window.
Beer cans rolled out of the Lincoln onto the road.[1]

When her head began to clear, Hilda refused to be transported to a
hospital by ambulance, promising that she would have her injuries
checked at an emergency room, but *later*. For now, she declared, it was
imperative that she and Cornelius proceed to the ceremonies. The ambulance took Martyn and Kennedy to the hospital, and Peplau and Cornelius
took a taxi to the convention hall. Other than remembering that she got
there, Hilda did not later remember the opening ceremonies.[2] After the

ceremonies, she was taken to the hospital emergency room in the care of
two Air Force nurses. Arriving at the hospital a little after 11:00 p.m., it
did not occur to her to use her name and status as the executive director
of the American Nurses Association to receive speedy treatment. Instead,
she waited impatiently until 2:30 a.m., and then decided her condition
could not be too serious since she was still sitting up and because no one
seemed to be paying any particular attention to her. The Air Force nurses
concurred in her assessment that probably nothing was broken, and perhaps indeed she would be better off in her Plaza Hotel bed than spending
more hours after an exhausting day in the hospital emergency room.[3]
Because as executive director she had myriad responsibilities at the convention, and because her campaign for president was well under way,
Peplau refused to return to the hospital the next day. Black and blue
bruises were spreading across her back, thighs, and legs, but she could
move, and she could think, and that was all she needed. Since she was
never x-rayed, she did not know then the extent and seriousness of her
injuries, nor could she have imagined the eventual long-term consequences of this traumatic assault on her neck and spine. For the remainder
of the convention she was beset with excruciating headaches and suffered
lapses in memory. She found it difficult to stand for any length of time.
As it turned out, these were conditions that would persist over the next
several years.[4]

Her campaign for the presidency, however, was in high gear and well
organized—complete with buttons, posters, slogans, and pennants. Beverly
Hoeffer of New Jersey, the national chair of the Peplau campaign, and
Grayce Sills from Ohio, the campaign coordinator, together with the New
Jersey delegation, were in charge of orchestrating the nomination from
the floor of Hildegard Peplau for the presidency of the American Nurses
Association.[5] The campaign group had coordinators for the larger states
and regions drawn from among psychiatric nurses from all over the country.[6] All those years working in the state hospitals and serving on national
boards and committees were paying off. As the outgoing executive director, Peplau received invitations to all the many receptions hosted at the
convention by state associations, pharmaceutical firms, publishers, and
exhibitors. She distributed these tickets to the psychiatric nurse campaign
workers who used them to fan out and gather intelligence. At midnight
each evening, they would meet with Grayce Sills and Beverly Hoeffer to
assess the information and plan for the next day. The next morning, Sills
and Hoeffer would brief Peplau. Hilda managed to get to some of the
early morning delegate caucuses before the day's proceedings opened
with a House of Delegates meeting (when she would have to be on stage),
but evenings were spent lying exhausted and in pain on her bed. Because
she did not share with anyone the effect that the accident had in fact had
on her, few realized the extent of the pain she was experiencing.

During the convention, Hilda remained dazed and in distress. Grayce
Sills kept asking, "Are you okay?" She would reply, "Yeah, I'm okay"—
but she wasn't. The last night in Miami, Sills caught sight of Peplau's leg,
which was one solid hematoma. Her bruises had begun to turn green,
and her dizziness increased. She could barely stand, but she carried on.[7]
Although she was at the center of a convention of several thousand nurses, no one other than Sills seemed to notice Hilda's physical distress. In
retrospect, Hilda felt deep disappointment recalling the apparent indif-
ference of her colleagues in nursing to her condition.

Initially there were eight candidates for the ANA presidency, the greatest number to compete for the position in ANA history. Some of these
candidates were promoted in an effort by ANA staff members to split the
Peplau vote.[8] While the official leadership looked on askance, however,
the rank-and-file delegates rallied. By the final ballot on May 8, there
were three candidates remaining. Out of the more than 1,000 ballots cast,
Peplau won by 14 votes.[9] Never had an ANA election been so contested.

There would be no time after the convention for Peplau either to recu-
perate or to seek medical attention. She left Miami on May 8, after a particularly stressful ANA board meeting. By May 11, Peplau was back in
New York removing her personal pictures and files from the ANA offices
and turning over her keys. It was not a particularly happy nor gracious
occasion. Her successor was openly hostile, informing Peplau that since
as executive director Hilda had rented out any extra office space, there
would be no space for her to use at ANA headquarters during her term as
ANA president.

Nonetheless, at first it appeared that the presidency would be a much
more personally satisfying experience than her stressful tenure as executive director had been. By May 15, the flowers and letters of congratulations were pouring in. Typical of the many letters Hilda received is this
one from Eloise Lewis, dean of the College of Nursing at the University
of North Carolina at Greensboro:

> The American Nurses Association never has had a president held in
> such high esteem by the practicing nurse or one to whom so many feel
> so near. As a person, teacher, and practitioner, you have always cared
> enough to give unselfishly of your time and talents . . . I personally am
> very grateful to you for the courage and wisdom that marked your
> tenure of office as executive director . . . thank you, for all of us, for
> your willingness to assume leadership in these troubled times.[10]

That the office was an important one is evident from the fact that letters
of congratulation were received not only from William Cahill, the governor of the State of New Jersey, but also from President Richard Nixon, and
United Nations Secretary General U Thant.[11] Similarly, the New Jersey State
Senate and Assembly passed resolutions lauding her election to nursing's

highest position. In June, a testimonial dinner was held in her honor at the Manor in West Orange, New Jersey, but what Peplau remembered above all else of this festive occasion was the physical pain she endured while sitting through the long dinner and equally long tributes to her. This interlude in her life should have been a time of celebration, a time to let the compliments roll, and to recognize that her efforts on behalf of the ANA had not gone altogether unappreciated. What should have been a tour of triumph, though, became instead a haze of pain to be endured.[12] She would write, "Where before I enjoyed receptions, speeches, and activities that required standing but got me among nurses, I now abhor them, and find the work increasingly difficult."[13] Still she felt she had neither the time nor the energy to seek medical help and forced herself to keep going. She went to all the receptions planned for her and attended all the meetings already on the calendar for the president of the ANA. She also began an odyssey she had set for herself; namely over the course of her presidency to visit each of 50 State Nurses Associations. Neck pain kept her awake at night, and if she stood for any length of time—and all the receptions and talks required that—she was in agony for days afterwards. Years later, Xrays revealed several collapsed vertebrae.[14]

A bright spot in the early summer was a surprise party at her home organized by former students. Hilda had gone to Summit Hospital for the one and only session of physical therapy she allowed herself, and the organizers descended on her home. Flowers and a cake were delivered, the champagne was iced, and food was brought from Nathan's Delicatessen in Brooklyn. She was given a ring of pale blue turquoise surrounded by diamonds, and a gold pin holding three delicate birds. The ring she would wear for years, until arthritis made it difficult for her to wear any rings at all. As she explained in her thank-you notes to the celebrants, "Pins, as we say in Pennsylvania 'stick friends'—and our friendship has 'come a long way and will surely continue.'"[15]

The joy of the surprise party faded as the hard work of the office began. Not only was the ANA staff in New York difficult, so was the board. As a whole, it would tend to ally itself with a return to a status-quo director in opposition to a president whose broad popular base and militant vision for the professionalization of nursing made them uneasy.

AN ACTIVE PRESIDENCY

Peplau's first board meeting was indicative of things to come. Minutes of that August meeting indicate that 40 to 50 staff members were in and out of the meetings, suggestive of a degree of staff disorganization and distraction that is hard to imagine.[16] Peplau had to leave immediately after that board meeting because she had again agreed to spend Mondays at

Rutgers, and the fall semester was beginning. It was ANA practice that the 2-day board meeting be followed by 5 days of committee meetings, thus extending the meetings through an entire 7-day week. In August, Peplau left for Rutgers after the first 2 days, thus missing the ANA committee, division, and section meetings that followed.[17] In writing to compliment her conduct of the board meeting, Philip Day commented, "As I expected, you did a masterful job—and very real thanks for your efforts," but then went on to observe that after she left, "The board discussion of the National Fund for Graduate Nursing Education turned into an Alice-in- Wonderland nightmare, and I'll discuss it over a lunch with you some day."[18]

Peplau's presidency was nonetheless an active one. Archived files are full of announcements and news accounts of her travels around the country during her term. Wherever she went, Peplau stressed that organized nursing could make significant improvements in health care delivery systems through the united efforts of professional nurses. For example, she continued to work with the American Medical Association's joint-practice commission to seek ways in which nurses and physicians could cooperate to enhance health care across disciplines and professions. This was work in which she eagerly participated, but it was work about which the ANA Board was most suspicious.[19] She was also deeply involved with government officials and representatives of allied health organizations on every level in discussions related to expanding roles for nurses.[20]

Her position as ANA president offered Peplau a great deal of visibility nationally, but within the organization itself, she soon found that the board would frustrate her every step of the way—seldom making a decision, never having enough information, constantly referring every matter for further study.[21] Nonetheless, as 1970 drew to a close, Peplau refused to be shackled. Instead, she again marshaled her strength, determined to make her presidency count. She would visit every state, listen to nurses at every level, and exhort those willing to hear at every point. She perceived herself to be near the end of her career, and she resolved to give nursing her all before going into the supposed sunset of retirement. She was determined to rekindle enthusiasm for the work that had so long consumed her energies. She would be intently focused on visiting, listening, and hearing the membership at large. Hilda was aware that, historically, the ANA president was considered to be a figurehead, not a policy maker or maker of agendas. Peplau, though, was temperamentally unable to play the role of figurehead, and, by her own assessment, she was not a politician. She had goals, things she wanted to accomplish: professionalization, advancement of educational standards, and encouragement of nursing research. She would use the position as best she could, but she could not play the political game.

A PRESIDENCY COMES UNRAVELED

By January 1971 Peplau knew that her mission to professionalize nursing would continue to be an uphill battle, but she willed herself the physical strength and endurance to continue to fight. In retrospect, she noted that

> Once I got into ANA, I got the idea that this was THE professional organization [for nurses] and that it needed to be professionalized . . . And there were a lot of things I didn't know about it. I didn't know that it was [essentially] a labor union, although it had been since 1947.[22]

The pressures thwarting Hilda's intentions and draining her energies came at her from every direction. She had been inundated with Christmas cards in 1970 and gamely was trying to respond to every one. She had absolutely no staff support from the ANA, and very little at Rutgers, since she had turned the administration of the graduate program and the secretary assigned to it over to Shirley Smoyak. Peplau had insisted that all ANA mail addressed to her be sent to her for answering. But the executive director insisted on reading the mail addressed to the president, and decided whether to answer it or to send it on. Since Peplau was seldom satisfied with the answered mail sent out in her name, she specifically requested that *all* mail addressed to the president come directly to her.[23] The director persisted in deciding what should be sent on and what she could handle herself, however. In exasperation, Peplau wrote to her early in January 1971 to object to a letter that had been sent to the Kentucky State Nurses Association in Peplau's name and to other related incidents:

> There is another aspect you need to consider. I had asked early on in our working relationship that all mail addressed to me be forwarded to me, and that when you reply *at my request* this should be indicated in the letter. I was not consulted about this letter but your reply does not show this . . . I must express serious objections to this procedure and insist that *all* mail addressed to the president be forwarded . . . I also insist that *all* replies show clearly whether I am responding or whether you are in my behalf. As for the reply to Mrs. Kemp—it is long winded and not at all to the point . . . There is quite evidently a problem within ANA regarding information processing and response. Many items that I send to you are not heard about again unless I ask about them. This puts the burden of keeping track of details upon a volunteer fully employed elsewhere and is a great burden, especially in light of my well-known effort to use face-to-face contacts to increase confidence and membership.[24]

There follows a long list of 17 specific complaints and illustrations of mishandled or non- handled items. Peplau ends, however, by trying to ease the brunt of her criticism and engender cooperation. She seemed to have had no sense that the force of her letter was likely to have had the opposite effect. After stating the facts, Hilda wanted to offer some encouragement:

> Enough of this! You must surely know that you have had my full and complete support. I have tried to be direct and honest with you and have come directly to you, rather than to any other ANA staff member. I have made every effort to recognize that your style of working is different from mine and to work with rather than belittle the difference . . . But, there is in my mind a lingering impression that the President is not viewed as the elected leader to be consulted freely and informed fully.[25]

She just could not leave it alone, just yet, though. There then follows of list of 7 more items sent on to ANA headquarters for which no action had been taken or about which no information has been forthcoming. Not surprisingly, the director continued to answer mail and then send it on to Peplau as she saw fit in case she "might also want to answer or respond too."[26]

One of Peplau's intentions as ANA president was to pursue her goal of establishing within the profession a process of certification for master's prepared clinical specialists in nursing practice. At Peplau's insistence and with the support of other leaders in psychiatric nursing, the ANA finally agreed to call a national conference to discuss the certification issue. As Peplau walked through the conference hotel in Atlantic City in 1971, she noticed a large group of Rutgers graduates in deep discussion with an ANA staff member. The staff member was trying to persuade them to *oppose* certification. Peplau was aghast. She had used her position as president of the ANA to call the conference, and an ANA staff member was openly working to undermine its purpose. Peplau took a deep breath and marched up to the group. She told them right there that they should just go ahead and set up a mechanism for certification on their own, and not wait for ANA to see the light. The New Jersey group did just that, setting up a state certification process that took effect in 1974 and continues to the present.[27]

On the road Peplau was invariably a phenomenal success. Letters of appreciation flowed in from all over the country, but dealings with headquarters continued to deteriorate. By the time of the April 1971 board meeting, it was obvious that much of Hilda's work on the road was being undone in New York. At the January 1971 Board meeting, no audit report had been available. When Peplau questioned this, the executive director assured her she would "have the audit report in ample time for the May meeting." On April 2, however, the Arthur Young company wrote to Peplau as president of the ANA to inform her that the auditors were "now off the assignment because various materials required for their examination was not ready or available."[28] Peplau requested that they nonetheless make recommendations to help the organization become more efficient. In June, Arthur Young sent her a three-page letter of specific recommendations, that, if adopted, would make the ANA more professional in billing and accounting areas. The letter concluded with the observation, that "While there has been significant improvement during the last year due to your influence, it is quite obvious that there is a great deal of work remaining to be done."[29]

A battle of wills was now evident. Peplau, in her capacity as president, sent a steady stream of requests to the ANA headquarters in regard to correspondence with SNAs on various issues, new items for meeting agendas, her own travel arrangements and reimbursements, and so forth. Her requests were met with long, formal responses, generally explaining why the staff did not have time to respond to or do what was requested. Presumably to demonstrate how disrespectfully she was being treated by the staff, Peplau sent a whole packet of this material to the board. If the board was sympathetic, there is nothing in the record to so indicate.[30]

In line with her determination to be both an activist president and to move the profession forward, Peplau succeeded in getting the board to endorse her call for a national "forecasting conference" to project where nursing should be in 10 years time. After the initial approval, however, she found herself frustrated at every turn. First she tried unsuccessfully to get the *American Journal of Nursing* (AJN) to conduct a survey of ANA membership on "Forecasting Nursing for the Decade Ahead," but such a survey was never conducted.

Peplau's level of frustration rose even higher when she received a letter from Rozella Schlotfeldt, an innovative dean at Case Western Reserve University. Schlotfeldt expressed concern over the fact that the AMA was then defining the scope of practice for a new category of healthcare worker, to be called physician assistant (PA).[31] Schlotfeldt warned that the AMA was gathering in under its own wing much of what nurses in fact do, although nursing had never actually delineated its own scope of practice. Schlotfeldt was pleading that the ANA take the lead in doing so and soon was joined by many other nursing leaders in voicing concern. Peplau urged that rather than oppose the PA movement, nursing finally declare its own specializations as defined by clinical expertise. For this reason alone, she hoped the importance of the proposed forecasting conference would be underscored. By March it was evident to her that this project too would be sabotaged by the ANA staff. In some frustration she wrote to the executive director on March 3, 1971:

> I have a carbon of S[hirley] Burd's letter to you that she will not participate in the forecast. She, like Dr. Field, indicates that information was

not given or not made clear . . . It wouldn't be difficult to infer that the forecasting experiment has been set up to fail—what with delays and inattention to detail. And that's too bad for it suggests that only staff-controlled within ANA projects are possible. Needless to say, I am greatly distressed at that thought.[32]

This letter must have crossed one sent to SNA directors on March 5 from ANA. It was not exactly an endorsement of the conference, nor a ringing call to serious discussion and reflection about the future of nursing at the end of the 20th century. Quite the contrary—

ANA has a very modest budget for this endeavor and regrets that it cannot arrange for meetings with each SNA. If an SNA wishes to send comments on nursing and its direction in the decade(s) ahead, the president and the board would welcome the information to add to its collection of principal ideas to be included in the forecast.[33]

On March 26, insult was added when the ANA sent another letter to the SNA presidents, this time requesting that material be sent to ANA headquarters for the forecasting conference by March 19—a week *before* the letter went out![34]

Without input from the SNAs, or from nursing at large, what could be salvaged of a conference was held at the University of Connecticut on April 2, 1971. Lacking wide participation and with an agenda of limited scope, the forecasting conference would be one of the greatest disappointments of Peplau's presidency. The event, or nonevent as it was, served notice, should she have needed it, that everything possible would be done to see that Peplau failed in her goals while in office.[35]

In spite of all this, however, it remained clear that among rank-and-file nurses there was wide appreciation for Peplau's efforts. The files are replete with scores of letters of thanks for all she was doing to reestablish the credibility of the ANA as a professional organization relevant to a broad spectrum of nurses. She received appreciation for speaking across the country to SNAs, to student meetings, and on university campuses on the general theme of "Trends in Nursing."[36] Lacking support for her efforts from either the ANA Board or staff, she nonetheless persisted in urging nurses to look ahead. A typical letter to Peplau reads;

At long last I was able to view the video tape of "Trends in Nursing." Your candid answers to questions on the nurse-doctor relationships, physician's assistants, dual appointments, and career ladders are both stimulating and informative to the viewer. I think we are quite fortunate at the University of Virginia to have captured you forever on our campus on video tape. The natives of Virginia are still remarking on the thrill of having you speak throughout the state; the feedback I have heard has all been extremely positive both in terms of your person, and the content of your addresses.[37]

Fatigued after the disappointment of the forecasting conference, but not defeated, Peplau tried to set up a committee on nursing research. Although she would eventually succeed, at this time she was informed that there was no money for ANA committee expansion.[38] The continuing financial disarray had other consequences. Much to her chagrin, the ANA was in arrears in its dues to the International Council of Nurses (ICN), an organization that Hilda firmly supported as important to nursing worldwide. Finally, after much work on her part, the board agreed to make a token payment of $617 toward its dues of nearly $4,000 to the ICN, attributing the small amount offered to "the financial cycle at ANA."[39]

In response, in part, to the continuing financial crisis, the ANA board had begun in late 1970 to investigate a move of the headquarters offices out of New York to the new Crown Center in Kansas City, where rent would be more affordable. The board had begun this exploration many months before Peplau's term as executive director ended, but did not make a final decision until May 1971, well into her presidency. Unfortunately, the staff had not been consulted and thus the decision came as a shock to many staff members who assumed, incorrectly, that the recommendation for a move had been made by Peplau. The board did nothing to counter this impression, thus greatly increasing the tension between the staff and the ANA president.[40]

For the remainder of 1971 meetings were long and complicated; dozens of staff members drifted in and out, handing out reams of paper. Motions were piled upon motions, motions to amend already amended motions were passed, motions were withdrawn. In all the parliamentary maneuvering, very little seemed to get accomplished. In the May meeting, a report from the Membership Promotion Committee was accompanied by 20 motions, and 15 substitute motions and motions to amend.[41] Peplau gamely kept trying to summarize and bring the discussions to a conclusion, but the discussions simply went on and on and on.

In her diary account of the May board meetings Peplau recorded that there were a few questions and no real answers in regard to the ANA financial situation. She noted rather sadly, "I say little—my power being nil." There had been no financial reports since January in spite of the board's policy that "the comptroller will prepare and the executive director will send monthly financial reports to the Board."[42]

On May 24, 1971, an emergency board meeting was called to deal with staff distress over the move to Kansas City. As Peplau noted in her diary, "There has been no effort to prepare the staff for the psychological trauma of relocation." Further, she wrote, the "attitude is—you can't have that information."[43] Peplau asked for a closed board meeting without any of the staff present, but only one other member of the board supported her motion.[44] At the May 24 meeting Peplau also urged that an ANA advisory committee be established to represent the views of the state nurses associations to the ANA Board on various matters. Having traveled the country meeting with SNAs, she knew they would welcome coordination and direction as the healthcare system developed and changed and an increasing number of resulting issues affected nursing. For Peplau, her recommendation was an attempt to open channels of communication and to give SNAs a stake in ongoing ANA work. The ANA Board, though, simply could not come to terms with the idea of such a body. There were endless questions about what kind of advice would be sought, where it would go, who would determine where it went, and what standing such advice would have. In the end, predictably, nothing at all happened on this front.[45] By the end of May, the board was openly hostile to Peplau, not giving her complete agendas for the meetings over which she was to preside and not telling her when and where committee meetings were scheduled. She was not given copies of items added to the agenda nor told what new business might be brought up. When she raised objections she was ignored.[46]

Although it was fairly common for ANA presidents to serve two terms, Peplau decided after the May 1971 board meetings that she would neither seek nor accept a second term. Hilda, in her disappointment and frustration, was by that time near a breaking point, as is clear from the following entries in her diary:

> I'm not paranoid, but I have made the right decision for me not to run again, for I surely do not have the confidence of the board and I suppose of the staff . . . I just won't play the dirty political game to beat this system. I hope I can control my feelings . . . There really isn't any insight on the board that I can make and after today's power showdown [the rejection of Hilda's request to have a closed board meeting to discuss the headquarters move], I see no constructive effect to my opening the situation for discussion on any level with anyone. I am terribly weepy (i.e., helpless) about the whole thing. I've worked terribly hard to change ANA and the members' perception of it, and just possibly all I've done is to raise hopes [that won't] be realized and thus made the situation worse than ever . . . Staff sit and watch with what seem to be grim and mask-like faces. These are days when I truly wish I wasn't president, hoping thereby I wouldn't know whether things at ANA are truly better or worse.[47]

By June 1, Hilda's spirits were somewhat revived by a trip to Texas where she was feted in grand style. The depth of her fatigue, however, was evident to her. She complained in her diary of "the handicap of physical exhaustion . . . My neck aches. My thinking is belabored. I am bothered by being [recorded] without being asked. The tapes reflect my total and spreading exhaustion."[48] Wherever she traveled, the dinner parties were many and, she noted, "belabored—they really don't know what to talk about with me."[49] It was at this point that her old friend from Texas, Bill Field, with whom she had worked with Shirley Smoyak in the Albuquerque family therapy workshops, began to pressure her to make videotapes. The concept was to capture the Smoyak, Field, and Peplau contributions to ongoing workshops in nurse psychotherapy. Hilda knew she was simply too tired to participate and only very reluctantly agreed to contribute "what she could." Field, however, had no idea how literally true that was, and from that point on would nag her to get going on her contribution.[50]

On June 9 Peplau was in Reno, Nevada, where she taped a joint interview with the president of the AMA, which she considered "a real coup—the only one of my term."[51] Although she acknowledged having a good time, Peplau still complained of exhaustion. From Reno, she went on to Las Vegas where she taught a course, did more videotaping, and attended more receptions, breakfasts, and dinners held in her honor. By June 14, she was back in Albuquerque participating in the family therapy workshops with Shirley Smoyak and Bill Field.

The explanation for Hilda's unremitting exhaustion is not hard to find. When she was not in tension-filled and disheartening ANA Board meetings, Peplau was traveling about the country. After the Albuquerque meetings in June she returned home just long enough to switch wardrobes and head back to Washington, D.C., and a 5-day trip through the state of Virginia, that included appearances in Arlington, Richmond, Roanoke, Charlottesville, and Norfolk. On June 24 she was in Minneapolis, Minnesota; on June 25 she was in Rochester, New York; and then it was back to Washington on June 27.[52] Her life was a constant stream of interviews, press conferences, banquets, and receptions, all requiring remarks and talks.[53]

In the middle of the June ANA activities, she went to a National Institute of Mental Health event in Washington: "So good to see Bob Felix. I owe him so much. And Dr. Westermark too."[54] Peplau went directly from the NIMH celebration in Washington to the ANA's 75th Anniversary Dinner. Although Peplau was to preside over the festive occasion, she had not been involved in the planning, and her role was completely scripted by staff. She was given no opportunity to speak, or even to make remarks on her own. She was too exhausted from her injuries and her schedule to protest. She simply did as she was instructed, and read her lines. The fact that Hilda acquiesced in this manner is indicative of both how exhausted she was, and of how far the relationship had deteriorated between her and the staff that had worked under her direction just a year earlier.[55]

The extensive international travel that had begun some 6 years earlier when Peplau was appointed Nurse Consultant to the U.S. Surgeon General continued apace through the summer of 1971. In early July, still suffering from weariness and now vertigo as well, Hilda attended a 4-day workshop in Puerto Rico. She was home on July 14 in time to pick up Tish, who would travel with her to England and Ireland. In England, Hilda made a sentimental trip to Winchester and Bournemouth, where she spent so many romantic days with Mac during World War II. But both places had lost their magic for her. Hilda reported being "disappointed" and a little sad.[56] Other than that, there are no notations in her diary to suggest the importance of these places in Hilda's life. The diary simply records the hours that she and Tish woke up, what they ate, and what they saw. There are no personal reflections at all.

Travel with Tish always revived Hilda's energies and by July 26 the two were in Ireland where Hilda would be attending the meetings of the International Council of Nurses. As president of the ANA, Peplau was the official American country representative. She appreciated the level of competence and professionalism she encountered at ICN, which tended to restore her faith in her profession. Hilda loved the ICN. Its mingling of younger and older nurses of every color and nationality, its many spoken languages, and all the pageantry that accompanies international meetings greatly appealed to her.

Hilda was home for one day, August 3, before flying off to Anchorage, Alaska, on another Air Force tour. In her position with the office of the surgeon general she held the temporary rank of major-general, which assured red-carpet treatment at Air Force hospitals around the world. From Alaska, she flew to Japan and the Philippines. By August 26 was back in New Jersey getting ready for another year at Rutgers.

On September 2, Peplau was featured on the morning *Today* show with Barbara Walters. While thrilled with the interview, Peplau was annoyed that Dean Chapman had not notified the Rutgers faculty, or the university's public relations department. Notwithstanding, nurses across the country were excited to see one of their own on such a popular national television show. The fact that Peplau was articulate for nursing, and that Walters was clearly impressed, generated a flood of complimentary letters.[57] The enjoyment of such favorable fame was short-lived however. For then it was back to reality and the endlessly floundering ANA Board meetings in New York. In December, Hilda enjoyed a brief moment of relief during a trip to Geneva. She returned in time to go to the White House on December 23, to be present when President Nixon signed the National Cancer Act.[58] Hilda could not have helped but note that the White House was a long way from Reading, Pennsylvania, and the little house where she was raised a block from the railroad tracks.

In her 1971 Christmas letter, Peplau recounted that in the course of the past year she had seldom spent a night in her own bed.[59] She had visited 25 of the 50 states she vowed to visit over the 2-year term of her ANA presidency. She'd been to Alaska, which she loved, and to which she vowed to return. She'd had also visited Puerto Rico, Grand Bahama Island, Ireland, Switzerland, France, and England, and gone on to Tokyo and Singapore and back again via Hawaii and California.

THE FINAL YEAR

The year 1972 began well with a visit from Grayce Sills, who always raised Peplau's spirits, but the weeklong ANA Board meetings at the end of January brought back the reality of her situation. She noted on January 28, 1972, "By today I was exhausted—totally. I had such pressure in my head and difficulty swallowing and great pressure in my speech center. No one cared or even noticed."[60]

In February, Peplau flew to Memphis for the Tennessee SNA convention, where she stayed with one of her former students, Shirley Burd. Being with Shirley brought back a pleasant memory. Traditionally at the opening ceremonies at ANA conventions there would be a long procession of past and current ANA presidents and executive directors, all dressed in long evening gowns. (Hilda participated in this pomp and circumstance, but privately, she jokingly referred this event as "Nursing's Miss America Pageant.") When Peplau was installed as ANA president in 1970, Shirley Burd and Annie Laurie Crawford, another colleague and professional friend, assessed her wardrobe and decided that for this occasion Hilda needed something that had not been previously paraded. Almost overnight, Annie created a lovely new gown, and Shirley made an elegant gold cape to go with it.[61] As this event illustrated, the rigors of dressing appropriate to her position as ANA president was quite a departure for Hilda. In her personal life, at home on the weekends, she was likely to be found wearing slacks and a tee shirt. She dressed appropriately for her professional duties at Rutgers, but when she became a spokesperson for the ANA, she felt obliged to be exceptionally well dressed. After her election to the presidency, she bought an entirely new basic wardrobe and found a talented dressmaker who made several suits and another evening gown for her. While the parade of formal gowns at ANA conventions was not at all Hilda's style nor consistent in any way with her vision of the nursing profession, she went along with the custom. By the time of her retirement, she had a closet full of long gowns.[62]

In March, Peplau continued her traveling, attending SNA meetings, keeping her promise to visit all 50 states. She continued to complain of neck pain and to express frustration that her physical situation limited her ability (in her opinion) "to be responsive or sharp."[63] She reported to the April 7 meeting of the Executive Committee of the ANA Board that she had visited with the leaders of many nursing organizations, including those associated with the Veterans Administration, the Military Nurse Corps, and Nurses for Political Action among others, and suggested that the leaders of the major organizations related to nursing be invited to meet with the ANA Board to discuss the need for a united stand for nursing.[64] She just could not give up trying, in spite of her intellectual understanding of the basic futility of the effort.

In April Peplau noted that ANA Board meetings had become "just a ritual" and that the 3-day Finance Committee meeting held April 20–23 was a "waste of time."[65] The 1972 President's Report was presented at the April board meeting, which was to be Peplau's last in her capacity as president. This report revealed both the broad scope of her activities and the depth of her continuing frustration. The report made recommendations, but the wording is such that it was clear she did not hold out much hope for action.[66] Her own efforts to compress the schedule notwithstanding, she noted that board and committee meetings still consumed as much as 7–9 days out of the month. She complained that the ANA Board tolerated "such an unbusinesslike approach to work—I wonder how they can waste so much time?"[67] Hilda's one accomplishment at this meeting was to persuade the board to do an annual evaluation of the executive director. This process would begin in 1973, when Peplau would no longer be president, so it would be clear this was a professional evaluation, not a personal vendetta. Writing about this board meeting Peplau expressed exasperation that the board gave her a piece of jewelry as a tribute to her leadership while driving her nearly to the brink with its dithering. She complained that "the rituals are getting to me. I am practically hysterical. I'll never make it. The board enjoys my suffering—it seems to improve their humor."[68]

While Peplau continued to receive letters from nurses expressing appreciation for her efforts, ironically it was the letters from the SNAs beseeching her to do various things on behalf of nursing and to speak out for various causes, that caused her the greatest frustration. She brought these issues, which often centered on matters of certification of levels of practice and definitions of clinical specialties, to the board, but was not able to get board members to focus the discussion, to summarize, and to treat a question rationally and bring it to a conclusion.[69] Any issue of this nature introduced by Peplau sent board members off on tangents and in several directions simultaneously. And any issue raised by Peplau on behalf of the SNAs was in addition to the many motions forwarded to the board from the House of Delegates. Instead of organizing these motions into coherent recommendations, the staff simply forwarded them all to the board for action. The flood of motions from the House of Delegates, absent thoughtful staff consolidation and recommendation, left the board immobilized and assured it could not cope with more from Hilda Peplau.[70]

"IF ANYTHING CAN GO WRONG, IT WILL"

With Hildegard Peplau at the podium, presiding as president, the 48th ANA convention, held from April 30 to May 5, 1972, in Cobo Hall in Detroit was a disaster. On the surface, it should have been a high point of Peplau's career. Peplau and Margrethe Kruse, the president of the ICN, were to be feted. Hilda had a stunning silk gown and cape to wear, made for her by Annie Laurie Crawford and Shirley Burd from material brought from Thailand by Grayce Sills.[71] A report on the scope of nursing practice, or more accurately "extended roles for nurses," was to be presented at a plenary session. Peplau hoped this presentation would at last generate goals defining and extending the boundaries of nursing practice.[72] Further, there was a proposal to establish a National Academy of Nursing to honor excellence in the profession.[73] Hilda approached the convention with an unrealistic optimism.

She perceived from the opening night, however, that it would be a very rough convention. Nothing on the stage was in order: The microphone did not work; there were no chairs for the invited guests; and there was no program on the podium for Peplau to follow as she presided over the opening ceremony. At her insistence, the parliamentarian came to her room at 10:30 that night to go over the agenda for the following day. Peplau's agenda was in one order, the parliamentarian's in another, and the backup materials contained in a separate book matched neither. They spent the night getting the two books and the supporting documents coordinated, not finishing until 8:30 the next morning.

In spite of their effort, however, nothing was in order during the meeting. While Peplau's agenda now agreed with that of the parliamentarian, the delegates had a completely different agenda and incomplete backup information. The result was pandemonium on the platform, with much whispering in ears and frantic running back and forth. Peplau ordered all the ANA staff off the stage, so that she and the parliamentarian could try to run the meeting. According to Peplau, though, the parliamentarian began to break under the pressure, and the staff whispering continued, only now on the floor directly in front of the podium. It was all very distracting, and the delegates reacted with predictable hostility. The proposal to create an Academy of Nursing was attacked for its elitism and referred back to committee, the paper on extended roles for nursing digressed into a discussion of "caring," and suspicion was voiced that this was yet another way to change educational requirements.

On May 4, Hilda noted in her diary, "All I want now is for it to end."[74] She recorded that, "The mood of the house is puzzlement. More people are sitting in the bleachers to watch the fun. The word is out that the Board is giving me the works."[75] At a reception held at the end of the convention, however, Hilda was overwhelmed by the length of the line of well-wishers waiting to speak with her. Clearly there were many among the SNA delegates who appreciated her courage and leadership.

Peplau was not alone in her assessment of the convention. Even *Nursing Outlook* acknowledged some of the difficulties in its editorial concerning the convention:

> ANA President, Hilda E. Peplau, was at various times tough, unrelenting, overwhelmed. She managed to keep the House of Delegates under control—no mean task—and even to hold on to her sense of humor . . .
>
> It was a convention marked by preoccupation with the nurse's expanded role and the preparation for it; and a convention marked by an unusual amount of procedural and parliamentary difficulties . . . Even tougher sailing was ahead when, on Wednesday morning, the subject of including the *American Journal of Nursing* as an ANA benefit came up. The topic itself, plus the parliamentary hassle that evolved from the discussion made very high waves indeed. Another stormy session resulted from the delegates' discovery that the use of voting machines precluded write-in votes. The best word for their reaction is "outraged."[76]

This convention experience marked the end of Peplau's 2-year term as ANA president. She would remain on the board as second vice president for another 2 years. At a luncheon for the new board, one of the newly elected members commented that she hoped that during Peplau's remaining term on the board, "people are going to lay their knives down."[77] After the convention, Peplau was so exhausted she did something she had not done in 2 years: she spent 5 days in bed. On May 17, 1972, she paused to try to regain her perspective. She wrote in her diary that it had been 25 years since she started the nurse-patient studies at Teachers College, and now "whole roomfuls of psych nurses are certified. It is a great joy to realize I had something to do with their being there."[78]

Although Hilda's tenure as president of the American Nurses Association had been discouraging and disappointing to her on a personal level, to many others in nursing, outside the leadership clique at ANA headquarters, Peplau's role as a highly visible leader in her profession had been strong and effective. She had made a real effort to travel the country, to meet nurses where they lived and worked, and to raise issues with them that were important both to them and to the profession. She never talked down to nurses, and they responded more and more enthusiastically as the year went on. As Grayce Sills remarked, "It was exciting to watch."[79] Peplau's activism, however, was not exciting to the ANA Board. The board treated her as though she had committed a crime. Her own analysis was probably close to the truth: In an interview in 1994, Peplau looked back at her career and made the comment that, "politically I was not a good President. It was a political role—I was supposed to be just a figurehead. It took me a while to understand that. I am not a politician."[80]

At the end of May, she admitted, "I am wearying of it all. I can't bear to be a symbol without substance."[81] That June she received her second honorary degree—this time from Boston College, which was particularly nice because it afforded her the opportunity to visit Tish who was now in her fourth year of graduate school at Harvard. Although physical complaints continued to plague her, she nonetheless looked forward to another trip to Alaska that summer. On her return, she found a letter from Kay Norris, one of her first students and now a good friend, who wrote attempting to explain reality to Hilda:

> I heard it was rough—but it's not clear what made it so. I'm glad you are out of it. The people in the system have a couple of generations of know-how about how to manipulate it to their own ends. They used you when they needed you, you may be sure—but they knew how to make you powerless when they wanted to. I had hope for a while because of your tremendous ability, but could see the system closing around you once you were not in the executive director's chair.[82]

July was a restless month. She was exhausted, but something more was pulling at her. Her childhood friend, Betty Kreiger Price, was much on her mind. In the spring, Hilda had learned that Betty had been in a deep depression since the death of her husband, Ted, the previous year. Betty's sister, Natalie, kept Hilda informed and in July reported that Betty was not rallying, that she did not want to see friends, she was not eating, and had no interest in living. Hilda promised to come later in the month, but Natalie discouraged her. On July 20, Hilda telephoned and got Natalie's husband, Wayne Gormis, who told her that Betty was in the hospital. Hilda was on her way to a meeting of the National Federation of Business and Professional Women in Atlantic City the next day, but promised to come to Reading immediately after that. In Atlantic City, Hilda could not get her mind off Betty. She began to relive all the early years, the teenage years when Betty and Natalie's home was her refuge, the fun years of dating, the early years of Betty and Ted's marriage, the bands, Betty's wonderful voice and nightclub singing. Increasingly uneasy, she left the convention early and first phoned Tish, finding all well there. Then she called Reading. Betty had died the day before, July 22, 1972.

Betty's death put a final period on Hilda's youth. Betty was buried in Reading on July 26, but Hilda did not go to the funeral. The burial was very private—only the immediate family. This was Betty's specific wish.

She had shut out all her friends in the last year of her life, and did not want them mourning her without her Ted. Natalie urged Hilda to come and spend the weekend after the funeral, but Hilda felt there was no point in that. She knew Betty had needed her in the last year of her life, but she had not gone. She could not bear to go now that it was too late.[83] With Tish grown up and Hilda's own childhood circle of family and friends slipping away, she was beginning to feel not only alone, but very lonely.

Peplau had decided that she would retire from Rutgers at the conclusion of her term on the ANA Board. She had no wish to return to Rutgers, where she understood yet another dean was in trouble, but retirement was still two years away. She applied for and received a reduced teaching load, and it was understood she would retire after the 1973–74 academic year. In September Peplau found that more students than ever were seeking admission to the Graduate Program in Psychiatric Nursing. Those who were beginning their first year in the program were disappointed to learn Hilda Peplau was essentially on leave and would retire before they completed their own graduate work under her direction.[84]

October began on a somewhat higher note. Hilda was in Washington, D.C., for government committee meetings the first weeks of that month and noted in her diary that people seemed friendlier than usual, "even the ANA crowd."[85] The weather was lovely and the city looked beautiful. For the first time in a long time Hilda seemed able to enjoy things—food, the city itself, even the receptions. While there, she managed to schedule an interview for three members of the board and herself with the secretary of Health, Education and Welfare (HEW), Elliot Richardson. Peplau prepared an agenda of 15 major points she hoped to make. At the appointed time, she and the others were ushered into the secretary's office, where they sat for 10 minutes before Richardson entered, mail in hand. Every time Peplau started to talk, he'd start looking at his mail. She could have understood this if it were 20 minutes into the meeting and it was clear the nurses had no real agenda, but at the beginning of a meeting she thought his inattention showed only disrespect. Whether that was disrespect for women in general or disrespect reserved for a delegation of mere nurses, she was not sure. In a gesture of controlled frustration, Hilda picked up her purse and dumped its contents on Secretary Richardson's desk, explaining that while he looked at his mail she would sort her purse. That got his attention. When the meeting was over Richardson walked Hilda to the door, and thereafter was unfailingly gracious when their paths crossed. He invited her to a state dinner and to several Washington luncheons after that, seeming to enjoy her company and valuing her input.[86]

The next week Peplau was in Kansas City for an ANA Board meeting in the new headquarters. Almost immediately the back pain and nausea started again. As recorded in her diary: "Typical ANA—lousy staff work, long meetings, no results."[87] Nothing pleased her. She found the new headquarters in poor taste, with red carpets and chairs in the reception area and clashing plaids in the meeting room. Although she was determined to make her 2 years on the board less exhausting than the 2 years of her presidency, this too had its cost in terms of draining her strength.

> I decided to play it cool . . . I have a pretty clear idea that my views are not exactly welcomed. I came late, arrived alone, am not available for dinner, and limited my comments to brief and few remarks. I was rewarded with great solicitousness. [The executive director] apologized because my name was the only misspelled name on the Committee on Committees Report. I hate games. I am letting the Old Guard maximize their power and take the consequences. There's less tension, less real work done, an unfinished agenda . . . Home at 2:00 a.m. Vomiting and back pain.[88]

In the last months of 1972 and into 1973, Peplau remained on the move. From the middle of September until Christmas 1972, for example, she spoke in New York, Boston, Chicago, Minneapolis, Atlanta, Memphis, Miami, Albuquerque, Chapel Hill, Los Angeles, and Indianapolis, rarely with more than 2 days at home between trips. When she was home, she was unavoidably involved in Rutgers business. On the road, she appeared as a guest lecturer at meetings of the nursing honorary society, Sigma Theta Tau, at college graduations, and at State Nurses Association meetings; she delivered papers to the American Psychiatric Association, the ANA annual meetings, and local and annual meetings of psychiatric nurses; she was the keynote speaker at a conference on changes in mental health benefits; she prepared papers and gave talks for many smaller, more specialized nursing groups. She again went to Nigeria as the external examiner, and she attended ICN meetings in Switzerland.

In her role as second vice president of the ANA Board, Peplau halfheartedly but persistently pressed the Board to move ahead with certification, to be assertive in keeping all regulation of nursing with nursing's professional organizations, and to develop an academy to recognize excellence in nursing. Board meetings continued to be chaotic, with between 40 and 50 staff members present at any given point in time. The staff also began to grow again, with 10 new positions created early in 1973.[89]

Despite her decision to cut back, Peplau's schedule was again seriously out of hand. Her determination as president to visit every state's SNA had been punishing, and the choice to continue on without medical treatment after a serious accident undoubtedly had consequences that undermined her health and sapped her strength. Nonetheless, she continued to travel—seeing this as her remaining opportunity to speak out for change, to work to ignite the spark wherever it might fall. Still, she found that everything was an extraordinary effort. The physical exhaustion just would not lift, and the depression she had battled for the better part of 2 years was almost debilitating. Contemplating retirement, however, made her uneasy. So, Peplau decided to seek support for a position on the ICN board. This, she believed, would keep her involved in formal nursing, working with women in international nursing whom she'd come to respect and admire. She wanted to retire from the sources of her frustration, Rutgers and the ANA, but not from nursing itself nor from her efforts to elevate the standing of nursing as a profession.

THE FINAL INSULT

In spite of her 1973 New Year's resolution to lay low, keep quiet, and try to recapture her credibility at ANA, Hilda just could not do it. Keeping quiet when she saw a need for action was not in her repertoire. She continued to write long letters to the ANA about what it should do about various matters of national importance, ranging from healthcare legislation to research support, as well as matters of importance specifically to nursing such as certification and self-regulation.[90] She also continued to urge the ANA Board to act on such issues—and they continued to avoid doing so.

As 1973 began, she was concerned that congressional funding for traineeships for nursing would cease, and that this would have tremendous consequences for nursing education at the university level. In spite of her urging, the ANA declined to act, considering funding to be primarily an issue of interest to universities and thus their responsibility.[91] Working with her friends in Washington, D.C., and on non-ANA committees, Peplau did help to save the traineeships. Congress approved the renewed funding in June.[92]

In many ways Peplau's final disillusionment with the ANA leadership came in May. As the board meeting began the morning of May 1, 1973, both board and staff members seemed to Peplau unusually cheerful and friendly. Just before noon the five board members who served on the Committee on Committees, of which Peplau was a member, were asked to meet over lunch to deal with a few "quick" matters. As the committee settled down for the lunchtime meeting, a legal brief dated April 30, 1973, from the ANA's legal counsel, Edward W. Kriss, was distributed. The brief was entitled "Legal Implications of Appointing a Member of the Advisory Board of *Nursing '73* to the Board of Directors of The American Journal of Nursing Company."[93] *Nursing '73* was a popular monthly magazine, and Peplau served on its board as a favor to one of the editors.[94] For many years it had been the practice that the outgoing president of the ANA be appointed to the board of the AJN. Peplau had been looking

forward to this appointment, as she hoped to upgrade the quality of the
AJN, making it a journal of scholarly rather than simply professional
record for nursing, as many other journals were for their professions.
Peplau sat in stunned disbelief as the committee voted unanimously to
refer this matter to the full board immediately after lunch. Peplau did
not participate in the ensuing brief committee discussion, and could not
believe the full board would endorse such an unfair and obviously personal vendetta. After all, the appointment of the outgoing ANA president
to the AJN Board was all but a pro forma proceeding. Never had it been a
controversial one.

She was in for a shock, however. Almost immediately after the full
board convened, the legal brief was distributed, and the lawyer, who just
happened to be on the premises, was called in to present the brief in person. Clearly this had been and would continue to be a scripted proceeding. In summary, the brief stated,

> The Committee on Committees of the ANA has recommended to the
> Board of Directors of ANA that Y [i.e., Hilda E. Peplau] be appointed to
> the Board of Directors of the *American Journal of Nursing* Company. It
> has come to the attention of the Committee that Y is listed as one of five
> Chief Advisors on the Advisory Board of a monthly magazine, *Nursing*,
> which is a competitor of *American Journal of Nursing*. The Board of
> Directors of ANA has requested that General Counsel advise it as to the
> legal implications of the appointment of Y to the *Journal* Board and
> whether such appointment will result in a "conflict of interest situa-
> tion" with regard to Y's performance of her duties as a member of the
> *Journal* Board.[95]

The brief then went on to discuss corporate law with regards to conflicts
of interest and the fiduciary duties of board members, offering appropriate case citations, and concluding that "the courts have developed the
general rule that directors may engage in independent enterprises, but
they cannot compete with the business of the corporation."[96] After
reviewing conflict of interest law, the brief concluded,

> The cases summarized above involved specific transactions by or
> involving a director with conflicting interests. There is no specific trans-
> action to analyze with regard to Y and the *Journal* Board. In short, since
> Y has not yet assumed her duties on the Board of the *Journal*, no claim
> can be made that Y has breached a fiduciary duty . . . At this juncture,
> the most that can be said is that if Y is seated on the Journal Board a sit-
> uation is created that is ripe for abuse of fiduciary duty . . . the state-
> ments and votes of Y while sitting on the *Journal* Board would be open
> to question—was Y acting with only the best interests of the *Journal* at
> heart, or was Y acting in such a manner so as to benefit *Nursing* or her

own interest in connection with *Nursing* . . . Further, the fact that other members of the *Journal* Board know of Y being on the Advisory Board of *Nursing* would have a stifling effect on deliberations of the *Journal* Board . . . A board of directors cannot function properly if board members cannot fully discuss and disclose the affairs of the corporation in front of another board member because of the possibility that such information may be of benefit to a competitor . . . the dual directorship role would be most uncomfortable for the . . . Board and for Y . . . Good business practice dictates that preventive law be practiced, and that Y not be appointed to the *Journal* Board.[97]

When the vote had been taken, Hildegard Peplau became the first and only president of ANA not to be appointed to the AJN Board.[98]

Instead of seeing this as the political maneuver that it was, Peplau chose to see it as an attack on her integrity.[99] She was not so outraged at the vote itself as by the fact that she had been blindsided. No one had alerted her to the issue or discussed it with her. She could not believe—if "conflict of interest" was actually a concern—that no one had brought that to her attention. Nor had anyone asked what she wanted to do about it. Instead, they had solicited a legal opinion from the organization's lawyer. She had not been given advance notice and had not been offered the obvious option of resigning from *Nursing '73*, which she could easily have done. Rather she had been humiliated at the ANA Board meeting. To Hilda, the most outrageous aspect of the whole affair was that her integrity had been questioned, as was implied by the assumption in the brief that she would act in a way to harm the AJN. Peplau did *not* see that her often expressed goal to "raise the standards" of the AJN would be perceived as threatening to an establishment that resented her own widely admired publications and that strongly resisted her progressive advocacy for the professionalization of nursing. She did not understand the maneuvering to keep her off the AJN board as a political move, and thus she seemed to miss the core of the issue. As Hilda herself analyzed the situation,

> The intent was to embarrass me . . . I couldn't believe it was happening. This is what went on in high places in nursing! I'm not a politician, I can't turn around and make things nice. It was a character issue. I didn't expect them to change their votes—just to be decent, to ask questions, to have an open discussion. I wasn't the best President in the world. I am not a politician. But, I am honest, open, and forthright. They could have asked me.[100]

After this heartbreaking board meeting, when she learned conclusively that she had few friends among the leadership at the ANA, Peplau went on to Mexico City and the meeting of the ICN Board. At this meeting,

Dorothy Cornelius was elected president of the ICN. Peplau felt tension whenever she was around members of the American delegation, and noted in her diary that "I play the game badly."[101] The tension was somewhat relieved when Tish arrived to join her mother on a tour of the Yucatan. Before leaving Mexico City, however, Peplau was pitched headfirst out of a taxi when it started to pull away from the curb as she was preparing to exit. She did spend the week touring with Tish, but experienced agonizing back pain and had swollen thighs and many bruises. She arrived home after a month of traveling, unpacked, changed clothes and went to the Rutgers Medical School for a lecture by her old friend from Nigeria, Dr. Adeoyo Lambo, who had become president of the World Health Organization.

When Hilda entered the lecture hall, Lambo was well into his lecture. When he spotted Peplau, he interrupted his presentation, bounded up the aisle taking the steps two at a time, and gave her a big bear hug, much to the amazement of the president of the medical school, Stanley Bergen, and much to the detriment of her badly injured spine. After the lecture, Bergen invited Hilda to join a group for dinner, but she had already accepted an invitation to the Smoyak home, and knew that her aching back would inhibit her enjoyment of the company. During the reception that preceded the lecture, the medical school's vice president, Charles Vivier, had invited her for drinks, dinner, and conversation later in the week. As she noted wryly in her diary, "The sudden popularity was full of opportunity, it was sad to miss."[102] From this point on, it would be clear that recognition of Peplau's contributions to nursing would far and away outstrip her lack of popularity at the ANA headquarters and the persistent insider fighting at the Rutgers College of Nursing. But it was still too soon for her to appreciate this fact.

In June, Hilda headed for Europe, where she would participate in a NATO-sponsored conference on anxiety. Tish, who was then completing her PhD in social psychology, had been invited as a guest and was able to attend many of the sessions. The conference was held at a lovely resort hotel in the German Alps, at the time of the region's annual asparagus festival. Mother and daughter rented a Volkswagen, and squeezed in several trips into the countryside. This would be their last opportunity to travel together before Tish moved to Los Angeles to assume a faculty position at UCLA.

January 1974, found Hilda entering her final semester at Rutgers and her final 6 months on the ANA Board. At this point, she was too weary even to revise the nursing chapter for the *Comprehensive Textbook of Psychiatry*, a piece she had enjoyed contributing since 1965, primarily because it kept her current on the literature and kept nursing included in this leading psychiatry textbook. She wrote, suggesting others who might be willing to write the chapter.[103]

In February, the Council of Psychiatric Nurses proposed to the ANA Board the establishment of a Hilda Peplau Award to be given for outstanding contributions to psychiatric nursing. The ANA Board informed the council that a person must be deceased before an award could be established. Later that same year the board established the Jessie Scott Award, however, and Jessie Scott was still very much alive at the time. It wasn't until 1990 that the ANA established the Hildegard E. Peplau Award for contributions to nursing research, and presented the first award to Hilda Peplau, who was also still very much alive.

In June, Hilda attended the ANA convention in San Francisco. President Gabrielson's customary presidential speech reviewed the saga of the ANA debt and the necessity to fire long-time employees. Peplau commented in her diary, "People kept watching me to see if I'd walk out, but I stayed to the end."[104] The next day was spent politicking for the position of ANA third vice president, for which she had been nominated by the states of Washington and Pennsylvania. Peplau was pleased to have been nominated, but ran against her better judgment. She did not think she could win. Nonetheless, she was shocked to lose by a two-to-one margin. The margin was so overwhelming, at least in part, because a very popular Black nurse from Ohio had been slated by the nominating committee to run against her.[105] Peplau, though, took the defeat as a final attempt to discredit and humiliate her.[106] She nonetheless acknowledged that in the course of the conference she had been given "lots of awards. Some nice, some silly . . ." She noted with irony that one was in recognition of her work at Teachers College.[107] Thus, the ANA chapter drew to a close. This chapter, like others, would leave her with a sense of profound disappointment.

Although discouraged professionally, Hilda nevertheless looked forward to the remainder of this particular trip. Hilda had been joined in San Francisco by her beloved sister, Bertha Reppert, and Bertha's daughter Susannah. At the conclusion of the convention, Hilda, Bertha, and Susie flew to Los Angeles and stayed with Tish at her apartment in Santa Monica. From there, the four women set off for a nostalgic cross-country journey. This time, in contrast to Hilda and Tish's first cross-country trip in 1957 in the ailing, old white Ford, they traveled in Tish's new, blue Volvo sedan, purchased with Hilda's help when Tish's own old Volkswagen coughed its last gasp that spring. From Los Angeles, they drove to Palm Springs and spent a day in the Joshua Tree National Monument, then on to Las Vegas. They went to on to Zion, Bryce, and the Grand canyons the next day, then went on through Navajo country and Monument Valley to Durango, to Silverton and Ouray, and into Colorado Springs to see the Air Force Academy. Then it was on to Kansas and through Missouri to the final stop in Mechanicsburg, Pennsylvania, to drop off Bertha and Susie and the many treasures they had accumulated along the way. Leaving

Hilda at home in Madison, Tish travelled on to Boston to continue work on a longitudinal research study she had begun while a graduate student at Harvard. Peplau worked through the months of July and August in her office at Rutgers, conscientiously sorting through files and putting them in order. She was torn between the pull of a sense of duty to do it, and the temptation to simply walk away. She stayed in her office.

On Peplau and Leadership

What are we to make of the fact that Peplau experienced such intractable resistance and hostility in her 4 years in leadership positions at the ANA, while at the same time, and subsequently, her contributions to nursing were repeatedly recognized with the profession's highest honors?[108] Peplau never fully understood that leadership does not devolve upon an individual merely because that person is qualified, sensible, and responsible. Peplau came to the ANA interim executive director position as an undisputed leader in psychiatric nursing, lauded for her pioneering work with graduate students and her dedication to clinical care. Her talents did not lend themselves so naturally, however, to leadership positions in an established corporate, or institutional, culture. Hilda believed instinctively that a leader must be worthy of being followed—more disciplined than others, more committed, more able. She assumed she met these criteria. As she saw her role, it was to set goals, to motivate, to create a sense of urgency and mission, to lead and influence others to follow where she led.

In her work as a teacher of psychiatric nursing, her leadership was evidenced through her role as mentor to generations of students, encouraging them to aspire to high standards of professionalism. Through her endless workshops she extended her ideas and visions to nurses across the country. In so doing, she inspired many nurses to return to school, many others to adopt professional ambitions, and still others to become leaders in their own right. In this she was remarkably effective. When Peplau attempted to transfer these skills to the ANA organization, however, she was confronted by a very different kind of culture, one that she did not understand. There her strengths—embodying as they did a vision for change—were perceived not as a call to action but as a very real threat to an established order. At the ANA she would find that she was a leader without followers.

In her clinical work Peplau understood at a very fundamental level the importance of understanding how others perceived their world and finding there something that would respond to her encouragement. Ironically, the woman who introduced interpersonal relations to nursing could not transfer these insights to her own leadership of her profession. She understood but did not respect the underlying ethos of the ANA Board and staff. More fundamentally, she understood the necessity to change that ethos if nursing were to attain the stature of other major clinical professions, but she did not recognize the threat such change would pose to its entrenched leadership. She did not use her skills in interpersonal relations to identify and tap into strengths in her ANA staff that she might use in attaining her goals. She found it difficult to understand the tenacity of an established corporate culture that, in its own self-interest, would circle the wagons and form otherwise unlikely alliances in defense of the status quo. She relied, instead, on the logic of her views to carry the day. Studies of leadership styles in business schools and by psychologists have shown that the most effective leaders switch flexibly among various leadership styles (authoritarian, mentor, coach, facilitator, etc.) as needed.[109] This she could not do. Effective leaders are sensitive to the impact they have on others and adjust accordingly in order to get results. Peplau understood this in regard to working with patients in mental hospitals, but she seemingly could not transfer those skills to her ANA leadership positions.

It was as a teacher and mentor, and as a reformer in clinical psychiatric care, that Peplau would be recognized in the future. Her difficulties with the ANA and the defeat of her agenda there would be largely forgotten in the years ahead. As the 1960s ended and the 1970s began, factors other than the hostility of nursing's corporate leadership would circumscribe Hilda's vision for professional nursing. These factors would include the continued increase in unionization among nurses, the continued diversity of educational entry points for nursing practice as community college nursing programs continued to grow, and the decline in federal funding for nursing education and research. Further, increased opportunities for bright women in other professions would deplete nursing's intellectual capital. These factors were clearly beyond Peplau's control and in no way a reflection on her leadership.

What the ANA presidency did do was to afford her the opportunity to travel to every state in the nation advancing the cause of nursing education, nursing research, and professionalization. Her impact among rank-and-file nurses, and outside the sequestered environment of the ANA headquarters, proved to be enormous. The ANA positions she held, for all the personal anguish she endured, afforded her yet another platform, another pulpit, from which she was able to speak. For this too she would be remembered.

ENDNOTES

1. Interview, Hildegard Peplau, March 2, 1992.
2. Ibid.

3. Diary entry, May 13, 1970, in Diary #2 for 1970, in Box 8, #242.
4. Interview, Hildegard Peplau, February 10, 1992, and Peplau diaries from 1970–1974.
5. Anne Patterson, President of the New Jersey State Nurses Association, placed Peplau's name in nomination from the floor on May 5, 1970. *New Jersey Nurse* May–June, 1970: 3. For details of the campaign see typed, unsigned notes found in Box 2, #28, and materials in Box 32, #1243.
6. Letter from Grayce Sills to Barbara Callaway, February 13, 1999.
7. Interview, Grayce Sills, June 15, 1996, in Washington, D.C.
8. Interviews, Martha Rogers, March 14, 1993, in Phoenix, Arizona, Grayce Sills, June 15, 1996, in Washington, D.C.; and Anita O'Toole and Suzy Lego, September 14, 1996, in Sewickley, Pennsylvania.
9. On the final ballot, Peplau received 395 votes, Eleanor Lambertsen 379, and Lucie Young 230. See news clippings in Box 2, #27. Other details of the campaign and Peplau's physical condition may be found in Box 2, #49.
10. Letter from Eloise Lewis to Hildegard Peplau, May 19, 1970, in Box 33, #1238.
11. See Box 2, #27, for the letters from Nixon and U Thant, and Box 32 #1248 for letter from Cahill.
12. Descriptions of her pain and the frustrations it caused her are included along with clippings of an endless array of events in Box 2, #27–49.
13. Notes found in Box 2, #49.
14. All of this was much to the frustration of the lawyers for the insurance company representatives in Miami who were trying to settle up after the May 4 automobile accident. At their insistence, Peplau did see a Dr. McClellen in Summit, New Jersey sometime after returning from Miami. He prescribed a neck brace, that she refused to wear because she thought it would not project a good image for the president of the ANA. The lawyers were pressing her to get a complete physical and report from the doctor, but she was too stressed and too exhausted to pursue it. During May and June, as the bruises got greener, she simply took aspirin and lay abed when she wasn't walking or standing.

In July she finally did go for a session of physical therapy at the Summit Hospital near her home, but this was not something she felt she could continue, for the demands on her time were simply too great. Through most of July and August, 1970, the lawyers continued to plead with her to get an "adequate report" of the accident. They chided her for not seeking consistent, constant medical attention. As the lawyer assigned to her case, Lennard Robbins of a law firm in Hollywood, Florida wrote, "a continuity picture is most important, and we do not have it in this case." A couple of weeks later, in response to her plea of no time and endless demands, he wrote in obvious frustration that,

> I really don't like to be difficult, but find that we seem to have some problem in communicating the need for substantiation . . . I must have more cooperation in order to effect any kind of a satisfactory settlement. I don't know how I can impress this on you, but hope this letter will serve that purpose. (Leonard Robbins to Hildegard Peplau, July 25 and August 15, 1970, Box 2, #49)

Still later, Robbins wrote to demand that she "get the requested items, information, and reports to me forthwith." (See letters to Hildegard Peplau from Leonard Robbins of the law firm Abrams, Anton, Robbins, Resnick and Schneider of Hollywood, Florida written between June and November, 1970, in Box 2, #49.) Peplau did write to the Morristown doctor, pleading for the appropriate report, but simply did not have the energy to pursue it beyond this. Thus, nothing came of the settlement, and the case was simply closed. Although this was before "pain and suffering" settlements became common cause after automobile accidents, it is clear that Peplau had a strong case, even in 1970. What she did not have was the energy to pursue it. The consequent physical debility would cost her dearly during her entire ANA presidency. Because she shared her physical distress with so few, few knew the physical toll the ANA presidency would take.

15. Unsigned and undated letter found in Box 33. The party was orchestrated by Janice Manaser, Fern Kumler, Ann Lazaroff, and Kay Harrison. Joe Geller brought the champagne and Shirley Smoyak brought the cake. Friends came from far and near and filled her home with laughter, music, good cheer, and heartfelt good wishes. The party was a bright spot in an otherwise dismal month of pain.

16. See Board Minutes in Folders 14–15 in the ANA Archives, Mugar Library.

17. There are five standing ANA committees—By-Laws, Committee on Committees, Credentials, Finance, and Membership. There are four Commissions—Economic and General Welfare, Nursing Education, Nursing Research, and Nursing Service. Finally, there are five Divisions of Practice—Community Health Nursing Practice, Geriatric Nursing Practice, Maternal and Child Health, Medical/Surgical, and Psychiatric and Mental Health Nursing Practice. All met that August for the convenience of the board member liaisons to the committees.

18. Letter from Philip Day to Hildegard Peplau, August 31, 1970, in Box 40, #1460.

19. See questioning of her participation in the Joint Practice Commission on the part of Board members in Box 34, #1260.

20. See materials in Box 2, #27.

21. Ibid.

22. Letter from Hildegard Peplau to Grayce Sills, November 25, 1997. Also, see Grayce Sills, "Peplau and Professionalism: The Emergence of the Paradigm of Professionalization," *Journal of Psychiatric and Mental Health Nursing 5* (June 1998): 167–171. In this article, Sills summarizes Peplau's paradigm of professionalization as self-regulation of nursing practice focused on the examination of its clinical work. The professional society (which Peplau thought ANA should be) "must identify the phenomena of concern in relation to the society, define the scope of the professional practice in that domain, set the standards for safe practices and certify to the public that the conditions for the trust of the public have been met" (Sills, op cit, 168).

23. The enormous amount of ANA correspondence and the 1970 Christmas volume may be gleaned by a look through files in Box 35, #1328–1336.

24. Letter from Hildegard Peplau, January 14, 1971, Box 35, #1281.

25. Ibid.

26. Letter to Hilda Peplau, February 9, 1971, Box 35, #1282.

27. Interview, Hildegard Peplau, February 11, 1992. Once New Jersey led the way, the ANA saw the light. (See correspondence from Janice Geller to Hilda Peplau in Box 5, #193, in regard to the progress of establishing certification in New Jersey.) Certification brought in revenue. So, after several years the ANA established certification centers, thus bringing a significant source of revenue into the organization.

28. Cover letter from Arthur Young and Company to Hilda Peplau, April 2, 1971, Box 35, #1301.

29. Letter from Arthur Young and Company to Hilda Peplau, June 7, 1971, Box 35, #1301.

30. Box 35, #1302 contains the packet of material sent to the Board of this one-sided correspondence.

31. Letter from Rozella Schlotfeldt to Hilda Peplau, February 21, 1971, Box 35, #1303.

32. Letter from Hilda Peplau, March 3, 1971, Box 35, #1297.

33. Letter from ANA to SNAS Presidents, March 5, 1971, Box 35, #1297.

34. Ibid, March 26, 1971.

35. See Box 35, #1308, for a verbatim report of the "Conference on Forecasting Nursing for the Decade Ahead," University of Connecticut, April 2, 1971.
36. For many such letters, see Box 35, #1286.
37. Letter from Mary Reres, Dean, University of Virginia College of Nursing, to Hilda Peplau, August 18, 1971, in Box 35, #1292.
38. See Box 35, #1300, for documentation of the effort to set up the Committee on Nursing Research.
39. See Box 35, #1324, for correspondence with ICN's in regard to dues. ICN's frustration with ANA is expressed in correspondence found in #1288. In Box 34, #1260, there are Board minutes that indicate Peplau was *pleading* with the Board to honor its commitments to ICN. That the ANA president found herself in such a position at all is indicative of the strained relations between Peplau, the staff, and the board.
40. Minutes of Board meeting of May 27, 1971, when this decision was made, and Peplau's recordings of staff reactions, may be found in Box 35, #1299 and #1304.
41. These minutes were found in Box 35, #1299.
42. Diary entry, May 12, 1971, Box 8, #243.
43. Diary entry, May 24, 1971, ibid.
44. Diary entry, May 24, 1971, ibid. The lone Board member who supported Peplau was Jackie Smith.
45. See material in Box 34, #1260.
46. Minutes of Board meeting, May 27, 1971, Box 35, #1299.
47. Diary entry, May 29, 1971, Box 8, #243.
48. Diary entry, June 2, 1971, ibid.
49. Ibid.
50. See packet of letters from Bill Field to Hilda Peplau in Box 26, #960, and in Box 28, #1053.
51. Diary entry, June 10, 1971.
52. See Peplau's personal calendar in Box 35, #1326.
53. Ibid.
54. Diary entry, June 30, 1971.
55. See Box 35, #1284, for preliminary planning, and #1325 for the 75th anniversary program and the script for Peplau.
56. Diary entry, August 3, 1971.
57. See transcript and photos of the September 2, 1971, *Today* show broadcast in Box 35, #1284, along with many letters received about it.
58. December 1971 Christmas letter, in Box 5, #197.
59. Ibid.
60. 1972 Diary, entry for January 28, 1972, in Box 8, #243.
61. Interview, Annie Crawford, September 7, 1995, at Elizabeth Carter's summer cottage on Lake Hapatong, New Jersey; also, Anne Peplau to Barbara Callaway, January 6, 1999.
62. Notes from Anne Peplau to Barbara Callaway, January 6, 1999.
63. Diary entry, March 7, 1972.
64. President's Report to the ANA Board, April 7, 1972, in Box 36, #1344.
65. Diary entry, April 10, 1972.
66. President's Report, April 1972.
67. Ibid.
68. Diary entries for April 1972.
69. See Box 36, #1339, for random materials and notes from ANA Board meetings and a collection of these letters.
70. Board materials in Box 36, #1349.
71. Communication from Grayce Sills to Barbara Callaway, February 13, 1999.

72. This report was the result of a committee on nursing practice appointed by the Secretary of HEW, at Peplau's urging. Peplau served on it in her capacity as president of the ANA. The other committee members were Rozella Schlotfeldt, Constance Holleran, Eileen Jacobi, and Eleanor Lambertsen. Schlotfeldt, Peplau, and Holleran had controlled the committee, and the report was one of which Peplau was proud. See Box 2, #28.
73. See materials on this convention in Box 2, #28.
74. See diary entries from May 1–5, 1972 and materials concerning the convention in Box 36, #1339.
75. Ibid.
76. The point at issue with regard to the *American Journal of Nursing* was the use of ANA dues. The largest part of ANA dues were by now supporting the union activities endorsed by the Division of Economic and General Welfare, by far the most important part of ANA for a majority of its constituent members. Peplau was trying to increase dues support to the AJN while upgrading the journal to a first class refereed journal of reference. These issues are discussed in correspondence between Hilda Peplau and Luther Christman deposited in the Schlesinger Library Peplau collection. The editorial quoted is from *Nursing Outlook* (Summer 1972): 75.
77. Diary entry, May 17, 1972.
78. Ibid.
79. Interview, Grayce Sills, June 16, 1996, in Washington, D.C.
80. Interview, Hilda Peplau, March 9, 1994, in Sherman Oaks.
81. Diary entry, May 27, 1972.
82. Letter from Kay Norris to Hilda Peplau, October 14, 1972, in Box 5, #196.
83. See diary entries for June and July, 1972.
84. See letters expressing alarm from present and potential students in Box 36, #1343.
85. Diary entry, October 7, 1972.
86. Interview, Hildegard Peplau, February 10, 1992, and diary entry, October, 1972.
87. Diary entry, October 14, 1972.
88. Diary entry, October 7, 1972.
89. See Box 75 for minutes of 1972 ANA Board meetings in the Mugar Library, Nursing Archives. Other minutes of Executive Board meetings are found in Paige Box 6 at the Mugar.
90. See letters from Hilda Peplau to ANA executive director in Box 37, #1354.
91. See agenda and notations in Box 37, #1351, of Board meeting of March 13, 1973.
92. See letter from Connie Holleran to Hilda Peplau, June 28, 1973, in Box 35, #1351.
93. This legal brief may be found in Box 37, #1351.
94. Interview, Hildegard Peplau, June 16, 1995, in Washington, D.C.
95. The legal memorandum, from Edward W. Kriss, to ANA executive director, dated April 30, 1973, may be found in Box 37, #1351.
96. Legal brief from Edward W. Kriss, 2.
97. Legal brief from Edward Kriss, 6.
98. Interviews, Grayce Sills, October 29, 1992, in St. Louis, and Catharine Norris, March 9, 1994, in Tucson, Arizona.
99. In fact, there was neither competition nor "fiduciary" conflict between the two journals. *Nursing '73* was a commercial news trade magazine, while the AJN was the official publication for a professional organization. In fact, during the time Peplau served on the Board of *Nursing '73*, it never met, and she had never been asked to review articles for publication. Interview, Catharine Norris.
100. Interview, Hildegard Peplau, March 2, 1992.
101. Diary entries, May 15 and May 17, 1973.

102. Diary entry, May 30, 1973.
103. Letter from Hilda E. Peplau to Dr. Alfred Freedman, January 5, 1974, Box 40, #1473.
104. Diary entry, June 4, 1974. Also, see presidential speeches in *One Strong Voice.*
105. Interview, Grayce Sills, June 16, 1995, in Washington, D.C. The nominating committee was chaired by Dorothy Cornelius. In the 1970 campaign this nurse had been a part of Ohio's support for Peplau. Once paired for mutual gain, they were now pitted against one another.
106. Another example of a matter designed to humiliate her leadership was the issue of a membership experiment initiated by the NYSNA. An individual nurse became a member of the ANA through membership in her local SNA. With Peplau's encouragement, NYSNA decided to organize itself on the ANA model, i.e., in New York the SNA would be a federation. Thus, any nurse who was a member of any nursing organization (an honorary society, an alumni association, a union) that in turn was a member of the SNA would be a member of ANA. Peplau had encouraged this experiment, and the ANA Board had agreed early in 1972 to go along on an trial basis. The ANA staff were most agitated, however, and in 1973 got the Board to renege, thus creating enormous ill will all around. Materials on this issue may be found in Box 37, #1350.
107. Diary entry, June 6, 1974.
108. For years after retiring, Peplau continued to send news stories concerning items they might want to address to ANA's leadership. She never received back so much as an acknowledgment. She continued to believe that only knowledge about clinical phenomena and interventions that produce beneficial outcomes would make a difference in professional recognition—not salaries. During the last decade of her life, the ANA honored her at every opportunity, awarding her every honor nursing had to offer, but the ANA staff still would not respond to her.
109. See, for example, Daniel Goleman, "Leadership That Gets Results," *Harvard Business Review* (March–April 2000): 78–90.

Retirement: "Psychiatric Nurse of the Century" **15**

People don't realize I am tired of it all, but [still] I would welcome, cherish intellectual discussion or analysis.

—Hildegard Peplau
November 1974

Hilda Peplau's final 2 years at Rutgers were neither happy nor fulfilling, even though her program was where she wanted it to be, her students were as bright and creative as she had ever hoped they would be, and she, herself, was at the top of her profession. Nonetheless, by the fall of 1973, Hilda had found it increasingly difficult to drag herself in to Rutgers. She expressed no interest in the politicking surrounding yet another dean's search and, indeed, distanced herself from the process, which culminated in the appointment of Eleanor Knudson as dean of the College of Nursing in early 1974. She found even the students to be exhausting. Writing in her diary, she remarked,

> The noise on the tapes, the interference of the MDs and RNs in the students' work and the outright sabotage have gone on for sixteen years, and for me that's enough. The students are novices—pure anxiety. It's exhausting . . . It's harder and harder to go to Rutgers . . . I have little control over anything . . . Faculty meetings are a fiasco.[1]

In retrospect it is clear that Peplau was in the throes of a deep depression, and that depression was linked to continuing, unremitting physical pain. Hilda had been in nearly constant pain since the time of the Miami accident. Although she did not know it at the time, she had suffered at least one collapsed/crushed vertebra and was beginning to develop osteoporosis. Even after she had seemingly recovered from the trauma of the accident, the chronic, relentless back pain would remain with her for the rest of her life. Whenever she stood to give a speech, stood in a reception line, or attended any kind of function that required standing, she was in agony. She never sought help, she never learned the techniques a rehabilitation specialist might have given her to deal with chronic pain, she never resorted to pain killers. Drawing deeply on her mother's German stoicism, she simply toughed it out. On really bad days, she might lie down for a while on her bed to seek relief, but she did not complain. Only occasionally did she mention her pain to Tish.[2] It is clear that no one seemed aware of Hilda's perilous physical condition and she confided in no one. It seems equally clear that Hilda did not let her daughter know how compromised her health was at this point, nor how fragile her psyche. Thus, the 1973–1974 academic year was for Hilda not a triumphal finale but a painful, staggering stretch to the finish line. This was simply not a year in which she could summon the energy for anything, including enthusiasm for her own considerable achievements.

On April 8, 1974, the Rutgers College of Nursing staged a "state of the art" conference as a tribute to Hildegard Peplau and her contributions to nursing education and to psychiatric nursing. This conference was a wonderful opportunity, one to which she normally would have responded with renewed vigor and intellectual challenge. She managed to work with Shirley Smoyak in orchestrating the conference, but rather than feeling stimulated, Hilda was tired, in pain, and just plain bored by the proceedings once the conference was under way. She had labored too long, too hard, and too intensely to have any energy left for simple relaxation and enjoyment of what she had wrought. Instead, she sourly found fault with all.

On May 7 she taught her last formal class, and the following evening a large retirement dinner for her was held at one of Newark's more posh restaurants, the Manor. It was a gala celebration of her career and an acknowledgment of her standing as the most eminent member of the College of Nursing faculty. While she appreciated the occasion, she could not help but note, "I really enjoyed it with a sense of sadness that these bright young people have more years with this pathological clique that run the college."[3] At home later that night, she wrote, "another major nose bleed . . . I am so weary . . . I am a walking case of ailments."[4] The many celebrations of her tenure at Rutgers that were held that spring had become a burden as she herself had come to view her retirement not so much as a triumphant exit as a sad collapse.

After the June trip west to the 1974 ANA convention in San Francisco and her leisurely drive back across the country with Tish, her sister Bertha, and her niece Susie, Hilda returned alone to her office in New Brunswick to go through her files and ready the many boxes of material to be sent to the archives in Women's History in the Schlesinger Library at Radcliffe College.[5] While initially she found a sense of accomplishment in reviewing her career through her papers, she was soon bored, then tired of the job. By the end of July, she exclaimed "What a mess. It's deadly work. I am exhausted by the conflict of whether to do it and get it done vs. walking away and saying the hell with it."[6]

On August 28, 1974, she finally finished. The desk was clear. "Lots of paper, instructions, data, grant background, etc.," had been passed on to Shirley Smoyak and "a great indolence has set in."[7] Hilda did not record a single relaxing day or activity during the entire month. She had not sat down to visit, to reflect, or even to watch a movie. "Indolence" is a misnomer. Peplau was simply exhausted from nearly 30 years of nonstop work—teaching, summer workshops, professional associations, committee work, national and international lecture circuits, and the endless frustrations of college and nursing politics.

Hilda turned 65 on September 1, 1974, and on that day she officially retired from Rutgers. Before taking on any other obligations or making any commitments, she had decided to give herself a month in California with Tish. Thus, on September 1, she locked the front door of her house on Shunpike Road and took off for the drive back to California with Tish—without setting foot again in the College of Nursing. She *felt* she had no good-byes to say, no friends to see, no colleagues with whom to reminisce. It was simply over.

For the 20 years she had been at Rutgers, Peplau had put more energy into her work than any other 10 or even 100 people combined. In those years, she had never taken a sabbatical—that ritual of academic life that affords a faculty member time to rethink, reflect, and renew both the mind and the spirit. She had been vilified through two incompetent deanships. During her final 4 years at Rutgers she had made a near superhuman effort to fulfill her faculty responsibilities while at the same time laboring to save the American Nurses Association (ANA). Even Hilda Peplau could not shoulder such an overload. It nearly broke her physically and psychologically. It certainly deprived her of the possibility of relaxing and enjoying her last year at the university, of receiving and absorbing the many honors and kudos that were at last coming her way.[8] Instead, she was overwhelmed with exhaustion.

In her own eyes, at the end of her academic career Peplau felt that she had largely failed to do what she'd set out to do—raise the level of nursing education, nursing practice, and nursing research through reforming psychiatric nursing. Perhaps her agenda was too broad in scope, her sights set too high, and her estimate of what was possible for one human being to accomplish, too unrealistic. At Rutgers, she felt she had failed. After 20 years, the College of Nursing was not much stronger than she had found it. The faculty was still largely an inadequately credentialed one in an increasingly more respectable public research university. The faculty was torn by dissension, without a vision of its future, and largely without the ambition to change and grow with the rest of the institution. Hilda found this discouraging in the extreme.

The Graduate Program in Psychiatric Nursing was too costly to sustain without the federal support that Peplau brought in. After her retirement, the program was eventually pulled into the other master's level programs being developed at the College of Nursing. By 1983 it had been watered down to the point that it simply disappeared as a freestanding program educating nurses to be clinical specialists.

AN UNEASY LEISURE

During the late summer of 1974, when she was cleaning out her office and files at Rutgers, Hilda yearned for the peace and rest she believed retirement would bring.[9] Peace she would find; rest would be only temporary. First, though, there was the drive back to California with Tish. The two took the southern route this time. Hilda traveled in style, riding in Tish's new Volvo, with Tish doing all of the driving. After stopping overnight with Bertha in Mechanicsburg, the two drove due south to Charlottesville, Virginia, where they visited Thomas Jefferson's Monticello. From there it was on to Asheville, North Carolina, to relive memories of their time there with Hilda's brother Walter and his wife, Anne, and then on to Nashville and a stopover with Shirley Burd at the University of Tennessee. From Tennessee, they drove straight across Arkansas and Texas to one of their favorite cities, Albuquerque, and a visit with Josephine van der Meer at the University of New Mexico. Then on through Tucson and Yuma to San Diego, and north to Los Angeles where Tish was on a career track as an assistant professor of psychology at the University of California, Los Angeles (UCLA).

On September 28, Hilda took an airplane back to New Jersey, glad to be home again in Madison. *Now* she planned to relax. She would catch her breath and finally pay attention to her aching body. She dreamed of a new freedom to simply do what she pleased. She had turned the graduate program at Rutgers over to Shirley Smoyak, and she steadfastly refused to be drawn back into it.[10] She refused Dean Eleanor Knudson's request that she stay on another semester "for the good of the program."[11] She wanted to be gone. Like many women who have crossed the boundary beyond middle age into that period in life for which we have no single satisfactory phrase, she was determined to decide what she wanted to do, relieved of the pressure of feeling obligated by duty. It wasn't exactly retirement that Hilda craved in 1974 but rather freedom from the demands and perceived inadequacies of others; however, she was not sure what form that would take. As soon would become evident, she had, to a certain extent, merely altered her life from its previous frenetic pace, which found her nearly every week in flight or on the road, to one still fast-paced, but paced with demands of her own choosing. Free from the unrelenting institutional pressures of the ANA and the university, she found that she could not entirely abandon her old ways. Nonetheless, she was determined to slow down, to pause, to tend to her house and her papers, and to find things she could enjoy, including, at least in her imagination, the peace and quiet of aloneness.

Before she could indulge in her anticipated rest, however, there were yet more parties. They began in October when she returned from Los Angeles. The New Jersey State Nurses Association outdid itself with a big one given at one of New Jersey's premier party sites. The New Jersey governor again paid tribute, many former students returned to attend, and nursing faculty from around the country gathered to celebrate the Peplau career. The event was, as she recorded in her diary, "too much. I am not a grateful receiver."[12] A red tribute book had been prepared for the occasion into which had been inserted letters of appreciation and congratulation. Hilda, who did not accept praise easily, found it difficult to read.[13] There was one exception, and it brought a tear to her eye. That was the letter written by her sister Bertha:

> What has Hilda done for me? To coin a phrase, let me count the ways. I would have to include all she did for our family, the new heating system, the medical care, vacations at Bennington, my prime source of second-in-line clothing, the fun of basking in her reflected glory. Counting the illimitable stars in the heavens would be easier. And yet there is one thing . . .
>
> A half century ago, more or less, my sister clipped from the *Reading Sunday Newspaper* a small article announcing a series of summer classes in Nature Study to be held during the summer months at the Reading Museum. She also gave me the 7¢ bus fare. In fact she gave me a quarter, no small feat in those depression days, so there would be enough for an ice cream cone too.
>
> I attended those classes that summer, studying everything from frogs to butterflies to mushrooms and more, walking the five miles to and fro every day, propelled by an enormous appetite for more of this great big wonderful world surrounding us. A city girl, product of a closely populated half street, I found here education and inspiration for a lifetime.[14]
>
> Enrolling in those classes opened my eyes to the most wondrous world, the unbelievable beauty and endless intricacies of our natural surroundings. It is an on-going love still growing, expanding to include home, family, business and organizational activities. A happier commitment is harder to imagine. All that I have ever done in preparation for

my present pursuits began with the Summer Nature Study Classes at the Reading Museum and Hilda's substantial encouragement.

The broad spectrum of natural sciences began to channel into the field of botany, then horticulture, now herbs, a natural evolution, the distillation of interest and continuing education. This pleasant specialty will hold me enthralled the rest of my life, I'm sure. I consider it a blessed calling—vocation and avocation combined. And for this, I thank you, Hilda.[15]

Although Bertha's tribute was special, the party itself was an ordeal. Not only did many of the words of praise ring false, but Hilda was tired and complained of continual back pain, nausea, and dizziness. In addition to the large fetes, there were other, smaller, parties organized by former students and colleagues whom Hilda had come to number among her friends. These were far more enjoyable and genuine occasions for her.

Soon, however, a sense of uneasiness began to set in. Hilda reported that life suddenly seemed "deadly quiet." She continued to receive innumerable requests, most inviting her to give papers. Most of these she declined with the admonition to "let somebody else do it." The suggested topics now bored her. There were seemingly unending phone calls, but these she found more annoying than welcome. For the most part, the callers phoned to gossip or pass the time of day rather than discuss issues of substance. "People don't realize I am tired of it all, but [still] I would welcome, cherish intellectual discussion or analysis," she noted in her diary.[16] She did agree to work with the National League for Nursing on trying to differentiate what nurse practitioners could do that other nurses could not, and she continued to help Janice Geller and other former students working to establish joint-practice guidelines in New Jersey. These chores, however, were undertaken out of a sense of obligation rather than out of true interest.[17]

Hilda went back to the family home in Reading in November to attend the wedding of the son of her foster brother, Johnny. The excursion provided a festive reunion. Hilda gave a reading at the wedding, and then went on to Wernersville State Hospital to see her sister Clara, whom she had not visited in many years. She was surprised to find her older sister totally lucid for the first time in over 40 years.[18] From Reading and Wernersville she went over to Mechanicsburg to spend Thanksgiving with Bertha and her family, returning to Madison "with neck and every bone aching."[19] December found her collapsed, recouping for Christmas, when Tish would return for the holidays.

By January 1975 she was somewhat refreshed, and more than a little restless. Tish had been home for Christmas, and in February Hilda visited her in her new home. Tish had left her apartment near the Santa Monica beach, and, with Hilda's help, had bought her first house over the hills from UCLA in Sherman Oaks. While staying with Tish, Hilda taught a special course in graduate nursing at UCLA in the capacity of visiting professor. This was hardly fulfilling, however. She felt the undergraduate program there to be no more substantial than the program at Rutgers, and the graduate program prepared no clinical specialists. That February she not only taught a graduate course but also gave seminars at the Veteran's Hospital and held "fireside chats" for both graduate and undergraduate students, as well as for faculty at the UCLA Faculty Club. She also lectured at both the Los Angeles and Long Beach campuses of California State University.[20] Nonetheless, she complained of having "really nothing to do," and of being "totally bored and trapped."[21]

Anyone reviewing Hilda Peplau's life as her retirement set in would expect a sense of completeness, a sense that she had given her all, a sense that it was time to step away. Perhaps one would expect a sad resignation about her profession, and certainly her deep physical exhaustion can be understood. The truth is, however, that Hilda did not, could not, relax into a quiet retirement, satisfied that she had done her best. She retained her unshakable faith in steadfastness of purpose and in the necessity to undertake risks to work for chosen goals. True to form, she just couldn't sit still.

Peplau wanted new challenges, but wasn't sure yet where she would find them. She had made it clear she wanted and needed rest, peace, and quiet, but she found it unsettling that others seemed to be taking her literally. She was uneasy, and puzzled by her vague sense of dissatisfaction. At home in Madison she was taken at her word and left alone. The ANA did not call. She noted rather wistfully, "I am the only ANA president I am sure who one year later—off the Board as VP—has had not a single board or presidential request to do anything, or to serve on a committee, especially the nominating committee, which is certainly unusual."[22]

SEEKING A FOCUS

After returning from Los Angeles in early March 1975, Hilda continued to complain in her diary about a "deathly silence" where anything important was concerned.[23] She was not being asked to serve on national committees, and while she was invited to present scholarly papers at academic conferences, she was not asked for position papers on national nursing issues. Restless to be active in spite of her resolve to "leave it to others," she began to focus her interest on international nursing. During most of her career, she'd been totally consumed with U.S. nursing, and, although interested, she had not been notably active in the International Council for Nursing (ICN). As president of the ANA, she had attended her first ICN meeting in Dublin and was immediately impressed. Here, for the first time in her career in professional nursing, she had met a body of women in leadership roles whom she deeply respected. She was subsequently elected to the ICN Board and would remain on the board for 8 years.

Thus, in 1975, Peplau turned to the ICN to renew her sense of worth, of doing something of value. She had long been interested in international nursing practice, beginning with her first expert advisory position with the World Health Organization in 1948, but had never had the time to become involved at that level. This interest had never abated, and, after 6 months of uneasy retirement, she found in the ICN the focus she sought for her interest and remaining energy. She continued to serve as a board member and then as third vice president until 1983, when she moved to Los Angeles—in effect retiring a second time. Although she declined to seek the ICN presidency when asked, she did persuade the first two non-European, non-U.S. nurses to run. Both, Muringo Kiereini of Kenya and Mo-Im Kim of Taiwan, were subsequently elected to the office of president.[24]

In mid-March, 1975, she was off to a conference in Saarbrucken, West Germany, where she found the physicians no more impressive than were nurses when it came to substantive contributions. From the conference she went to an ICN Board meeting in Geneva. From there Hilda flew to Madrid to join Bertha and her daughter Nancy for a tour of Spain. Nancy Reppert had been a Spanish major in college and was fluent in the language, which greatly facilitated the trip. In April, she went to Bertha's for Easter, and began planning another visit with Tish in Los Angeles followed by a July trip to Asia. She continued to feel dispirited and oddly out of sorts, though and continued to complain of "having nothing to do." Her mood changed dramatically for the better when Dorothy Hall, the WHO representative in Copenhagen, called her from Europe on April 23 to ask if Hilda would consider accepting a WHO assignment in Belgium at the Catholic University of Leuven. Within a week, Peplau had accepted the assignment and agreed to move to Belgium the following September for the academic year 1975–1976. Her life again had a focus; she again felt stimulated.[25]

First she made a return trip to Iceland in June, again with Nancy Reppert, where she presented a paper on "The Role of Nursing in Primary Health Care" at a conference in Reykjavik, before embarking by herself on the planned tour of Asia, visiting nursing programs and sightseeing.[26] The Asian trip included a week of teaching and touring in Japan, and 12 days of ICN meetings in Singapore. On August 13, 1975, Peplau left Singapore for her first vacation alone, visiting Indonesia, Java, Jakarta, Bali, and Bangkok. She was bothered by the noise and pollution of Bangkok, and the contrast between rich and poor in Jakarta, but she thoroughly enjoyed traveling by herself.[27]

All during this time, Bill Field, her colleague from the summer work-shops in New Mexico, was after her to tape additional lectures for the Peplau/Smoyak/Field (PSF) series, even sending her lists of suggested topics, and persistently urging her to do more.[28] Although this was a project in which she had lost interest, she did not have the heart to turn him down. Clearly Field believed that without new material from Peplau, the series would die out. Never one to do things the easy way, Peplau did not dig out old papers on the suggested topics and read them into a tape recorder as suggested. Instead, she wrote out new ones in long hand, and then read them aloud, once for practice and once for the tape to send to Field.[29] She found this burdensome, and constantly complained of the onset of back and neck pains when engaged in this narration. Over the next 2 years Bill Field continued to plead with her to immortalize her work through making tapes for PSF Productions. Field never seemed to realize how much work Hilda put into the 16 new tapes she did make for him.[30] Hilda could not simply talk into a tape recorder as Field wanted. Thus, she firmly but unequivocally put him off, but he continued to try: "You could supplement your retirement income nicely if you just would."[31]

Nonetheless, between taping for Field, teaching at UCLA, lecturing, traveling, and the ICN, it is clear that Hilda had plenty to do. It was just that she felt that other than the ICN, what she was doing was either frivolous or unimportant, and she yearned for something of "substance."

Peplau returned from her Asian trip the first of August 1975 to find that her sister Clara must leave her home of over 40 years in the Wernersville State Hospital and return to Reading, where her family would have to arrange alternate care. On June 26, 1975, the U.S. Supreme Court had ruled that non-dangerous patients in state mental hospitals must be released to their communities.[32] Bertha agreed to take responsibility to find an appropriate place for Clara in Reading and found that in the West Reading Nursing Home. Clara would live for only a few more years, disoriented and devastated after losing her place in the only home she had known for over 4 decades.

As for Hilda, she had only 3 weeks before leaving for Belgium, and immediately began preparations for what would become a 2-year assignment, but not before again wondering why she was not sought out by her U.S. professional association. "It puzzles me that almost nothing has been asked of me. I used to be so sought after. Why?"[33] In fact, she was in considerable demand, often asked to present papers at academic meetings or to lecture in universities.[34] But Peplau had been engaged at a policy-making level for the past decade, and it was these assignments she missed. It is curious, however, given Peplau's emotionally exhausting years with the ANA as executive director and president, that she should now wonder why her successors there did not seek her out. It was with a sense of enormous relief, then, that she welcomed the April call from Copenhagen and the prospect of a year in Belgium. Here she hoped she would again feel engaged, feel that important work was being done, feel that she had a mission.

BELGIUM

The WHO assignment quickly became multifaceted. If U.S. nursing had driven her to despair, the Belgium assignment offered her new life. In addition to teaching, Peplau had agreed to help develop a Training Program for Nursing Leaders at the Catholic University of Leuven. The Catholic University of Leuven was actually two universities, one French and one Flemish. Her affiliation would be to the Flemish speaking branch of the university. While there Peplau would also be the adviser to a Working Group on the Role of Nursing in Psychiatric and Mental Health Care, which met under WHO's auspices in Copenhagen four times during 1975–1976.[35]

It was a new life in more ways than one. Peplau had left her comfortable home in New Jersey for life in a medieval Belgian city, full of massive Gothic buildings and old, narrow cobblestone streets.[36] She arrived on an evening flight and was met at the airport by two of her new younger colleagues and soon to be graduate students, Agnes Roelens and Luk Cannoodt. They had collected keys from the beguinage, where she would stay, but they did not know to which apartment Peplau had been assigned. Peplau did not know what a beguinage was, and when they arrived it was dark, cold, and drizzling, and she could not see. They entered through a thick wall, and the narrow cobblestone street terrified her: She feared falling and renewing her body's aches and pains. A seemingly rude concierge finally agreed to show them the way to the top and the allotted apartment. The apartment itself was cold and dirty, and there were neither sheets nor blankets for the bed. After much hassling with the concierge, both were grudgingly produced. Later, the concierge would become a good friend.

Peplau's assignment was not an easy one. The Kingdom of Belgium shares its borders with the Netherlands, Luxembourg, Germany, and France, and has a population of about 10 million people. It was a part of the Netherlands until 1930. Flemish is spoken in the north, French in the south, and German in the east. In government bureaucracy, in education, and in all manner of social institutions, the country's linguistic divisions are reinforced. During the 17th century, a semireligious order of women known as the Beguines opened the first school to train religious nursing sisters, but the inquisition was still very active and greatly disrupted the natural progression of what most likely would have become the nursing profession in Belgium. It wasn't until the 19th century that hospitals began to train nurses.[37]

After 1957 nursing programs in Belgium began moving from hospitals into the universities, but they remained under the jurisdiction of medicine. In the 1960s, the Katholic Universitat Leuven divided into two parts—Leuven for Flemish speaking students and Louvain in Brussels for French speaking students. Both branches of the university began developing programs in "Hospital Sciences" to prepare certificate nurses to qualify as nurse teachers and administrators and asked permission to establish master's level programs for nursing.

As Hilda's friend Dorothy Hall, the regional representative of WHO in Copenhagen, explained to her, Belgium had funds deposited with WHO intended for use in recruiting someone to help them develop Europe's first graduate nursing program in Belgium.[38] Peplau had served on a number of WHO advisory committees and knew several Belgian doctors involved in the nursing effort, including Dr. Peter de Schauwer, who specifically requested that she come in order that he might have someone with whom he could argue.[39] The politics, Hilda would discover, were Byzantine, but the setting was charming.

The morning after she arrived, Hilda descended the steep steps from her attic apartment and entered the enchanting world of the beguinage. It was a world she would come to cherish, a world that provided her the physical surroundings and the quiet space where at last both mind and body would begin to mend. Walking the steep streets of Leuven, buying fresh fruits, vegetables, delicious cheeses, and 10-grain bread on her way home, she exercised more and ate a healthier diet than she had in years. There was a long tradition of taking care of women in the beguinages of Belgium, and Hilda Peplau felt pleased to be part of that tradition. She took care of herself in a setting where women for hundreds of years had come for support and nurturing. The walking, buying, and carrying groceries, climbing stairs, and eating well helped mend her body (although she continuously complained of the difficulty of walking on cobblestones). The ambiance of the beguinage mended her soul.[40]

The beguinages of Belgium trace their origins to the year 1118 when the Bishop of Liege, Lambert le Begue, established a religious order for women, who then built enclosed compounds, known as beguinages. Beguinages for centuries provided sanctuary for women joined together to devote themselves to prayer and good works, to live apart from the world, but without taking vows to leave the world altogether.

As did nuns, Beguines took vows of chastity, hard work, and obedience to a mother superior—but their vows were temporary and reversible, did not include poverty, and the mothers superior were elected for terms of 2 or 3 years, thus making the beguinage among the first quasi-democratic institutions of medieval Europe. Upon entering the beguinage, the Beguines retained their personal property and some measure of personal autonomy. They paid no revenue to the church, and institutional and vocational self-sufficiency were emphasized. Finally, the Beguines were free to leave the beguinage and resume their old lives when their husbands returned from war, or when they felt safe in the world. Inside the beguinage they lived in a community of women, making candy and lace to sell, baking hosts for Holy Communion, and in general learning the satisfaction and pride that comes from being self-supporting. Perhaps partly as a consequence, the beguinages ran afoul of the church, and in the 14th century they were outlawed by the pope, until the bishop of the Netherlands interceded on their behalf. Hilda Peplau felt very much at home.

Peplau's first impression of the beguinage in Leuven had been of an old and cold place. Her second impression was one of beauty, peace, and quiet, where the presence of the past was easily felt. In part this was because the beguinages are enclosed spaces surrounded by high brick walls that seem to keep the Middle Ages in and the 20th century, with its noise and speed, out. When Hilda ducked in through the gate of the outer wall of the beguinage, the rumble of traffic disappeared; the only sound was the tolling of the bell of the serene chapel in the corner of a lovely garden.

If the beguinage was a blessing, the university was a nightmare. Lectures were to be written out, word for word, and given to students. Obsessive and conscientious as ever, Hilda would produce over 600 pages of handwritten lecture notes, translated into Flemish by a brilliant, compulsive, and equally obsessive former priest.[41] Peplau's lectures were dense, deep, and complete. Reverting to the habits of a lifetime, she worked until the wee hours of the morning every night, producing prodigious amounts of material, trying to condense, organize, and present all that she had learned in 44 years of nursing.[42] When she wasn't writing lectures, Peplau was writing friends and deans in the United States asking for books for the Leuven library, and for teaching materials. She was energized by the experience, and was again completely absorbed by her work, which was both engrossing and exhausting. Because she was so conscientious, her effort was no doubt much more exhausting than it needed to be, but half-measures were not her style.

At the university, Peplau worked closely with Dr. Jan Blanpain and the other physicians, whom she respected, but nonetheless ran into obstacles nearly everywhere. Not surprisingly, she did not understand the politics of this very political university, and thus was sometimes mystified as the year unfolded. Her students ran into unexpected roadblocks as they developed their research proposals or tried to put together committees to supervise their dissertations. The interrelationships and politics between the Belgian and visiting academics escaped Hilda, and thus she often inadvertently trod on toes. As she wrote rather ruefully to Dorothy Hall after her first year at Leuven, "JB is ostracizing me now, even though I don't have a clue as to why. There are two classes at KUL—the controllers and the controlled—and I fit neither of them, so am in limbo most of the time . . . I am 67 now and have to really concentrate to keep anything straight!"[43]

Thus, although she welcomed the challenge and the involvement, and although she loved the beguinage and could feel her body mending, there was also an undercurrent of self-doubt here—doubt that her enormous investment of intellectual energy would pay off, the sense that covert sabotage lurked around every corner, and the suspicion that the lecture/note taking/exam format would not produce independent thought and strong direction for nursing in Belgium.[44] Although her mind was engaged by the challenge and even though the Paul Harvey news on the one English language radio station kept her up on major news from home, she soon found herself plagued by a sense of isolation and aloneness. At the same time, the absence of outside demands, the rainy weather that kept one indoors, and the quiet peace of the beguinage contributed to what she thought was probably her best work in regard to classroom teaching.[45] Although she thought she and her work were appreciated, she came to believe that nursing in Belgium would not be greatly affected by her effort. She wrote to Shirley Smoyak along these lines, describing the "childish" politics of manipulation and avoidance and expressing doubt about her long-range impact: "I do my work as best I can, but I know it's such a small drop in this enormous pool of childishness . . . Here, maybe as a function of my age or there being only me, I don't see any real effect—immediate or long range."[46]

By the end of 1975, Hilda was eagerly awaiting a visit from Tish. By this time Tish had indeed become Hilda's best friend, as well as her traveling companion. This Christmas they would go on a safari in Kenya, organized through the ANA. At Hilda's request, Tish had collected boxes and boxes of books to donate to the university's small nursing library. Hilda had written her in great detail about her day-to-day life at Leuven, about her lectures, and the intrigues she could not comprehend. In her daughter she had found the professional friend she had always wanted. Tish, too, was now an academic enmeshed in institutional politics at UCLA, so the two could share on a professional level in ways they had not done heretofore. With the aid of Tish's insights, Hilda began to understand the patriarchal triumvirate (physicians, clergy, and lawyers) that stood in the way of nursing's development in Belgium. When she combined this insight with her own belief that only by developing clinical specialties could nurses hold their own in the health professions, she began to get a clearer picture and a deeper understanding of nursing's problems at home. In retirement now, she had the time and distance to reflect and could share these reflections with Tish, who always gave her a serious and thoughtful response. It was one of the best gifts she could receive from her daughter.

After the Christmas trip to Africa and the good visit with Tish, Hilda returned to Belgium in the late winter of 1976, refreshed and philosophical. She finished the academic year and returned to her home in Madison in April in a good frame of mind. The Smoyaks met her at the airport and took her home for a family dinner before depositing her in her freshly cleaned and aired home on Shunpike Road. Refreshed and energetic once again, she immediately accepted an invitation to attend the 1976 summer ANA convention in Atlantic City as a guest of the association. At this convention, the ANA was to issue a "Statement on Psychiatric and Mental Health Nursing Practice" and sent her a copy for comment. Before going to Atlantic City, Peplau read this statement with disbelief, and then wrote a 4-page response, consisting of 78 questions.[47] She was thanked for her "valuable time and input," and invited to sit on the platform while the statement was discussed, but not to speak nor voice her concerns. The ANA strikes again, she thought. At this convention, however, she was beginning to be recognized for her lifetime contributions to nursing, and this seemed to outweigh the discomfort she caused by her usual attention to detail and the thoroughness and challenge of her preparation. At this convention, she felt feted for the past, but ignored in the present.[48] It would take another decade for her work and contributions to the ANA to be fully appreciated—and for Peplau to appreciate the appreciation.

Before attending the ANA convention, Hilda planned a whirlwind trip up and down the East Coast that was reminiscent of those of earlier years. The central event was the awarding of another degree, the honorary doctor of science from Duke University. That she was once again herself is confirmed by her itinerary. She would fly from Newark to Philadelphia on May 2 to participate in a seminar at the University of Pennsylvania, then fly on to Columbus, Ohio, to speak to graduate students on May 3, and then to Washington, D.C., to speak to a Sigma Theta Tau meeting. Only then would she fly to Raleigh, North Carolina, to be a guest of Ruby Wilson, dean of the College of Nursing at Duke and be feted by the nursing faculty before receiving the honorary degree at a ceremony on May 9. From there it was on to Atlanta, and then another week in Columbus, Ohio, where she would visit and speak at the undergraduate nursing graduation ceremonies before returning to Madison. She was home only briefly to share a few meals with the Smoyaks and other friends before going out to California to spend some time with Tish.[49]

Hilda returned to Belgium in September for a second year, considerably rested and eager once again to throw herself into the effort to make a significant difference. By now, she better understood the obstacles and had a clearer idea of the work to be done. In her last year there she would devote much time and effort to her students, urging them on to complete their degrees and to move into clinical doctoral work. Interdisciplinary PhD work, however, required the support of several other university departments, and institutional politics would throw every conceivable roadblock in the way. The difference now was that Peplau accepted her time was limited, as was the contribution she could make. She put her energy into revising and expanding her lecture notes in order to leave behind a substantial body of work and into assuring that her two doctoral students completed their dissertations. She worked incredibly hard, and felt good about it. She was intrigued by Belgium and its history, and began to truly enjoy the experience of living in another culture, along with the return of her physical health. During this time she wrote long, detailed letters to Tish and Shirley Smoyak outlining the constant intrigue within the university and the difficulty she experienced in trying to get her job done, but also her pride that despite all, her students were advancing. Nonetheless, when Hilda was asked to stay for a third year, Tish wrote in some exasperation, "Say no to Belgium next year. You can't save them. Do say NO immediately. You've done your altruistic/martyr bit. Enough. Come to L.A. Luv, Tish."[50] This time Hilda was able to say no. She was content as her work at Leuven ended in the knowledge that she had done the best she could have done and to leave it to others to carry on.[51]

Being in Europe, however, did give Hilda opportunity to work more closely with the ICN. Dorothy Cornelius was then president of the ICN. Never one to give up, Peplau began sending long, handwritten letters to ICN's executive director, full of suggestions, the principal one being the suggestion that ICN establish a Council of Nurse Researchers.[52]

In December 1976 Tish joined Hilda in Egypt where the two visited Cairo and floated up the Nile as part of a deluxe tour Hilda had selected for their winter holiday. From there they went on to Ethiopia where they spent Christmas, joining pilgrims from many places visiting the ancient stone churches of Lalibella and narrowly missing a dramatic coup d'etat in Addis Ababa. In addition to sightseeing, Hilda met briefly in Addis Ababa with leaders of the Ethiopian national nurses association. They returned by way of Athens, with a side trip to the Oracle at Delphi.

WORLD TRAVELER

Hilda was then completing her 2-year commitment to the Catholic University of Leuven, and had become deeply involved in the planning of the 1977 ICN Congress to be held in Tokyo that spring. Her responsibility for these arrangements accelerated considerably when, overwhelmed and out of her depth, ICN's executive director suddenly resigned in December 1976. It soon became apparent that not much was in order for the Tokyo meeting. Peplau quickly jumped into the breach, working closely with Cornelius, the board, and the ICN staff to "save" the Tokyo meeting. Her assistance was acknowledged by the new executive director, Barbara Fawkes, after the May 29–June 23 conference: "The success of the Congress in Tokyo was to a large part due to your preparatory work . . . thanks to your solutions to the many problems, many individual nurses arrived in Tokyo with proper credentials and were able to enjoy and benefit from attendance . . ."[53] In Tokyo Peplau was reelected third vice president of the ICN, and successfully drafted the first Asian nurse to serve as the ICN's next president, Mo- Im Kim of Korea.[54]

After the Tokyo Congress, Hilda returned to California to meet Tish and proceed on to a long-planned Alaskan cruise. The spectacular Alaskan landscape totally captivated Hilda, but she did not enjoy life aboard a luxury cruise ship: too much dressing up for dinner and too little content of an educational nature. "I learned cruises are not for me."[55] After the Alaskan trip, Peplau spent a week at the Menninger clinic where she was honored for her lifetime contributions to psychiatric nursing. She enjoyed both the praise and the workshop participation but was not tempted to reenter the fray: "I consider myself happily retired from gainful work— and it's a great feeling."[56]

The fall of 1977, Hilda finally allowed herself a real period of relaxation following purely personal rather than professional pursuits. She remained in California with Tish for a month, then returned to Madison and threw herself into household renovation—painting, sanding the floors, sorting out the books, rearranging the library. Tish was home for Christmas and to help her welcome 1978. Hilda celebrated her new life of leisure by taking her daughter out for Christmas dinner. No cooking, no dishes!

In March 1978 Hilda went to Geneva for a meeting of the ICN Board and returned home to prepare for a trip to the ANA convention in Hawaii. In Hawaii she was the guest of the ANA and the newly formed Council of Advanced Practitioners in Psychiatric and Mental Health Nursing, which was sponsoring a "Symposium Honoring Hilda E. Peplau."[57] At this symposium Grayce Sills and Dorothy Gregg presented moving testimonials, and a panel discussed Peplau's contributions to psychiatric nursing.[58] The room was filled—standing room only—with nurses from all over the United States wanting to express their affection for Peplau and appreciation for her work.[59] From this time forward, Hilda Peplau would be treated as a revered nursing leader, and old hostilities gradually were forgotten.

Having been out of the country for nearly 2 years and thus out of the loop in American nursing circles, Peplau was not involved in the politics of the convention, and had no desire to even hear the gossip. On this trip she seemed able, finally, to leave past disappointments behind, and thoroughly enjoy the attention and lack of stress. Relaxed as she was, she took full advantage of the island paradise in the Pacific. While in Hawaii, she had a reunion with Ann Clark, one of her few friends from the Rutgers years. She loved the islands, the pace of life, the beautiful days, and spectacular sunsets. "It was a great trip and a very pleasant cap on a career," she later recalled.[60] Finally, she was feeling a sense of closure on the past.

After the Hawaiian odyssey, Hilda returned to Los Angeles and spent July with Tish before venturing back to Alaska and a highly anticipated automobile journey through parts she had not yet seen of that beautiful state. This trip more than lived up to its expectations. Hilda was truly awed by the magnificence of Alaska's limitless landscapes. Her traveling companion was Beryl O'Neil, a longtime friend.[61] They began their trip by driving north from Los Angeles, through the redwoods of Northern California, and on up the coast to Vancouver, where they boarded a ferry which took them through the inland passage, to Haines, Alaska. From the deck Hilda watched the whales and soaked up the vistas. The two then flew in a small plane over Glacier Bay, and pronounced it a natural wonder of the world. The weather was perfect, and the scenery continued to be breathtaking. They retrieved the car and with Mary McKenzie, another academic friend from the Rutgers days, drove over the Dalton Trail and through the Chilkoot Pass into the Canadian Yukon Territory, reveling in the lovely unspoiled beauty of the place. The small creeks, the wildflowers everywhere, and the exquisite quiet all moved Hilda profoundly. The magnificent and huge Kluane Lake left her literally speechless.

Then, on August 6, 1978, this trip of a lifetime came to sudden and climactic end. On a beautiful, cloudless clear day in the wide expanse of the Yukon Territory, in a great land of beauty and peace, a car came roaring around a curve, seemingly from nowhere, and hit the three travelers, knocking their car off the road where it rolled down an embankment. Hilda Peplau, at nearly 70 years of age, was once again the victim of a serious automobile accident. This time she was saved by Canadian Mounted Police. Enduring excruciating pain from new injuries, Hilda scarcely remembers the 5 days it took to get to Anchorage where she finally was able to see a doctor and where she then stayed for 3 weeks at Mary McKenzie's home gathering what strength she could for a flight back to Los Angeles.[62] Tish and Steven Gordon, the handsome sociologist Tish would later marry, met Hilda at the airport with a wheelchair. Hilda stayed with Tish until she was well enough to return to Madison in late September.

She spent the next 3 months in intensive self-rehabilitation. She ordered a new mattress, prescribed rest and fluids for herself, and consulted a physical therapist. The routine seemed to work, but the old untreated injuries made recovery difficult and full of agony. Shirley Smoyak was on hand to tend Hilda's garden and assure that she ate well. Christmas 1978 was far more solemn than she had anticipated, but by the middle of January, when Tish, who had come for Christmas, left to return to UCLA, she was beginning to feel much more upbeat.

In March 1979 Peplau declared herself "rehabilitated," and left for the ICN Board meeting in Geneva, and then a return visit to Belgium. She returned home to await the end of the semester at UCLA, when Tish joined her for another spectacular trip, this one to Morocco, where they were joined by Tish's good friend Gail Gulliksen, a U.S. foreign service officer then stationed in Paris. The threesome toured in style, hiring a Mercedes and a driver for seeing the country, staying in first-class hotels, and eating in the best restaurants. They visited Casablanca, Rabat, Meknes, Tangier, Fez, and Marrakesh. Hilda loved the North African country, and added it to her list of places to which she vowed a return.[63]

Her travel for the year was not finished. By the end of August Peplau was off on a 3-week safari through Kenya. She loved the magnificent endless blue skies, the gentle climate of the Kenyan Highlands, the jacaranda trees, the people, the food, the sounds of the night. Hilda Peplau was confirming what she had long known deep down: She was a true world traveler. She had come a long way from Reading, Pennsylvania, where she first dreamed of someday seeing Egypt. The trip ended in Nairobi, where the ICN was meeting for the first time in Africa. At this meeting, Peplau convinced the young president of the National Nurses Association of Kenya to run for the ICN presidency at the next ICN Congress. E. Muringo Kiereini accepted the challenge, and 2 years later wrote to Peplau,

> If I may say it again, it was simply great to have an opportunity of working with you in the ICN Board . . . You always had a smile when I came to you for guidance . . . You gave me a lot of encouragement and confidence in realizing that even as a young nurse my leadership and contribution to the ICN meant something even to the more experienced and older nursing colleagues like yourself. You are truly gifted in developing people . . . I would not be here today were it not for you . . . Thank you for your many kind deeds. They are most appreciated and treasured by me."[64]

In spite of her best intentions, however, Hilda was not really ready to live what she described as a life of "self-indulgent leisure" when she returned home in the fall of 1979.[65] She could not resist the innumerable calls to concern herself once again with national nursing issues. She began to travel the country speaking at meetings of Sigma Theta Tau, the nursing college honorary society. She felt hope that the younger generation would not only listen but act upon the matters she chose to address (primarily continuing concerns that nurses undertake serious research, serious redefinition of their work, and the importance of clinical specialization and self-regulation).[66] The ICN was scheduled to meet in Los Angeles in 1981, when her term as third vice president would conclude. Hilda greatly appreciated the fact that Sigma Theta Tau had decided to sponsor a program about nursing research in her honor during the ICN meetings. She felt that her efforts had begun to pay off. Muringo Kiereini would be presiding at the meetings, and research symposia would be a part of the program. Now, at last, she began to feel that her work had been worthwhile—and that she could truly retire.

The year 1981 brought an end to Peplau's official role in the ICN. She went to Geneva for her last ICN Board meeting in the spring, and then on to Belgium to visit her former students and colleagues there. The ICN 1981 Congress in Los Angeles that summer, June 28–July 3, would be a celebration of her years on the board and as a key figure in ICN work over the past decade. There were many receptions to fete her, and she was presented with a certificate and plaque in recognition of her 1973–1981 service on the ICN Board.[67] Constance Holleran, the new executive director, thanked Peplau profusely: "Only those close to the scene can appreciate the amount of work, long hours, and extraordinary dedication that have gone into your role as a board member."[68]

When the congress ended, Hilda and Tish took a 2-week trip to Alaska, continuing what Hilda now dubbed "my perpetual vacation (called retirement)."[69] The highlight of her third trip to this vast state was flying over the Pribiloff Islands, noted for their birds and wildlife. She spent most of the fall of 1981 at home in Madison with the exception of a trip to Pennsylvania to spend Thanksgiving with Bertha and her family. Then it was off to Los Angeles to visit with Tish and her husband Steve Gordon, whom Tish had married in a quiet, civil ceremony in Santa Monica in June 1980.[70]

THE ANA—ONE MORE TIME

There was, however, one continuing challenge that Peplau could not resist. It was important enough to effectively bring her out of retirement and plunge her back into ANA issues. In early 1979 the phone call she had yearned for 10 years before finally came. At the urging of Anne Zimmerman, now president of the ANA, Peplau agreed to chair an ANA Task Force on the Nature and Scope of Nursing Practice and Characteristics of Specialization in Nursing. Here at last was a chance to define nursing in such a way as to permit it to grow as a profession in the years to come. How could she resist such a challenge? Peplau could not and she did not. She threw herself into the work of the task force with a vengeance, feeling she had one last opportunity to influence the way nursing thought about and defined itself. Not surprisingly, in addition to chairing the committee, she became the primary drafter and reviser of the committee's work. She made endless drafts, and there are many, many pages of her work in the archives to attest to how hard she worked at developing the document that would define nursing practice into the 21st century.[71]

The resulting document, *Nursing: A Social Policy Statement*, was adopted during the ANA convention held in Houston, June 8–13, 1980. It defined nursing as "the diagnosis and treatment of human responses to actual or potential health problems." The 37 page statement attempts to delineate the nature and define the scope of contemporary nursing practice, as well as to describe the characteristics of nursing clinical specialization. It has remained to the present day the definitive statement on professional nursing practice. Finally, nursing had an open-ended definition of itself broad enough to encompass the whole of nursing practice, and yet specific enough to distinguish it from other health professions. One of Hilda Peplau's greatest legacies to modern nursing is the *Social Policy Statement*.[72]

The *Social Policy Statement*, although adopted, was not uncontroversial. The main objection was that with its emphasis on "diagnosis and treatment," rather than on "care," nursing was limiting its scope.[73] Never one to run away from controversy, Peplau accepted many opportunities to speak on the *Social Policy Statement* during 1981, emphasizing wherever she went that far from limiting the scope of nursing practice, this statement placed the emphasis on self-definition and self-regulation of nursing, a profession dedicated to health maintenance (not disease).[74] It implied authority and autonomy to practice independently of other professions, and placed value on clinical nursing research.

At this time, issues of credentialing and certification of nurse specialists had become controversial, and there was great debate within nursing as to where credentialing authority should rest—with state boards or with professional organizations. Peplau had always taken the view that it was essential that all credentialing above the basic license to practice (the RN) be done by the national professional nursing association, that is, within the ANA, and not by politically appointed state boards of nursing. The basic nursing license, as defined in the nurse practice acts of each state, provided the foundation for the state boards of nursing to set rules and regulations concerning that basic license, she argued.[75] Beyond that, however, the credentialing and certification of specialists—those who by education and training were more advanced than the basic RN—should be the responsibility of the ANA. The *Social Policy Statement* was meant to lay to rest the question of "What is nursing?" by providing a simple umbrella statement, and then proceeding to lay out the guidelines for certifying clinical specialists under this general umbrella. Basically, Peplau argued, the statement "provides a formulation to help the profession move forward another notch."[76] By the 1990s, the ANA, having adopted Peplau's position, had moved into credentialing in a major way, but without agreeing on basic educational criteria. That issue would remain a muddle.

A QUIET TIME

Peplau's professional life had truly quieted down considerably by 1982, and her personal life finally began to take precedence. Tish and Steve's son, David Eric Gordon, was born April 12, 1982. Because David arrived about a week earlier than expected, Hilda missed the birth, but arrived within the week and stayed on through May to help Tish. David soon became a very important part of Hilda's life. He made his first annual photo appearance with her on her Christmas letter that very year, nestled in her arms. That spring the last of her childhood friends, Natalie Kreiger Gromis, died in Reading. Hilda had lost touch after the death of Natalie's sister, Betty, although the two exchanged Christmas letters and an occasional short note. On May 24, 1982, Natalie's husband Wayne wrote to inform Hilda that a massive heart attack on April 25th had taken Natalie's life. Natalie and Wayne had been married for 55 years, and Wayne was bereft. Hilda, for the first time, began to think in terms of life truly winding down.[77]

She returned to Los Angeles for 2 months in the fall of 1982 "so as not to miss David's struggles to learn and master crawling."[78] Hilda seemed content at last to settle into a life of reading and contemplation, playing the role of a grandmother, taking a trip or two a year, and giving half a dozen or so talks a year, usually to a Sigma Theta Tau meeting and state nurses conventions. She still attended the annual meetings of the ANA, where she inevitably presented a paper and where generally she was honored in one way or another, such as a special plenary session on her work, a research colloquium in her honor, or an award of one sort of another. In November 1982 Peplau returned briefly to Belgium for Therese Rodenbach's doctoral orals. Not wanting to be pulled into the intrigues, quarrels, and politics still rampant there, she made her own arrangements and stayed in a hotel rather than accept university hospitality. She spent a pleasant evening with Dr. Blanpain and accepted a large medal cast in her honor.[79] She also visited with two former students, Agnes Roelens and Luk Cannoodt, who had married in the intervening years and parented a son, Steven, and a daughter, Hildeke, named after Hilda. Peplau thought highly of Agnes Cannoodt and felt she had the emotional stability to overcome the institutional obstacles at Leuven and to help move nursing forward there. Thus, she managed to extricate Agnes and Luk from Leuven by arranging for them to come to Rutgers and New York University on fellowships in order to complete MS and PhD degrees.[80]

Peplau returned from Belgium before Thanksgiving and went immediately back to Los Angeles, where she renewed her relationship with her fast-growing grandson and gave the first lecture in a new annual distinguished lecture series at the UCLA College of Nursing. At the conclusion of the lecture, she was genuinely surprised to find herself participating in a reception to honor her career. In addition to speeches and kudos, the

Nursing Services of the UCLA Neuropsychiatric Institute presented her with a very special (and very heavy) bronze plaque. This plaque aptly summarized her career and gave testament to her reputation 10 years after her official retirement. It read,

HILDA E. PEPLAU
PSYCHIATRIC NURSE OF THE CENTURY[81]

Hilda was back in New Jersey in time for Thanksgiving with Bertha's family. In December, the Slack Publishing Company published a set of her many her many as yet unpublished papers in a *Collection of Classics in Psychiatric Nursing,* edited by Shirley Smoyak and Sheila Rouslin, both former Peplau students and proteges.[82]

At the new year, January 1983, Peplau began her last large research project, a genealogical study of the Peplau family. This was primarily for Tish and David, but also for Hilda's nieces and the next generations of the family. This work would occupy her for the next decade. During this time, Hilda relied extensively on invaluable help from her niece, Marjorie Reppert, who spent a week or two for many summers helping to sort and organize the materials Hilda had accumulated. The genealogy also took Hilda on several trips to Europe and introduced her to many relatives she had not previously known.[83] This journey back into history made her marvel all the more that her parents had managed to escape the ravages of Europe, and she grew more appreciative of their early fears and struggles in this country.[84]

The highlight of 1983 was another honorary degree—this one from Columbia University. Such sweet revenge! No one from the miserable Teachers College days was around to appreciate the irony, but Peplau did, and she enjoyed it to the fullest. Then she was off to Kenya again, this time to lead a summer workshop with Shirley Smoyak for Kenyan nurses. Then she set out on yet another safari, organized as a continuing education trip for psychiatric nurses. While on safari she was in another automobile accident. In this one she was not hurt, but it was a serious accident and a jarring experience nonetheless.[85]

In September 1983, the Rutgers College of Nursing inaugurated a lecture series endowed by Smith, Kline and French in her honor. The series honored the nurse who had made their best- selling feature film ever, and who had been their most reliable consultant. Dr. Letitia Anne Peplau was invited to give the first lecture. Rutgers President Edward J. Bloustein wrote,

> . . . I wanted to congratulate you on . . . the lecture series . . . endowed in your honor. You should be justly proud of that honor, for it reflects so well on you and your many achievements and upon this great University of which you will always be a part.[86]

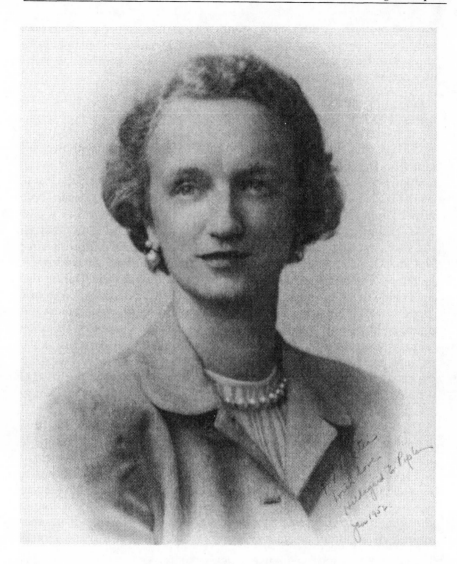

Hilda in 1951.

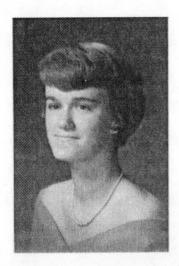

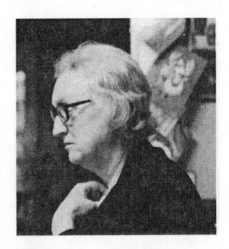

Tish's high school graduation photo, 1963.

Hilda 1973.

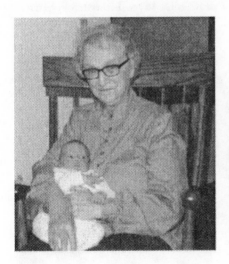

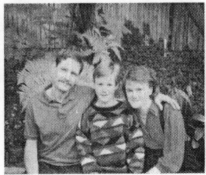

Hilda rocks her grandson David, 1983.

Steve, David, and Tish.

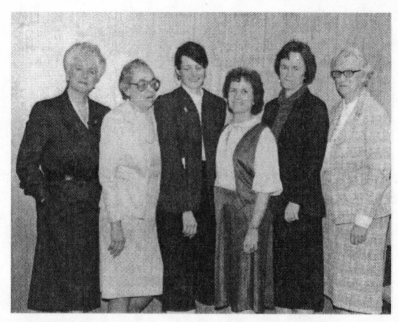

Conference on Graduate Nursing Education, Rutgers University, circa 1973.
Left to right—Dorothy DeMaio, Martha Rogers, Joyce Fitzpatrick, Shirley
Smoyak, Letitia A. Peplau, Hildegard E. Peplau.

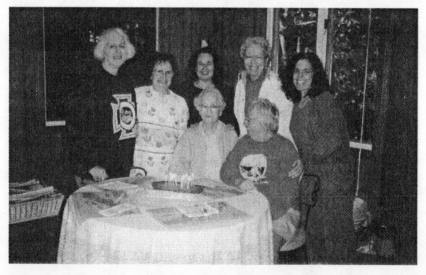

Hilda's birthday, 1988. Hilda is surrounded by Master of Science degree
graduates of Rutgers. Standing left to right—Ann Lazaroff, '62; Shirley
Smoyak, '59; Sheila Rouslin Welt, '61; Fern Kumler '63; Karen Hediger, '80.
Seated—Hildegard E. Peplau, Elizabeth Carter, '62.

That winter, just before Christmas, Hilda decided to do something whimsical to begin the new year in 1984: She sent a handwriting sample to an address she found advertised in *McCall's* magazine. On March 1, 1984, Peplau received the results. Had she done this earlier in her life, and had she given credence to such an exercise, she might have gained insights that would have helped her in her torturous years at Rutgers and in the ANA:

> You are a person of taste. In spite of symptoms of depression and a tendency to be discouraged, you have an extraordinary ability to cope. You have great sensitivity, with repressed latent aggressiveness. If you control your sometimes overcritical nature, you will have better success. You are impatient, but have great determination and energy.[87]

THE MOVE TO LOS ANGELES

In September 1983 yet another serious automobile accident brought home to Peplau that she was indeed moving along into old age, and was doing it alone in New Jersey. As she was turning into her driveway on Shunpike Road in Madison, her car was rear-ended by a loaded dump truck coming down the road. Her car was demolished, and again Hilda was badly hurt: She had another serious concussion, and injured her neck and back for the third time. She did manage to get to Los Angeles for Christmas, but she was in great pain. Once there, and with Tish's urging, she decided it was time to move to be near Tish, and to play a role in David's formative years.

She returned home to put her house in Madison on the market, and sold it in a week. Closing day was set for June 20, 1984. Hilda then spent 6 months sorting, selling, giving away, packing, and cleaning. She sent her remaining papers off to the Schlesinger Library, shipped her belongings, and flew to Los Angeles for good. The town of Madison planted a dogwood tree in the town plaza in honor of their departing distinguished citizen.

Hilda was never one to move slowly once she made up her mind. A few days with a real estate agent in Los Angeles, and she had bought a house on a tree-lined street in Sherman Oaks, within 5 minutes drive of Tish's home. Sherman Oaks, just across Beverly Glen Canyon from UCLA, Westwood, and Beverly Hills, is one of the most desirable of the Los Angeles "valley" communities. Hilda had spotted a street she'd liked, directed the agent to it, and immediately saw a house for sale. The sign had been up for 1 hour. Peplau went through the house quickly and liked the floor plan. She didn't look around too closely, but was pleased with the area and the street. She made an offer that was accepted. Hilda lived with Tish, Steve, and David from June until November 1984, while the closing on her new house proceeded. In November, on the day of the closing, she *really* looked around and was rather appalled. The house was basically solid, but needed a great deal of work. It featured a yellow shag rug that hadn't been cleaned in years, and chipped 1940s tile in the bathroom. The termites were so dense the house had to be tented to exterminate them. So, she hired a contractor and started in, beginning with peeling off paneled wallboard, which in turn was covering eight different layers of wallpaper. The contractor ripped up the rug, started spackling and painting, and sanded and varnished the floors. Then she moved in. Once there she discovered she couldn't stand the kitchen, and quickly hired another contractor who redid it in 1985. She also added a patio and a new roof. She wasn't finished, however. She decided to add a "family room" that would double as a library for her and a playroom for David. Then she added a new back porch and had the house re-stuccoed. For 2 years, she virtually lived the life of a building contractor. She was up every morning at 6:00 to supervise each step as the house was cleaned, stripped, fixed, painted, and stuccoed. She continued to live in the house as the work progressed, personally checking on every single detail. When it was finished, she had lovely hardwood floors, a remodeled kitchen and bathroom, a new brick patio, and finally a newly constructed library and family room to share with David.

Sorting, packing, moving, and renovating were not all Hilda did during 1984 through 1986, however. In the spring of 1984 she wrote and delivered nine professional papers—three in Canada, two in Switzerland, two in France, and two at the ANA convention. In February she had been asked by the ANA to serve as a consultant, meeting with the various divisions within the ANA "to assist in clarifications of terminology essential to the Association's leadership role and . . . assist with an annual assessment of progress on implementation of *Nursing: A Social Policy Statement*." On March 5, 1984, Peplau accepted the assignment, thus assuring some level of continued participation in professional nursing, courtesy of the ANA.[88]

That summer of 1984, at the age of 75, Hilda Peplau received the ANA Honorary Recognition Award at the New Orleans Convention for Pioneering the Development of the Theory and Practice of Psychiatric and Mental Health Nursing. She was cited for introducing the now historic one-to-one nurse-patient relationship studies that had changed the foundation of both undergraduate and graduate nursing curricula in the United States, while also changing the psychosocial component of all nursing practice.[89]

In 1985 and 1986 Peplau accepted appointments as a visiting professor at Ohio State University, where Grayce Sills was serving as a long-term interim dean of nursing, spending a month there each year. In the fall of 1986, she was also a visiting professor at the University of Washington.

While there, her brother Harold passed away. Travel arrangements from Seattle were quite complicated, and the timing was such that she could not get to Reading for the funeral. Johnny and Bertha stood in her stead.

In the spring of 1986 the ANA asked Peplau to prepare a position paper on clinical specialists. Peplau always took these assignments seriously, and spent nearly a year writing the paper. She looked at other professions to compare specialization in nursing to specialization in other fields. She again tried to alert nursing to the challenge coming from the state boards, emphasizing that the issue of specialization should be the profession's business, not the government's. After all her work, she was told "what a nice paper." No action resulted, except that the ANA printed an edited version of her paper, cutting out what Peplau considered to be the most important points.[90] Her New Year's resolution was "This is going to stop!"[91]

When her house was completed to her satisfaction in 1987, Hilda settled into her "real life" in retirement—the life of a grandmother. David took center stage and became her most consistent and nearly constant visitor. For most of the next 10 years, Tish brought him to Hilda's house several times a week, at first just to play, then to see if she needed any help, then to raise his vegetables in her garden, to do his science experiments, feed the squirrels, care for the great white and soon fat cat that took up residence in the patio, and to visit, watch television, do his homework, and, sometimes, just keep Hilda company. He was a great companion, a great friend, and the light of her life. Hilda bought David a series of bicycles—first a red tricycle, then a red bike with trainer wheels, and eventually a black two-wheeler. The bikes were kept in Hilda's garage at the "Blue House," as David called his grandmother's home. Hilda cherished these days of getting to know the bright, precocious boy—Tish's son, her grandson.[92]

Content to tend her garden, watch her grandson grow, read, contemplate, and reflect, Peplau gradually developed a "community of friends in practice," a small group of professional friends around the country and the world with whom she constantly exchanged ideas, reprints, articles, and reflections—mostly about developments in the study of mental illness and/or the state of the nursing profession. By 1990, Peplau subscribed to and read nearly 50 journals and magazines. She read through each rather thoroughly, clipping out relevant or just interesting material, and nearly every week sent out a mailing of selected materials to Suzy Lego and her husband Lee Spray; to Anita and Richard O'Toole; and to Sheila Rouslin Welt, Grayce Sills, and Shirley Smoyak among others. Each responded to her, and she circulated the materials sent and comments received on to the others. This community of friends in practice became a very large and a very satisfactory part of her life. The group had formed gradually as each corresponded with Peplau and then found themselves drawn together by interests that were both social and professional. They used one another as sounding boards. Through correspondence, Peplau achieved something she had always craved: a group of friends for whom thinking mattered. They shared a mutual concern about nursing and its future, and a yearning for someone to talk to about it. Through their informal exchanges of articles and information, each continued to grow professionally, and all learned from each of the others. Into the 1990s Peplau looked forward to the annual meetings of the ANA or the American Psychiatric Nurses Association (APNA), where she now regularly met with her informal "community of practice."[93]

The networking was enriched in the late 1980s and 1990s by what became annual gatherings in September of many of her former Rutgers students at the summer home of Liz and Jim Carter on Lake Hapatcong in New Jersey. Soon, these annual gatherings became biannual gatherings as the group reassembled in December for a Christmas party at the Carters' 78th Street apartment in New York City. After 1993, Hilda ceased to make these trips east, but the friendships were nurtured as "the group," as her former students began to call themselves, made twice yearly phone calls to their mentor.

Through Hilda's 70s and into her 80s, David was a constant joy in her life. As she approached her 90s, and the twenty-first century, David, as had Tish before him, began to go his own way. Hilda, however, was deeply grateful to have been able to share his boyhood, to have had the pleasure of watching him grow, and to have participated in his childhood without the worries, strains, and concerns that had marked Tish's growing-up years. As a grandmother, she found inner peace and personal content-ment. Other than her continuing chronic back pain and the inevitable dis-comforts of old age, life was good.

FELLED BY A STROKE

As she approached the last decade of the 20th century, sustained by her "community of friends in practice," Hilda was satisfied to give several presentations a year with accompanying trips, and, when she was home, to read and to tend her garden with David's help. She had reached a stage in life when she could simply enjoy each day. She was comfortable, her life seemed in order, and in a very basic sense, she was content. Then the unexpected happened.

On December 13, 1989, she arose as was her custom at 6:00 a.m., went to the kitchen, opened the refrigerator, and poured a glass of orange juice. As she was setting the glass on the table, she dropped it. She tried to pick up the glass, but could not feel or grasp it. Her left hand and arm sud-denly were nonfunctional, and she was overwhelmed with a pervasive sense of utter fatigue. At that minute, the phone rang. She picked it up and told the caller, Sheila Rouslin in New Jersey, "I think I've just had a stroke." She described to Sheila what she was feeling, then hung up, cleaned up the orange juice with her good arm and hand, and only then did she phone Tish, who arrived within the hour to drive her to the UCLA hospital.[94] The hospital experience was not a good one. There, in a state of numb shock and terrible exhaustion, she was put through 3 hours of tests, which required getting on and off gurneys, being taken up and down floors, and moved from clinic to clinic, all of which she endured as though a zombie.[95] That process went on far into the night, concluding with the medical diagnosis of right cortical stroke. She was not a docile patient. She later wrote,

> When the technician was taking blood, Dr. Rho reminded him to leave in my vein a heparin lock, in case "you have bigger strokes during the night and we have to get into your veins fast." "No way, absolutely not," I said. Rho argued that awful things could happen now that I'd had this warning stroke and quick access to my veins would be vital. "No, absolutely not," I said—again and again—until the very large, but gentle technician said, "Lady, you don't want it, you don't get it," at which point Rho capitulated . . . Against my will, after all that high tech, I was admitted to NPI [Neuropsychiatric Institute] . . . It was by then quite late. In my utter weariness, I had the sidebars left up on the bed, and turned on my side to sleep. At that point, three to four RNs appeared, lined up at the foot of my bed, and one by one said their names, which I recall as the "60 minutes crowd"—"I'm Mike Wallace," etc. That was the last I saw of them.
>
> At 6 a.m. I awakened as usual, couldn't find a call bell, so I crawled over the side rails and went to the bathroom. No soap! In a hospital! No towels either. Luckily, I always carry a toothbrush and toothpaste in my purse, and had asked Tish to leave them on the bedside table. I got dressed—no easy task—and sat down to wait for breakfast or some sound of life. Breakfast finally came at 8:00 after which Dr. Rho visited, mostly to tell me that I'd be the subject of "rounds" by the neurology team around 9:00 a.m. They came. The "chief" and four to five medical students, and several interns and residents. The "chief" joked that I was "famous." He put a quarter in my left hand—to demonstrate that I couldn't feel it, asked "how are you," and they left. (I was billed for this M.D. visit.)
>
> Then the director of nursing came. She gossiped. The social worker dropped in and gave me her card. A nurse came in and folded my blanket, "in case you want to go back to bed." What I needed then was a professional to say: "Lady, you have a problem, but there are things you can do to help bring about some improvements." No one did. When Tish came, I insisted she take me home.[96]

At her own insistence, Hilda had stayed in the hospital only overnight, but the process of absorbing and dealing with the stroke took much longer. This was an experience that would affect the rest of her life. In her own analysis, the stroke had its origins with the 1984 accident, when her car had been rear-ended by the fully loaded 10-ton dump truck in Madison. Although she'd sustained no observable injuries in that accident, she did begin having pain in her right eye shortly thereafter. Each year the pain increased, and each year she went to the Jules Stein Eye Clinic at UCLA, where she had been seen by three different experts. Two had changed her eyeglass prescription, and the third, just a week before her stroke, had recommended cataract removal.

During her next visit to the Jules Stein Clinic after the stroke, a very young resident asked whether she'd had any symptoms before the stroke. When told about the persisting eye pain, the resident said, "oh yes, amaurosis fugax." "What's that?" she had asked. "A common precursor of stroke," was the matter-of-fact reply.[97]

Back at home, she had trouble coming to terms with the fact of a stroke. At first, she simply felt shock. She had suffered a stroke, and her life was now different, but exactly how seemed rather vague, something she could not quite comprehend. She also felt a terrible exhaustion, as though enormous effort was required for the simplest action. Worse yet , she felt there was no way she could convey to others either the nature of the shock to her system or the extent of her exhaustion. And, simmering just below the surface, was a lot of anger—anger that nurses did not seem to know what had happened or understand how she might feel. Here was something nurses could have worked to understand. Here was an area where they could make a difference. Hilda felt, however, that they had been as indifferent if not more indifferent than the technicians and physicians she had encountered. From Peplau's perspective, the UCLA nurses had not seemed interested in the phenomenon. No one inquired about her concerns and fears, nor had they forewarned her of the angers and frustrations that result from an unexpected and incapacitating event, such as a stroke. In fairness, it must be pointed out, however, that Hilda had stayed in the hospital only overnight. The director of nursing and presumably others nurses knew that Hildegard Peplau was there, but almost as soon as they learned of it, she was gone.

Be that as it may, what Hilda *felt* was disappointment and anger that her expectations and hopes for nurses had not been met. She began to explore her anger: It extended to the three opthamologists who had not pursued her eye pain, which Hilda felt might have led to an intervention that might have prevented the stroke. As she was confronted daily with what she could not do, the ramifications of what had happened began to sink in. She could not hold on to the soap, so bathing was an ordeal; she could not fasten her bra, so getting dressed was frustrating; she could not hold a plate, so fixing a meal or doing the dishes was impossible. She was a single woman, living alone. She'd had a stroke—but life went on for others as though nothing had happened. Tish came by every day, but she had a husband and a child and a career requiring her attention. To the extent that Hilda believed herself to be a burden on her daughter, her anger deepened.

She sought relief from anger through sleep. She slept long hours, trying to let go of her anger and her disappointment that neither the nurses in the hospital nor any of her nurse friends who called as the word of the stroke went out seemed to have any insight into or even interest in what she was actually experiencing. Hilda slept more hours than she was awake, day in and day out. Gradually, her anger subsided, and her analytical mind took over. She began to analyze her extreme physical exhaustion. She recognized the fact that extra vigilance was required for virtually everything she did. She could not feel hot or cold on her left side, so she had to be careful not to burn or cut her hand. She could not feel swallowing, so she had to be conscious not to choke on her food. She made a nursing diagnosis: "the exhaustion effect of vigilance." When she shared her insights with nurses, however, she felt they simply were not interested. No one seemed impressed, no one took her insights up as a research idea, no one promised to do something with this insight. Thus, once again she was depressed about her profession as she set about dealing with her physical limitations. Once again she felt virtually alone. Gradually she took charge of her feelings and began to reestablish her sense of self, her lifeline to rational recovery.

Help came from a nurse clinical specialist in neurology, Joan K. Austen from the University of Indiana. Austen discussed the symptoms Peplau was describing with her and directed Hilda to sources of information about strokes and recovery. Her sister Bertha soon weighed in with information concerning exercise and physical therapy that a stroke-victim friend had been given by a specialist. Tish brought home books from the UCLA Medical School library. Hilda wrote the National Stroke Association for information. Based on a principle she had long espoused, "use it or lose it," she began to force herself to use her left arm and hand in daily chores, no matter how frustrating or futile it seemed at first. By force of mind and will, she reached out with her numb left arm and hand. Even though she had no feeling in her hand, she would touch objects and try to imagine their feel. In the literature she learned that it is possible for the brain to lay down new nerve pathways around dead cell areas. She wanted desperately to find out *how* to assist that outcome, but was frustrated in her search to find someone who knew. She called the neurologist she'd seen at UCLA, but he was of no help. Her nurse friend, Joan Austen, didn't know.

Peplau tried different strategies on her own and began recording her observations and reflections to chart her coping and recovery. Ever the nurse educator, she hoped someone would publish them, that they would be of use to nursing practice. Austen offered to take Peplau's written observations and to try to find an appropriate journal.[98] Peplau noticed that when she was physically exhausted or fatigued, the dysfunction was worse. As she coped, she wrote out the strategies she used as advice nurses could give to stroke patients. It occurred to her that the flashes of light going off in her brain were not unlike the startled responses she'd seen on the faces of infants: The way ahead, she realized, was akin to the learning that occurs in infancy.[99]

She began to condition her mind to think such things as "pick-up," "hold," "hang on to," "carry," "don't drop," "don't spill," "don't touch hot," and so forth. Using what she remembered of learning in small children, she wrote out a protocol:

1. Concentrate intensely on the immediate task;
2. use both hands at first in all actions;
3. watch the object, keep your eyes on your hands, and glance at the destination; and
4. verbalize each message.[100]

Gradually, through willpower and concentration, and without the aid of a trained rehabilitation therapist, Peplau restored function to her hand, and then to her arm. Yes, her brain had been affected, but it could also be reprogrammed. After about 2 years of self-rehabilitation, she could manage heat and cold without disaster, could hold onto soap in the shower, and had learned to compensate for things she could not do.[101]

Because she either did not seek or refused formal rehabilitation, Peplau did not have the benefit of having rehabilitation personnel nor home health care nurses with her to share her efforts or to offer companionship and support. She sought but could not find subjective accounts of others' experiences with a stroke. Recording her own experience was her attempt to share her experience with others, and to help nurses to better understand the adaptations required for maximum recovery. Her efforts at analysis increased her sense of both physical and psychological competence, but she had lost her mobility. One of the things she could not do was drive. She had to depend on Tish to take her shopping or out to run errands. Always extremely independent, she now found herself dependent on her child. It was not an easy or comfortable place to be.

Peplau sought to analyze and organize her life to minimize this dependence as much as possible. She set aside a day for shopping and errands, a day now shared with Tish. From time to time she made up large batches of the soups she enjoyed and froze individual servings for a later day. She renewed her correspondence with vigor and invested large amounts of time in keeping her "community of practice" in touch and alive.[102] Her correspondence about subjects other than stroke began to grow once again.

By 1992 her life had settled into a routine. She still arose at 6:00 every morning and watched the morning news, had her coffee and juice, showered, and then dealt with her mail. She answered all the mail she received, paying all the bills the day they arrived. Because she answered all the mail, the volume continued to grow. The mail arrived just before noon each day, and in addition to a steady stream of correspondence generated by her willingness to respond and the steady flow from her "community of practice" group, news magazines and journals arrived daily. These she continued to read and clip, making small piles to be sent out with letters to members of her "community."[103] She fixed her own meals, and had someone come once a week to clean and do the laundry. Until he entered high school in 1996, Tish drove David two or three afternoons a week to Hilda's house do his gardening and his homework. David was also learning to make fresh vegetable soup from the peas, beans, and carrots that he harvested from the garden. He also learned to bake. His specialty was chocolate cake with homemade vanilla butter cream frosting. Tish continued to come once a week to take Hilda shopping, or occasionally to the doctor. Peplau did not own a microwave, never bought an answering machine, and had no computer. Nor did she own a typewriter. When typescript was required, Hilda wrote out her material in long hand, and Tish typed (and couldn't resist commenting), Hilda revised, and Tish retyped the manuscripts for her. In this way, mother and daughter continued their "professional" sharing of thoughts and ideas.[104]

A STRING OF HONORS

Well into the 1990s, Hilda Peplau continued to write regularly to the ANA, alerting them to issues on the horizon or making suggestions for panels or plenary sessions. Even 25 years into retirement she continued to attend the annual ANA and APNA conventions, almost always presenting a paper or appearing on a plenary panel herself. Hilda Peplau did not walk quietly into the sunset.

In 1992, the ANA Board of Directors established the Hilda Peplau Award in her honor. This was only the second award ever created by the ANA to commemorate a living nurse. The Peplau Award was established specifically to recognize outstanding contributions to nursing made by a psychiatric-mental health nurse. Hilda Peplau herself was the first recipient of this award, an event orchestrated by Liz Carter and Shirley Smoyak, and presented on June, 16, 1992, at the ANA convention in Boston.[105] Peplau was cited as a "clear thinker who has changed the field of nursing dramatically over the course of her career."[106]

In 1994, Hilda was notified by the Library of Congress that she had been selected as one of 50 prominent Americans to be honored at a special reception and exhibition on October 16, 1995, co-sponsored by the Library's Office of Scholarly Programs and Marquis Who's Who, publisher of *Who's Who in America*, the annual biographical reference publication. Among others selected to receive this honor were Walter Annenberg, the philanthropist and former U.S. ambassador to Great Britain; former president Jimmy Carter, the architect I. M. Pei, evangelist Billy Graham, author Saul Bellow, actor Paul Newman, General Colin Powell, cellist Yo Yo Ma, playwright Arthur Miller, singer and songwriter Bruce Springstein, and author Elie Wiesel. There was only one nurse: Hildegard E. Peplau. The 50 men and women selected, along with distinguished guests, and President and Mrs. Clinton, gathered on a starry Washington evening in the large exhibition hall at the Library of Congress. There were speeches and toasts, and a tour of the exhibit organized around the theme of the importance of biographical references as a mirror of changes and advances in all areas of American society. The exhibit graphically portrayed the notable achievements of the honorees in advancing the frontiers of knowledge, technology, and quality of American life over the previous 50 years. Peplau felt deeply moved by this unexpected honor. The recognition established that she was indeed an extraordinary woman, one whose achievements were acknowledged beyond the restricted circles of nursing.

In the years since her retirement in 1974, Peplau had been awarded nine honorary degrees. In addition to the Alfred University, Boston College, Duke, and Columbia University degrees, she received degrees from Rutgers University in 1985, the University of Indianapolis in 1987, Ohio State University in 1990, Indiana University in 1994, and the University of Ulster, Northern Ireland, in 1994.

A highlight among these proceedings had been the 1992 event when Boston College awarded her a doctor of science in nursing degree, one of the first such honorary degrees conferred on a nurse. There Hilda had stayed not with the dean of nursing but at the Sheraton Hotel in downtown Boston, where she was feted together with her co-honorary awardee, Adlai Stevenson. Hilda had long admired Stevenson and had been a staunch supporter of his candidacy for U.S. president when she was at Teachers College. The reception the night before the ceremony had been quite jolly; there Hilda discovered that there was nothing stuffy about the Jesuits. She enjoyed the occasion immensely. The graduation ceremonies the next morning were like an Irish festival. There was a sea of green gowns, with cardinals and priests in their bright robes and Hilda in her Columbia blue. She had no idea how she had been selected, but it was an occasion she treasured.[107]

After the Columbia award in 1983, came Rutgers in 1985, and that, she recalled, was "pretty neat." The dinner the night before was an elegant but informal catered affair in the home of a new dean, Dorothy DeMaio. Dean DeMaio had invited the women members of the Rutgers Board of

Trustees, who accepted, and had also thoughtfully arranged for Hilda's nieces—her sister Bertha's four daughters—to be there. Present and former faculty members, former students, and Rozella Schlotfeldt, who was a visiting professor that year at Rutgers, joined the faculty for the lovely, large, and totally relaxed party.

The next morning it got even better. To march into the Louis Brown Athletic Center, with the bands playing, the entire faculty in flowing multicolored gowns, was truly a thrill. With 27 schools, the Rutgers commencement is a huge affair. The institution had grown immeasurably since Hilda's time there. It was now truly a major public research university, and under the leadership of Dorothy DeMaio, the College of Nursing had grown into its status as an equal to other Rutgers colleges offering a full range of programs from the BS in nursing to the PhD. As he presented Peplau with her degree, the university's president, Edward J. Bloustein, kissed her. This was the first and only time she had been kissed by a university president! It was a moment to savor, and she did. It felt, finally, like a wonderful conclusion to her Rutgers career.

In August 1994 Peplau journeyed to Ireland to receive the honorary doctor of science degree from the University of Ulster, where she was again referred to as the "Mother of Psychiatric Nursing" and honored for

Being one of our great pioneers. Her influence and work has permeated all areas of nursing practice and transcended all cultural boundaries. While her career has been based within the USA, her influence on nursing as a science and an art has been worldwide.[108]

There was a special conference in her honor and Hilda was asked to present a paper. She had long had an interest in schizophrenia and decided to use this occasion to offer guidelines for identifying specific nursing strategies to use in dealing with schizophrenic patients. Thus, as she celebrated her 86th birthday on September 1, 1994, Peplau was still urging nurses to be scientific, to analyze and report on what they do, to record how they make a difference in patient care in ways that are unique to the profession.[109] This was her last trip across the Atlantic.

In the fall of 1994 she flew to St. Louis for the annual APNA convention, which that year featured a "Dialogue with Hilda E. Peplau" narrated by Dr. Claire Fagin, who had been a student of Hilda's at TC in the early 1950s. By this time Fagin had achieved acclaim as the dean of the School of Nursing and then as interim president of the University of Pennsylvania. Clearly at the top of her form, Peplau regaled the audience with stories from the early days in the back wards at Brooklyn State Hospital, but also raised issues continuing to challenge nursing's professional identity.[110] This would be her last contribution to a nursing convention.

In October 1996 after an APNA meeting in San Diego, Hilda and Grayce Sills headed out across the desert in a rented car to reflect on the meetings and to spend a few days in the desert gambling town of Laughlin, playing the slots. Hilda was exhausted from the meetings and the 5-hour drive from San Diego. After an early dinner and a few tries at the quarter slots, Hilda went to bed, but Grayce had gotten a second wind and continued to try her luck. At 2:00 in the morning Grayce hit the jackpot—the big one, 1 million dollars! She was kept up the rest of the night filling out forms, working out her tax liability, waiting for various casino officials to deal with the technicalities of actually giving her the money, and having her picture taken for the newspapers as reporters and photographers began to arrive. Tired but happy, Grayce returned to the room about 6:00 in the morning, to await a call from Hilda. Grayce and Hilda often traveled together, but always had separate rooms as Grayce was a reformed smoker and Hilda was not. The call came at 7:00, and as was their custom, Grayce went to get the iced coffee Hilda cherished first thing in the morning. At this point, Grayce had told no one of her incredible win. Her family on the East Coast was still sleeping, and she had not wanted to rob Hilda of cherished rest. Finally, the inquiry came: "Well, how did you do?" "Oh, I won a million dollars," said Grayce. "Yeah, we can still dream," said Hilda. Until Grayce went to her room, returning with a folder holding W-2 forms (the government got its money before Grayce got hers), instructions, options, etc., Hilda thought she was kidding. That night, they had a dinner on the town and both went to bed early. Sometime between 3:00 and 6:00 a.m. Hilda had either turned over and fallen out of the bed, or tried to get up and fallen down beside the bed. She was never sure which; it may have been another, small stroke. But she was sure that she had once again injured her back and aggravated old injuries. Stoic as ever, however, she insisted to Grayce that she was "all right," that she did not want to see a doctor, and that they should both enjoy the day because they had paid for a third night. They drove back to Sherman Oaks the next day, stopping often for Hilda to get out of the car and smoke a cigarette. It was clear she was in pain, but she refused to take so much as an aspirin for it. Grayce returned to Ohio, shaken but much richer. Hilda would never be able to stand comfortably again.[111]

Although once again often in pain, Hilda continued to write professional thought pieces and to correspond with PhD students who had begun contacting her as they developed their dissertations. After her nine honorary degrees, the awards established in her honor, and the many panels celebrating her work and contributions, she at last could believe that in the competition for enduring ideas in the development of nursing clinical practice, patient care, and psychiatric nursing education, her work had stood the test of time.

In June 1997 Hilda Peplau made plans to attend the ICN meetings in Vancouver, British Columbia. She anticipated that this would be her last

ICN meeting. Her unrelenting back pain was making travel more and more difficult. She now required a wheelchair and Tish's help to get on an airplane, and as much as she loved the ICN, she felt she no longer had the energy or even the will to undertake long trips. Thus, this trip to Vancouver would be special.

Arriving with Tish she went directly to the Pacific Hotel next to the convention center in the Vancouver harbor. With green mountains rising directly from the water's edge across the bay, big tour ships anchored close by, and tourists and nurses mingling on the wharf, the setting was beautiful and festive. They checked into the hotel and were escorted to a beautiful suite on the 43rd floor, overlooking the water. Grayce Sills had gotten to Vancouver early and picked the suite. Beautiful bouquets from nurses far and near filled it with vibrant color and cheerfulness. After a short nap, Hilda requested a wheelchair and briefly visited the exhibits across the street in the convention center with Grayce. She was immediately mobbed with well-wishers, including a group of South American nuns who insisted on kneeling in front of her wheelchair and kissing her hands. This was too much for Hilda, and she quickly returned to her suite. As much as she wanted to visit the exhibits to see where nursing was going, she simply did not have the strength for protracted socializing. Shirley and Neil Smoyak stopped by to see whether or not she needed anything, and Suzy Lego and her husband, Lee Spray, came for tea. The phone kept ringing, as many former students and professional friends hoped to see and visit with her. At Hilda's insistence, Tish fended them off. Hilda complained that she was tired, very tired. She needed to conserve her strength. For at this convention Hilda Peplau was to receive nursing's highest honor, the Christiane Reimann Prize. The Reimann Prize is nursing's ultimate recognition, its equivalent of the Nobel Prize for nursing.

First, though, she would have dinner with Grayce Sills, Dorothy DeMaio—still dean at the Rutgers College of Nursing, and with Dr. Irwin Pollack, her old friend and former chair of Psychiatry at the medical school at the time of her retirement from Rutgers in 1974. It was a time for reminiscing, reflecting, laughing, and enjoying. What started out as a lovely evening became tiring and painful, however, as the service in the very elegant restaurant was excruciatingly slow. She endured, but arrived home after midnight, exhausted and thankful that she had the foresight to rest during the day.

The next day, she asked Grayce to push her wheelchair into the convention center, but once in the hall, insisted on standing to walk to the front and then onto the stage for the ceremonies. She did allow her old friend and colleague, Connie Holleran of the ICN, to help her up the steps, and she thankfully sat in the chair provided, awaiting the opening of the convention. As the delegates from around the world filed in wearing their national dress, Hilda remembered only the good in her long career. International gatherings of nurses always filled her with pride and optimism, and this one would be no exception.

With flags surrounding the stage, with an orchestra playing national anthems, with nurses young and old acknowledging her as they filed by, Hilda was able to simply enjoy the moment. A long citation outlining her career was read, the plaque was presented, flowers were placed in her arms, and a standing ovation commenced. Hilda shared the honor with Mo-Im Kim of Taiwan, and the slightly younger Mo-Im Kim made her acceptance speech a tribute to her mentor, Hilda Peplau. Feeling vindicated at last, Hilda finally accepted that her active life as a nursing leader was truly over. She had become a living legend, an icon, a grey imminence. She was no longer controversial.

ENDNOTES

1. Diary entry, May 7, 1974, Box 8, Schlesinger Library collection.
2. Notes from Letitia Anne Peplau to Barbara Callaway, July 31, 2000. According to Tish, until the last years of her life, Hilda only occasionally mentioned her back pain. She didn't want to burden others with her problem, and tried to focus elsewhere in order not to focus on her agony. "Only in the last year of her life was she willing to use a wheelchair as a way of protecting herself. People didn't expect someone in a wheelchair to be able to stand to shake hands or engage in idle chat.... Her way of coping was to minimize and conceal as much as possible."
3. Diary entry, May 7, 1974.
4. Ibid.
5. In 1999, Radcliffe College was absorbed by Harvard University and is now known as the Radcliffe Institute.
6. Diary entry, July 26, 1974.
7. Diary entry, August 28, 1974.
8. The Rutgers story reached its logical conclusion when Peplau was awarded an honorary doctorate by the university at its 1985 commencement, a full decade after her retirement.
9. See diary entries for July and August, 1974.
10. See diary entries for October, 1974.
11. Letter from Eleanor Knudson to Hilda Peplau, August 21, 1974, Rutgers Personnel File.
12. Diary entry, October, 1974.
13. Ibid.
14. Hilda Peplau's sister, Bertha Reppert, was a world-renowned herbalist. What Peplau was to nursing, Reppert was to herbalists. Operating out of Rosemary House in Mechanicsburg, Pennsylvania, Bertha Reppert was well-known for over 40 years for her herbs and explanations for their usages.
15. The red tribute book with Bertha's letter may be found in Box 28.
16. See diary entries for October and November, 1974.
17. Conference papers on differentiation in practice and the Janice Geller correspondence on joint practice are found in Box 28, #1050, #1054, and #1066.
18. Diary entry, November 30, 1974.

19. Clearly Peplau continued to suffer the aftereffects of the automobile collision in Miami, now nearly 3 years behind her. See diary entries for November and December, 1974.
20. See letters, notes, programs, and other material in Box 29, #1078.
21. Diary entry, February, 1975.
22. Diary entry, May, 1975.
23. Diary entry, March, 1975.
24. Ibid.
25. Diary entry, April 23, 1975.
26. This paper and notes about the trip may be found in Box 39, #1422, along with letters from Dorothy Hall concerning the Belgium assignment.
27. From Hilda Peplau's 1975 Christmas letter, found in Box 4, #121.
28. See Bill Field to Hilda Peplau, November 22, 1975, Box 29, #1076: "... We could do much better if you only would. Our original offerings have paid off handsomely, but it can't last much longer ... "
29. See Box 28, #1028 for copies of the handwritten tape notes, and #1053 for correspondence from Field.
30. As she wrote to Field at the time: "100 tea bags, 400 ice cube trays, 500 sheets of paper and dozens of sleepless nights later, I am mailing you the last of the 20 tapes of the series on psychiatric nursing." Hilda Peplau to Bill Field, August 10, 1973, in Box 28, #1022.
31. See notes from Bill Field in Box 30, #1120 and #1142. Box 41 contains 16 tapes made for PSF Productions:
    A Concept of Psychotherapy
    Orientation in Interviewing
    Manifestations of Anxiety and Intervention
    Testing Maneuvers and Interventions
    Concept of Self Systems and Related Problems
    Interviewing as Language Competence Development
    Criteria for a Working Relationship
    Problems and Strategies in Nurse Psychotherapy
    Termination and Use of Summary
    Personality Development
    Anxiety Development: Panic
    Withdrawal Behavior
    Dynamics of Delusions and Hallucinations
    Language and Its Relation to Thought Disorder
    Illness Maintaining Systems
    Basic Principles of Patient Counseling
32. See clippings on desinstitutionalization in Box 8, #475.
33. Diary entry, August, 1975.
34. See examples of requests of her in Box 29, #1079–1081.
35. For information on this project see box 39, #1421 and #1422. The other members of the training program included Professor Peter de Schauwer, MD, Dr. Jan Blanpain, Ms. Mieke Grypdonk, Ms. Agnes Roelens, and Ms. M. Therese Rodenback.
36. For pictures of Leuven see Box 29, #1076.
37. In 1937 a Higher Council of Nursing Schools was established to determine the requirements for a common curriculum. The next year a General Union of Belgium Nurses was established to coordinate four distinct nursing organizations in Belgium divided by language (French or Flemish), religion (Protestant or Catholic), and philosophy. Various decrees issued between 1921 and 1931 had set down criteria for admission, length of studies, and clinical experiences required for

nursing diplomas. Nursing courses were taught by medical doctors. A royal decree in 1957 established that the criteria for admission into nursing programs would be the same as that required for entrance into the universities, thus, for the first time in Belgium, giving academic status to students entering nursing programs. See Dame Sheila Quinn and Susan Russell, *Nursing: The European Dimension* (London: Scutari Press, 1989), 44–50.

38. Letter from Dorothy Hall to Hilda Peplau, April 18, 1975, Box 39, #1422.
39. Interview, Hildegard Peplau, March 9, 1992.
40. An album of photographs, and letters from Hildegard Peplau to Tish Peplau and Shirley Smoyak, may be found in the archives in Box 29, #1076. Many of the observations that follow were provided by Hilda Peplau in interviews in Sherman Oaks on March 9 and March 30, 1992. Material summarized here is also found in Francine Prose, *Ancient Beguinages of Flanders* (Boston: Ivy, 1990), 27–47.
41. Interview, Hildegard Peplau, March 30, 1992.
42. Notes for these lectures are found in Box 29, #1085–1087 and #1088–1091.
43. Letter from Hilda Peplau to Dorothy Hall, November 12, 1976, in Box 39, #1422.
44. See large collection of letters from Hilda Peplau to Shirley Smoyak regarding the Leuven experience in Box 29, #1086–1087, and in Box 4, #172–173, as well as letters to Letitia Anne Peplau in Box 3, #94.
45. Interview, Hildegard Peplau, March 30, 1992.
46. Letter from Hildegard Peplau to Shirley Smoyak, October 30, 1976, in Box 29, #1076.
47. This statement and Peplau's comments may be found in Box 37, #1357. Notes on this convention may be found in Box 30, #1102.
48. Interview, Hildegard Peplau, March 30, 1992.
49. See letter from Terry Sanford, President of Duke University, to Hilda Peplau, April 13, 1976, in Box 30, #1094. Other materials in this file lay out her itinerary before and after this trip.
50. Letter from Letitia Anne Peplau to Hilda Peplau, November 5, 1976, Box 3, #104.
51. Interview, Hildegard Peplau, March 21, 1994. Also, a complete record of Peplau's 2 years at Leuven is contained in sequentially numbered, very dense and detailed letters written to Letitia Anne Peplau from Belgium during 1975–1977. These letters are found in Box 3, #90 and #94.
52. Letter from Hilda Peplau to ICN, November 5, 1976, in Box 38, #1377. These letters also include many suggestions for making things move more smoothly at the Tokyo ICN Congress scheduled for the summer of 1977.
53. Letter from Barbara Fawkes to Hilda Peplau, June 27, 1977, Box 38, #1378.
54. Interview, Hildegard Peplau, February 10, 1992, and with Mo-Im Kim in Vancouver, Canada, June 17, 1997. In June, 1997, Mo-Im Kim and Hilda Peplau would share nursing's highest honor, the Reimann prize.
55. See notes written by Hilda Peplau in Box 4, #121.
56. Ibid.
57. Materials about the conference and on the Council of Advanced Practitioners in Psychiatric and Mental Health Nursing may be found in Box 37, #1359.
58. The tributes by Grayce Sills and Dorothy Gregg may be found in Box 37, #1358.
59. Interview, Shirley Smoyak, February 13, 1999.
60. Hilda Peplau, Christmas letter, 1978, in Box 4, #121.
61. Hilda Peplau, Beryl Palmer O'Neil, and her sister, Ruby Palmer, were classmates at TC in 1946, immediately after the Second World War. In 1953, in New York City, the three classmates shared several private-duty patients in common, each working a shift. The two sisters retired in Los Angeles in the 1970s and Peplau, who did not have many personal friends in L.A., often enjoyed their company. Their

friendship, however, did not survive the Alaska trip, and both sisters refused to be interviewed for this study.

62. Details of the 1978 Alaska trip and the accident may be found in Box 31, #1120.

63. An account of the Morocco trip is found in Box 4, #121.

64. Letter from E. M. Kiereini to Hilda Peplau, September 21, 1981, in Box 38, #1389.

65. See 1979 Christmas letter in Box 4, #121.

66. See a collection of these Sigma Theta Tau talks in Box 31, #1129.

67. This plaque and the ICN agenda are found in Box 38, #1389.

68. Letter from Constance Holleran to Hilda Peplau, July 27, 1981, in Box 31, #1149.

69. Diary entry, July 1981, Box 4, #121.

70. Letitia Anne Peplau married Steven Gordon on June 26, 1980, in Santa Monica, California. It was a private ceremony before a Justice of the Peace. Hilda held a reception for the couple in New Jersey in August that year. See materials in Box 7, #224, and 1982 Christmas letter, Box 7, #232.

71. The many working drafts and hundreds of pages of notes made by Hilda Peplau of what was to become the *Social Policy Statement* may be found in Box 37, #1363.

72. *Nursing: A Social Policy Statement* (Washington, D.C., American Nurses Association, 1981), reprinted in Hildegard Peplau, "American Nurses Association Social Policy Statement," *Archives of Psychiatric Nursing* 5 (1987): 301–307.

73. Interview, Rozella Schlotfeldt, April 5, 1995.

74. Although clearly publishable, these talks and papers were not submitted to journals. By 1981, Peplau had decided she had published enough. Now, wherever she spoke, she was inevitably recorded. As long as the recordings were available, she saw no reason to put the time and effort into revising these papers for publication, or to submit her work for review by others. In fact, she decided the time had come to truly concentrate on getting her papers in order and donated to the Schlesinger Library for Research on Women at the Radcliffe Institute in Cambridge, Massachusetts. Many of the recordings of talks given after 1981 may be found in Box 39.

75. A speech on this issue may be found in Box 32, #1173.

76. Copies of speeches on these issues may be found in Box 31, #1143–1150. These speeches were written out in longhand by Hilda Peplau and then typed by Anne Peplau. They are scholarly pieces, complete with plentiful footnotes.

77. Letter from Wayne Gromis to Hilda Peplau, May 24, 1982, found in Box 7, #230, with notations by Hilda Peplau.

78. See accounts in Box 7, #227.

79. See letters about the Belgium trip in Box 7, #227. This heavy pewter medal is in Box 42, #1520 at the Schlesinger, along with other awards, citations, certificates of appreciation, honorary degrees, keys to cities, Senate Resolutions in her honor, the Florence Nightingale Medal, and the very large bronze R. Louise McManus Award Medal.

80. See letters to and from the Cannoodts and Peplau in Box 4, #162.

81. This plaque may be found in Box 42, #1547.

82. Shirley Smoyak and Sheila Rouslin, *A Collection of Classics in Psychiatric Nursing Literature* (Thorofare, New Jersey: Charles A. Slack, 1982).

83. Materials related to the genealogical study may be found in Box 7, #222.

84. A complete copy of this rather massive genealogical study has been deposited in the Schlesinger Library. It is a major scholarly work in its own right.

85. The Kenyan summer workshop materials and papers are found in Box 32, #1176. The safari for the nurses was organized by the Park East Tour Company. As the seven vans of nurses came around a bend in the road, the first van, in which Hilda and Shirley Smoyak were riding, hit another van which was laying on its side in

the middle of the road. The van was carrying workers for a Abercombie and Fitch tour, many of whom were seriously injured. The nurses descended on the scene and did the best they could until help arrived, some 4 hours later. Without emergency first aid equipment, the nurses could only stabilize the injured. Several were already dead when the nurses arrived. Hilda told Shirley, "I am too old for this," and declared this her last trip. Interview, Shirley Smoyak, April 17, 1999.

86. Letter from Edward J. Bloustein to Hilda E. Peplau, September 9, 1983, in Box 31, #1169.

87. The *McCall's* Handwriting Analysis is in Box 7, #230.

88. See letters and other materials found in Box 37, #1367.

89. This award and citation are found in Box 37, #1365.

90. Interview, Hildegard Peplau, March 21, 1994.

91. Hilda Peplau Christmas letter, 1986, in Box 4, #121.

92. Peplau's annual Christmas letters after 1987 featured David Gordon and chronicled his boyhood as her friend.

93. See Thomas A. Stewart, "The Invisible Key to Success," *Fortune 134* (August 5, 1996): 173–176. In this article Steward discusses "communities of practice where learning and growth happen." In 1997, Hilda Peplau was delighted to learn that now there is a name for something she had been involved in for years. See letter from Hilda Peplau to Barbara Callaway, March 13, 1997. (All the author's correspondence with Peplau in regard to this biography will be deposited in the Schlesinger Library at the conclusion of this project).

94. The account in this paragraph is taken from a letter from Hilda Peplau to Barbara Callaway dated February 21, 1993.

95. Details of the stroke experience are found in a 10-page written memorandum, given to the author. This document will be placed in the Schlesinger collection at the conclusion of this project, along with a first person account and analysis done by a nurse neurologist, Dr. Joan K. Austen, Professor of Nursing at the Indiana University School of Nursing. Dr. Austen wrote a narration to go along with a personal account given her of this experience by Hilda Peplau. See Joan K. Austen, "Reflecting on a Nurse's Personal Experience with a Stroke," n.d., to be placed in the Schlesinger archives.

96. Ibid.

97. Amaurosis fugax refers to partial or complete monocular visual loss consequent to retinal ischemia and is also called transient monocular blindness. Although Peplau had complained of eye *pain*, it is not clear whether or not she also experienced a loss of vision that might have alerted the Jules Stein doctors to amourosis fugax. More to the point, perhaps, is the fact that Peplau was a lifelong smoker, which would have greatly increased her risk of stroke. It was also clear from tests done while she was in the hospital after the stroke in 1989, that her carotid arteries were partially blocked at that time and likely contributed to the stroke. In hindsight, in 1998, Hilda and Tish would wonder why the neurologist did not suggest carotid artery surgery to clear that blocked artery, which likely would have improved the quality of her last decade of life. Notes from Anne Peplau, January 28, 1999.

98. Although a finished copy of this proposed article is in the archives, the author was unable to find a published citation for it.

99. Letter from Hilda Peplau to Barbara Callaway, October 5, 1993.

100. Ibid.

101. Interview, Hildegard Peplau, April 6, 1992.

102. Ibid.

103. When asked to what journals she subscribed, Peplau recited the following list off the top of her head: *Atlantic Monthly, Harper's, Vanity Fair, New Republic, New York,*

Esquire, Ladies's Home Journal, National Geographic, Private Practice, U.S. News and World Report, Newsweek, Vacations, Los Angeles, Home and Architectural Digest, Journal Psychosocial Nursing, Nursing and Health Care, Elle, Gentleman's Quarterly, Psychiatric Nursing, The New Yorker, American Journal of Nursing, Journal Professional Nursing, Nursing Forum, Perspectives in Nursing, International Nursing Review, New York Times Book Review, The Economist, as well as *The New York Times, The Los Angeles Times,* and *The Washington Post.* Interview, Hildegard Peplau, March 21, 1994.

104. Notes from Anne Peplau to Barbara Callaway, January 28, 1999.

105. *American Journal of Nursing,* June, 1992, 15. The second recipient of the award would be a nurse long active in international nursing and the Dean Emeritus of Downstate Medical Center in Brooklyn, Illdura Murilla-Rhode. Murilla-Rhode had been a Peplau student in her last year at TC in 1953. Interview, Illdura Murilla-Rhode, March 2, 1993, in New York City.

106. *American Journal of Nursing,* ibid.

107. Interview, Hildegard Peplau, April 6, 1992.

108. Citation by Professor Jennifer Boore, Head of Nursing Department, University of Ulster, read in presenting Hilda Peplau to the Chancellor of the University of Ulster for the D. Science Degree, August 31, 1994, provided to the author by Anita O'Toole.

109. This synopsis of Hilda Peplau's paper on schizophrenia at Ulster was provided by Dorothy DeMaio and Shirley Smoyak, both of whom attended the Ulster ceremonies in conjunction with the ICN meetings, also held in Ireland in August, 1994.

110. The author was present at this event.

111. Letter from Hildegard Peplau to Barbara Callaway, October 23, 1996, and discussion with Grayce Sills, August 27, 2001.

Conclusion: "Well Done"   16

I had exceedingly few real friends in nursing. It just didn't turn out that way for me . . . Whether it was just nurses in academe or whether it was just a distrust of women in leadership, I don't know.
—Hildegard Peplau
March 1992

A slight smile on her lips, her eyes alert and taking in the scene, Hildegard Peplau sat quietly and unobtrusively in her wheelchair, dressed in a lavender pantsuit, Tish at her side, waiting for the ANA House of Delegates to come to order for its awards ceremony. Their state banners held high, the delegates sat behind her. In the aisles, nurses were lining up to have photographs taken with her. It was Saturday, June 27, 1998, in San Diego, California, and the American Nurses Association was preparing to bestow upon Hilda Peplau its highest honor, induction into the ANA Hall of Fame. At last, the ceremony was under way. Before the Hall of Fame formalities, the Hildegard Peplau Award for contributions to the advancement of nursing through research was presented to Dr. Judith Haber, who noted that Peplau's vision had shaped many a career and inspired 3 decades of nursing graduates *after* her retirement. Then a film was shown, highlighting Peplau's career, and the current ANA president, Beverly Malone, herself a former Peplau student, called Hilda to the podium. Hilda's long career and major contributions were cited, and it was noted that her ideas of the nurse-patient relationship were now at the core of every nursing specialty and every nursing curriculum. In the wake of a thunderous standing ovation, Peplau accepted American nursing's highest honor with these words:

I haven't been in the ANA headquarters in Washington, D.C., for several decades now. I don't know if there is a hall for the Hall of Fame. Or whether it is just a photo album. Or maybe it's just a folder in a Steelcase file drawer. Whatever. I thank you.[1]

Then she turned and slowly walked off the stage. The large audience was stunned at first, not realizing that this short recitation was the sum of Peplau's remarks—she planned to say no more. Then they were on their feet again, laughing and applauding as Tish met her at the bottom of the ramp and began pushing her in her wheelchair out of the auditorium. Someone rushed forward, placing a beautiful bouquet in her arms. Others pushed through, snapping pictures. Tish kept her eyes straight ahead, pushing Hilda through the well-wishers back to her room. Hilda did not want to stay in the auditorium. She was pleased with the award but remembered all too vividly the painful experiences of nearly 30 years earlier when she took up the crucible of leadership in this organization. She did not want to endure the hypocrisy of many who would come forward to congratulate her now.

Although it was not said, many in the crowd believed that had nursing organizations followed where she tried to lead so many years ago, the changes she sought would have changed nursing profoundly and moved it in the direction of a profession. The changes she proposed were of the same magnitude for American nursing as those that Florence Nightingale brought about with her writings and advocacy for nursing in Europe a century earlier. Although American nursing resisted this quantum leap in its development, Peplau's impact remains deep and lasting, as evidenced by her many honorary degrees and nursing awards. While Hilda Peplau's experience was primarily in psychiatric nursing, her influence on the profession is much wider than that.

Peplau's *Interpersonal Relations in Nursing* is generally recognized as the first modern nursing text with a theoretical perspective, and as such represented a major paradigm shift in nursing.[2] Her early work with psychiatric patients and psychiatric and mental health nurses, presented in that book, together with a collection of her selected papers, is now recognized as "revolutionary."[3] In this work, she laid the groundwork for creating the specialty of psychiatric nursing as a subfield within nursing that is distinct from medical psychiatry. Today she is acknowledged as "the mother of psychiatric nursing,"[4] and the interpersonal perspective she advanced has been widely integrated into all levels of nursing education.

Peplau's subsequent work helped transform nursing from a "science of doing" to a "science of knowing" by establishing creative links between nursing research and practice.[5] Her mid-20th century focus employed deductive and inductive reasoning, moving up and down the ladder of abstraction to construct new nursing interventions and a nursing-practice foundation based on interpersonal relations. Early on Peplau identified practice as the context in which nursing knowledge could develop. In Peplau's work, nursing practice gave to nursing research a body of data that was patient-oriented, participatory, and context sensitive.

Her work changed nursing curricula across the whole spectrum of nursing education and led to dramatic changes in care. Talking to patients is now taken for granted. Previously, nursing care meant simply doing things to patients—feeding, washing, or administering medications. After Peplau, the emphasis shifted toward valuing each patient as an individual through the provision of appropriate interventions and care.

Peplau believed nursing to be a profession equal to medicine, sharing common goals and settings with it, but with its own and separate contribution to make to health care and recovery. There was never any uncertainty about her identification with her profession, and she held steadfast in her efforts to push its growth to its full potential. Like Florence Nightingale, she brought about a sea change in her specialty of psychiatric nursing, but unlike Nightingale, she did not have powerful sponsors, nor the endorsement of a powerful medical profession, nor was she able to overcome the massive resistance of the nursing establishment. Today, it appears nursing has yet to define and secure its place in the health care system, still unsure of whether it is a profession with professional norms and concerns, or a labor force focused on economic security and safe sinecures.

Throughout her career, Peplau stressed that the whole profession would benefit from the nurse specialists' efforts to push forward the frontiers of nursing knowledge and practice. This theme is evident in all her writing as she sought to extend the concepts gained experientially in psychiatric nursing to other areas of nursing practice and urged nurses to move from the specific to the general in their own work. She had clear ideas about the central importance of hypothesis testing and research for the advancement of the profession as a whole, and for that reason was an early advocate (in fact, *the* earliest advocate) of graduate education and postgraduate specialization for nurses. The honors she received in retirement affirmed the principles that she fought for throughout her professional life.

In spite of her disappointments, Peplau never deserted nursing, never betrayed it, never suggested it was less than a serious profession, never let anyone get away with demeaning or devaluing it. She remained, as everyone recognized, deeply serious about the profession, its problems, and its challenges. She constantly pushed precisely because she did take the work of nursing so seriously. During her career, she never despaired about its professional possibilities. She remained, through long, hard, slogging, difficult years, an outspoken, uncompromising, boundary-crossing nurse. "She knew that the profession of nursing is a bit like an ocean liner—slow moving and slow to change course. She hoped it was the Queen Elizabeth II and not the Titanic."[6] While nursing as a profession was often disappointing to her, nursing as a career had been enormously fulfilling. While the Columbia, Rutgers, and ANA years were full of pain and disappointment, they were also years in which she was growing emotionally and intellectually. Although often frustrated, she had no doubt her career choice was right for her. In her own words, "I don't think I made a mistake. As a nurse, I pulled my whole family into the middle class. For me and many others, nursing was a way of getting out of the "marriage trap" or bypassing the convent . . . I must say, in spite of its limitations, I've loved every minute of it."[7]

A visionary, Peplau was always available to serve on various commissions, committees, and task forces. She was always a major contributor on the many such bodies on which she served. She did not make people comfortable. In spite of her many appointments and wide-spread recognition in nursing, late in her life she would still comment that

> I had exceedingly few real friends in nursing. It just didn't turn out that way for me. Maybe I would have had better friends in hospitals. Whether it was just nurses in academe or whether it was just a distrust of women in leadership, I don't know.[8]

In later years she would fantasize that if she could do it over, or if there were reincarnation, she would return as a full-time clinician.[9] She would work directly with patients, and avoid the institutional and organizational politics that she found so frustrating.

Obviously, Peplau's single-minded dedication to her profession was not without its personal costs. Because she was so able and so outspoken, it was perhaps inevitable that she would become a leader in her profession. Her high energy level, her restless mind, her incomparable service, and unrelenting practice of what she preached, made her both difficult and visible. Hence she was often thrust into positions of leadership by force of personality and intellect, only to be handicapped by an inability to inspire action—or at least the action she wanted. She was intellectually seductive to students and some colleagues, but she seemed unable to channel this following into professional reform.

At a meeting of the American Psychiatric Nurses Association (APNA) in San Antonio in the early 1990s, Shirley Smoyak asked Hilda Peplau what she would do, were she younger, to get psychiatric nursing, or the profession generally, moving again. The next morning, Peplau presented Smoyak with eight handwritten pages of suggestions. It is easy to see that such a response is both endearing and exasperating, if not intimidating. Along with her suggestions, there were also questions, including these: Why don't psychiatric nurses do and publish outcome studies of their psychotherapeutic work with patients? and What are the three or four critical directions that psychiatric nurses ought to examine, study, and determine *now* to safeguard and assure the future of this specialty? Who should be in charge of such inquiry.[10]

In spite of her perceived lack of friends in nursing, her contributions to her profession are both many and major, and in fact deeply appreciated. Peplau played a role in the landmark legislation that established the National Institute of Mental Health in 1946. Until recently the NIMH administered federal funding not only for research but also for training mental health professionals to work with the mentally ill. Peplau assured nursing was included in this funding. These funds played a significant role in drawing women into nursing, and supporting them as they pursued graduate education.

As an ambassador for graduate education in nursing, Peplau had no equal. As teacher, mentor, adviser, and sponsor she has inspired generations of students to great expectations and accomplishments. She introduced major innovations in graduate education and nursing research through her participation in government policy-making committees that set the guidelines for funding programs for nursing research. Far from debunking nursing, Peplau had a powerful vision. She constantly sought ways to move nursing forward as a profession. Her insistence that to move forward nursing must document what nurses do was rooted in her fundamental understanding that a profession must define itself and be able to demonstrate and explain its role.[11]

In the quarter of a century that followed Peplau's formal retirement there was steady growth in recognition of the scope and depth of her work. From the publication in 1952 of her first book, *Interpersonal Relations in Nursing,* to the present, her work has remained relevant. That book has been translated into six languages, reissued, and is considered a nursing classic. Over time, Peplau was able to see the conceptual framework and concepts for psychodynamic nursing that she developed in the 1950s incorporated into the baccalaureate nursing curriculums.

Well into retirement Peplau's continued conference presentations and occasional publications developed ever more intensive formulations of her earlier work. Thus, the structural framework of her work continued to grow and change, as she inserted new experience into it, not merely additively, but in ways that increased understanding as well as the content of knowledge in her field.

Despite her personal disappointments, Hilda remained the essential optimist, encouraging others to carry forth her causes. It helped that as the years went by, she did see progress. She lived to see the development of graduate programs in nursing at major universities across the country. She rejoiced as Rutgers developed its PhD program in nursing. She watched psychiatric practice move from straitjackets and lobotomies to more humane and effective treatments. She watched as nurses moved from being physicians' handmaidens toward more collaborative and more autonomous forms of practice. She also watched the slow development of nursing research and theory—never enough, in her view, but more each year than ever before. That the graduates of her programs struck out on highly successful careers of their own gave her enormous satisfaction.

As a result, in part, of Peplau's constant exhortation, psychiatric nurses have produced the majority of publications in nursing research journals. At the time of her retirement, the field was considered on the forefront of nursing knowledge, on the cutting edge of change for the entire profession. The pioneering clinical experiments in nursing practice she initiated stimulated clinical nursing studies in other fields, and today nursing programs in major research universities reflect her canons and her values.

As the years in retirement went by, the honors bestowed by professional nursing piled up, until, in 1995, Hilda Peplau was officially recognized as a "living legend" by the American Academy of Nursing. Her books were reissued and pronounced seminal. Her reputation was rehabilitated and her legacy recognized by the time nursing's highest honor, the Christiane Reimann Prize, was bestowed upon her in 1997, thus assuring her place in nursing history. In 1998, when she was finally inducted into the ANA Hall of Fame, she was the only living nurse to be so honored that year. She held honorary degrees from nine universities, and was the only nurse named one of "Fifty Great Americans" by Marquis Who's Who and the Library of Congress. By any standard, her career has been well acclaimed.

While Peplau's legacy in psychiatric nursing is assured, much of what she advocated is not. In an age of pharmacological treatment of mental illness, Peplau continued to believe that most psychological disturbances would respond to a giving, supportive, caring, and thoughtful environment. By 1980, after she was well into retirement, much of the mental health funding network that had so generously supported her work came unglued. It is ironic that when psychiatric nurses began to move into autonomous practice, the federally funded mental-health system itself floundered. The National Mental Health Systems Act of 1980 was meant to provide more comprehensive and responsive service systems for the mentally ill. Instead, patients were forced out of mental hospitals, with no safety net. The NIMH is no longer an independent agency; its research is under the National Institutes of Health, and its service components are under the Substance Abuse and Mental Health Service Administration.

Although she was venerated as the "mother of psychiatric nursing" and a pioneer in nursing theory, the cause to which Peplau devoted so much of her career, the cause of professionalization, remains the most troubling. The question of the appropriate point of entry for professional nursing practice continues to be one of nursing's most vexing, unresolved issues. In this area, Peplau's career has had little impact to date.

What accounts for the resistance Peplau encountered as she attempted to head the cause for professionalization within the ANA? In Peplau's case, the combination of high intelligence and the certainty of her own convictions made those who had risen to leadership positions in the ANA uncomfortable. Such intelligence and such self-confidence, when they are publicly exhibited, as they were in Peplau's life and career, seemed to instill a simmering indignation in even the most generous of colleagues.[12] Peplau could be criticized and even disliked on various grounds; she was often misunderstood, and was probably intimidating and made many people uncomfortable, especially those who lacked their own sense of purpose. The fact that she was completely dedicated to her profession, however, could not be questioned.

Added to the envy and misunderstanding of her intentions directed at Hilda personally, was the fact that psychiatric nursing, just as is true for psychiatry in medicine, was viewed with suspicion by others. People have a natural fear of those they think might see below the surface of things. Peplau's Germanic, no-nonsense approach to life made many around her uncomfortable, and when this was added to a more general discomfort with psychiatry and psychiatric nursing, it is easy to see why she may have made others uneasy, even had she not had low tolerance for social niceties and nonsense.

There is little doubt that Hilda's low mastery of social niceties did handicap her leadership ability. Peplau was very task oriented, and as a task leader she was efficient, direct, and knowledgeable, and she got the work done, whether it related to her graduate program or to the ANA. In this she was remarkably effective. The irony was that as the nurse who focused on nurse-patient relationships and brought interpersonal relations theory into nursing, Peplau had so much difficulty with the interpersonal aspects of group interactions. She was equipped with limited social leadership skills. Perhaps it is not surprising that the daughter of Gustav and Ottylie Peplau had little foundation upon which to build such skills. Always focused on a goal, Hilda often seemed oblivious of the importance of people's feelings in keeping the group running smoothly and harmoniously. Successful leaders need both task and social leadership skills. While Peplau excelled in task leadership, and while she could and did lead her graduate students into new directions, the interpersonal leadership skills needed to move nursing's leaders in nursing's organizations eluded her.

Although Peplau did not fully succeed in getting nursing to adopt the reforms she thought necessary to advance as a profession, she did redefine and enlarge psychiatric nursing, and she did force nurses into new and significant ways of thinking. Through her more than 200 publications, she continually enlarged the vision of nursing. She launched a large cadre of students who continued the work, and who understood her vision. She furthered, reaffirmed, and solidified the work she began in the 1940s, even in retirement. To the end, she continued to be herself, not to compromise, to bring her unmatched intelligence, her impeccable integrity, and her boldness of thought to all who would receive them. Hildegard Peplau made major contributions to her chosen profession as a teacher, scholar, practitioner, and nursing leader. She used her energy and her intellect to improve her world. It was a job well done.

POSTSCRIPT

After the ANA Hall of Fame induction in San Diego in September, 1998, Hilda felt tired beyond anything she had ever experienced. In October, Tish finally persuaded her to see a doctor. After a long series of tests and consultations at UCLA, she was finally diagnosed with a rare cancer of the body's fluids—one of only 88 cases ever recorded. Her cancer was untreatable. She grew weaker and weaker. On two occasions she had fluid removed from her abdomen to reduce the pain she felt from the cancer. To help with other medical problems, she had carotid surgery and a pace-maker implanted shortly before her death. Her mind remained clear and analytical to the end. She continued to send short notes to her friends in her community of practice and conducted an extraordinary correspon-dence with Suzy Lego, who was also fighting a losing battle with cancer. On March 17, 1999, Hildegard Peplau died quietly in her sleep at home in Sherman Oaks. She was 89 years old. Her sister Bertha died a few months later on June 7, 1999, and her sister-in-law Anne, Walter's wife, had died a few months earlier. A joint memorial service for the three remarkable Peplau women was held in Mechanicsburg, Pennsylvania, on July 18, 1999.

ENDNOTES

1. Hildegard Peplau, ANA Convention, San Diego, California, June 27, 1998, accept-ing induction into the Hall of Fame.
2. Anita O'Toole, "Hildegard Peplau: A Living Legend," read on the occasion of the American Academy of Nursing ceremony designating her "A Living Legend," in Scottsdale, Arizona, May, 1998. In part, O'Toole observed: "The application of Sullivan's interpersonal theories of psychotherapy to nursing practice moved nurs-ing from a spectator observation of the patient to a new paradigm: nursing became a participant interpersonal process where the patient is a subject in an interperson-al relationship rather than an object to be worked upon. Peplau directed nursing's attention to the need to develop a consciousness, that is a theory, about the nurse-patient relationship and to use that theory to guide nursing interventions."
3. Hildegard Peplau, *Interpersonal Relations in Nursing* (New York: G. P. Putnam and Sons, 1952), reprinted, New York: Springer Publishing, 1992, and Anita O'Toole, and Sheila Rouslin Welt, *Interpersonal Theory in Nursing Practice: Selected Works of Hildegard E. Peplau.* (New York: Springer Publishing, 1992).

4. In the last decade of her life, every honorary degree or prize Peplau received referred to her as "the mother of psychiatric nursing." See the citations read at the University of Indiana, 1994; University of Ulster, 1995; and for the Christiane Reimann Prize in Vancouver, 1997.

5. Pamela G. Reed, "A Treatise on Nursing Knowledge development for the twenty-first Century: Beyond Postmodernism," *Advances in Nursing Science 17*: (1995): 70–84.

6. Letitia Anne Peplau, "Hildegard E. Peplau: A Celebration of her Contributions," American Psychiatric Nurses Association 13th Annual Conference, October 29, 1999, Toronto, Canada.

7. Interview, Hildegard Peplau, March 16, 1992.

8. Interview, Hildegard Peplau, March 9, 1992.

9. Interview, Hildegard Peplau, April 25, 1992.

10. Handwritten notes on yellow notepaper from the La Mansion Hotel in San Antonio, Texas, given to the author by Shirley Smoyak, n.d.

11. See Hildegard Peplau, "Theory: The Professional Dimension," in Kay Norris, ed., *Perspectives in Psychiatric Nursing* (Kansas City: University of Kansas Press, 1969), and "Operational Definitions and Nursing Practice," in L. T. Zderad and H. C. Belcher, eds., *Developing Behavioral Concepts in Nursing* (Atlanta: Southern Regional Education Board, 1968).

12. In an interview on April 7, 1992, Peplau commented, ". . . you have to start with a premise . . . if you started with the premise that many nurses were abused or had low self-esteem . . . it's a good hypothesis."

13. In an interview on March 23, 1994, Martha Rogers conveyed these insights and concluded by saying, "she was the brightest thing to come along in nursing ever." Grayce Sills, too, often remarked that Peplau's intelligence and conceptual frame of mind made others uncomfortable. These themes were repeated in discussions with many of Hilda's colleagues at Rutgers—men as well as women, university administrators as well as nurse faculty colleagues.

Selected Publications of Hildegard Peplau

BOOKS

(1952). *Interpersonal Relations in Nursing*. New York: G. P. Putnam and Sons. (Reprinted New York: Springer, 1990, 1992, 1995.)

(1964). *Basic Principles of Patient Counseling*. Philadelphia: Smith, Kline and French. (Spanish Edition, 1968; Japanese Edition, 1990; 4th Edition, 1992.)

BOOK CHAPTERS

(1963). "The Clinical Specialist Role," in Shirley S. Burd and Margaret Marshall, eds., *Some Clinical Approaches to Psychiatric Nursing*. New York: MacMillan.

(1967). "Psychiatric Nursing," in A. U. Freedman and H. I. Kaplan, eds., *Comprehensive Textbook of Psychiatry*. Baltimore, Maryland: Williams and Wilkins.

(1968). "Operational Definitions and Nursing Practice," in Loretta T. Zderad and Helen C. Belcher, eds., *Behavioral Concepts in Nursing*. Atlanta: Southern Regional Education Board.

(1969). "Theory: The Professional Dimension," in Catharine Norris, ed., *Perspectives in Psychiatric Nursing*. Boston: Little Brown.

(1982). "The Work of Clinical Specialists in Psychiatric Nursing," in Shirley Smoyak and Sheila Rouslin, eds., *A Collection of Classics in Psychiatric Nursing Literature*. Thorofare, New Jersey: Charles B. Slack, Inc.

(1987). "A Historical Perspective," in R. Parse, *Nursing Science: Major Paradigms, Theories, Critiques*. Philadelphia: W. B. Saunders.

Articles

(1942). "Health Program at Bennington College," *Public Health Nursing* 34(10): 573–581.

(1947). "A Democratic Participation Technique," *American Journal of Nursing* 47(5): 334–336.

(1951). "Toward New Concepts in Nursing and Nursing Education," *American Journal of Nursing* 51(12): 722–724.

(1952). "The Psychiatric Nurses' Family Group," *American Journal of Nursing* 52(12): 1475–1477.

(1953, Feb.). "The Nursing Team in Psychiatric Facilities," *Nursing Outlook* I(2): 90–92.

(1953, Oct.). "Themes in Nursing Situations: Power," *American Journal of Nursing* 53(10): 1221–1223.

(1953, Nov.). "Themes in Nursing Situations: Safety," *American Journal of Nursing* 53(11): 1343–1346.

(1955, Dec.). "Loneliness," *American Journal of Nursing* 55(12): 1476–1481.

(1956). "Discussion: Psychology and Psychiatric Nursing Research," *National League of Nursing Exchange 18*, 400–410.

(1956, Spring). "Present Day Trends in Psychiatric Nursing," *Neuropsychiatry 111*(4): 190–204.

(1956, July). "An Undergraduate Program in Psychiatric Nursing," *Nursing Outlook 4*, 400–410.

(1957). "Therapeutic Concepts," *National League of Nursing Exchange 26*, 38–57.

(1957, July). "What is Experiential Teaching?" *American Journal of Nursing* 57(7): 884–886.

(1958). "Educating the Nurse to Function in Psychiatric Services," *Nursing Personnel for Mental Health Program*, Atlanta, Georgia: Southern Regional Educational Board, 37–42.

(1958, Sept.). "Public Health Nurses Promote Mental Health," *Public Health Reports 73*(9): 828–833.

(1960). "Talking with Patients," *American Journal of Nursing 60*, 964–967.

(1960, Jan.). "Must Laboring Together be Called Teamwork? Problems in Team Treatment of Adults in State Mental Hospitals," *American Journal of Orthopsychiatry 30*, 103–108.

(1960, March). "A Personal Responsibility: A Discussion of Anxiety in Mental Health," *Public Health Reports 80*, 14–16.

(1960, May). "Anxiety in the Mother-Infant Relationship," *Nursing World 134*(5): 33–34.

(1962, June). "Interpersonal Techniques: The Crux of Psychiatric Nursing," *American Journal of Nursing 62*, 50–54.

(1963). "An Approach to Research in Psychiatric Nursing," *Training for Clinical Research:Mental Health Nursing*, The Catholic University of America, 5–44.

(1963, Oct.–Nov.). "Interpersonal Relations and the Process of Adaptation," *Nursing Science I*(4): 272–279.

(1964). "Psychiatric Nursing Skills and the General Hospital Patient," *Nursing Forum* (2): 28–37.

(1964, Nov.). "Professional and Social Behavior: Some Differences Worth the Notice," *Public Health Quarterly 50*(4): 23–33.

(1965). "The 91st Day: A Challenge to Professional Nursing," *Perspectives in Psychiatric Care III*(2): 20–24.

(1965, April). "The Heart of Nursing: Interpersonal Relations," *Canadian Nurse 61*(4): 268–287.

(1965, August). "Specialization in Professional Nursing," *Nursing Science 3*(4): 268–287.

(1965, Nov.). "The Nurse in the Community Mental Health Program," *Nursing Outlook 13*(11): 68–70.

(1966). "Nurse-doctor Relationships," *Nursing Forum 5*(1): 60–75.

(1966). "Nursing's Two Routes to Doctoral Degrees," *Nursing Forum 5*(2): 57–67.

(1966, March–April). "An Interpretation of the ANA Position," *New Jersey State Nurses Association Newsletter 22*(2): 6–10.

(1966, May–June). "Trends in Nursing and Nurse Education," *New Jersey State Nurses Association Newsletter 22*(3): 17–27.

(1967, Feb.). "The Work of Psychiatric Nurses," *Psychiatric Opinion 4*(1): 5–11.

(1967, Nov.). "Interpersonal Relations and the Work of the Industrial Nurse," *Industrial Nurse Journal 15*(10): 7–12.

(1968). "Psychotherapeutic Strategies," *Perspectives in Psychiatric Care VI*(6): 264–289.

(1969). "Professional Closeness as a Special Kind of Involvement," *Nursing Forum 8*(4): 342–360.

(1969, Fall). "The American Nurses' Association and Nursing Education," *Utah Nurse 20*(3): 6–8.

(1970, Jan.). "ANA's New Executive Director States Her Views," *American Journal of Nursing 70*, 84–88.

(1970, Summer). "A Special Kind of Involvement with a Patient, Client, or Family Group," *Comprehensive Nurse Quarterly 5*(3): 66–81.

(1970, Nov.–Dec.). "Changed Patterns of Practice," *Washington State Journal of Nursing 42*, 4–6.

(1973). "Illness Maintaining Systems" (audio tape presentation), PSF Productions, San Antonio, Texas.

(1977). "The Changing View of Nursing," *International Nursing Review 1977, 24*(2): 33–45.

(1978). "Psychiatric Nursing and the Role of Nurses, *International Nursing Review 25*(3). 41–47.

(1980). "ANA Statement Defines Scope of Practice," *ANA Newsletter 12*(4): 1, 8, 24.

(1980). "The Psychiatric Nurse: Accountable? To Whom? For What?" *Perspectives in Psychiatric Care 18*, 128–134.

(1982). "Some Reflections on Care in Psychiatric Nursing," *Journal of Psychosocial and Mental Health Nursing 20*, 17–24.

(1984, Jan.–Feb.). "Internal versus external regulation," *New Jersey Nurse 14*, 12–14.

(1985, Feb.). "Is Nursing Self-Regulation Power Being Eroded?" *American Journal of Nursing 85*(2): 140–143.

(1987, Jan.). "Tomorrow's World," *Nursing Times* 29–32.

(1987). "Interpersonal Constructs for Nursing Practice," *Nurse Education Today 7*, 201–208.

(1987, March). "American Nurses Association Social Policy Statement: Part I." *Archives of Psychiatric Nursing 1*(5):301–307.

(1988). "The Art and Science of Nursing: Similarities, Differences, and Relations," *Nursing Science Quarterly 1*, 8–15.

(1988, Spring). "Peplau Responds," *Pacesetter* (Newsletter of the American Nurses Association Council on Psychiatric and Mental Health Nursing) 15(l): 1–4.

Index

Springer Publishing Company

Enduring Issues in American Nursing

Ellen D. Baer, RN, PhD, FAAN, **Patricia D'Antonio,** RN, PhD, **Sylvia Rinker,** RN, PhD, and **Joan E. Lynaugh,** RN, PhD, FAAN, Editors

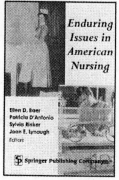

"A timely, important book that should be read by students and all practicing nurses...Provides background information and context for the most pressing issues facing our profession, including power, identity, and relationships with physicians and surgeons."

—**Elizabeth M. Norman,** PhD, RN, FAAN
New York University, Division of Nursing

This book presents nursing history in the context of problems and issues that persist to the present day. Each chapter provides a piece of the puzzle that is nursing. The editors, all noted nurse historians and educators, have made selections from the best that has been published in the nursing and health care literatures.

PARTIAL CONTENTS: I. Contemporary Issues in Historical Context • The Intersection of Race, Class, and Gender in the Nursing Profession, *D.C. Hines*

II. Identity: The Meaning of Nursing • Midwives as Wives and Mothers: Urban Midwives in the Early Twentieth Century, *L. Walsh*

III. The Nature of Power and Authority in Nursing • The Physician's Eyes: American Nursing and the Diagnostic Revolution in Medicine, *M. Sandelowski*

IV. The Nature of Nursing Knowledge • Constructing the Mind of Nursing, D. Hamilton • Delegated by Default or Negotiated by Need? Physicians, Nurse Practitioners, and the Process of Clinical Thinking, *J. Fairman*

V. Conclusion • Revisiting and Rethinking the Rewriting of Nursing History, P. D'Antonio • Appendix: Suggestions for Further Reading

2000 400pp 0-8261-1373-7 hard

536 Broadway, New York, NY 10012 • Tel. (212) 431-4370 • Fax (212) 941-7842
Order Toll-Free: (877) 687-7476 • www.springerpub.com

Springer Publishing Company

American Nursing
A Biographical Dictionary, Volume 3

Vern L. Bullough, RN, PhD, and
Lilli Sentz, Editors

Sharon Richardson, Bonnie Bullough, Olga Church,
Contributing Editors

*"For only a few of the nurses in this volume
was achievement an easy process. Their
lives emphasize what it was like to be a
nurse, what kinds of difficulties they
encountered, and how they overcame them.
The reader will certainly find out a great
deal about the nursing presence and about
what individual nurses have done to make
nursing what it is today."*
—**Vern L. Bullough,** from the Introduction

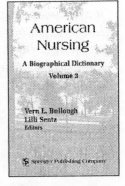

This exciting collection traces the development of the nursing
profession through the biographies of individual nurses since
1925. The list of several hundred names, compiled through the
help of nurse historians and volunteers from the American
Association for the History of Nursing, features notable nurses
Faye Abdellah, Virginia Henderson, Margaret Kerr, and
Thelma Schorr. It gives nurses a real sense of their history
which is not available anywhere else. The contributors of the
biographies, in an act of scholarly devotion, preserve a sense of
the profession's past.

American Nursing: A Biographical Dictionary, Volume Three
is an invaluable reference work for students and librarians.
Fully illustrated with many one-of-a-kind photographs.

2000 328pp 0-8261-1296-X hard

536 Broadway, New York, NY 10012 • (212) 431-4370 • Fax (212) 941-7842
Order Toll-Free: (877) 687-7476 • *www.springerpub.com*

Springer Publishing Company

Nurses in the Political Arena

The Public Face of Nursing

Harriet R. Feldman, PhD, RN, FAAN,
and **Sandra B. Lewenson,** EdD, RN

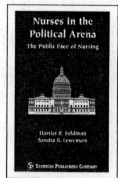

"The thrilling stories in the book tell of the way nurses work and the way they bring their experiences and knowledge to bear on political issues...The background presented in this book and the wonderful stories it tells will inform, stimulate and inspire current and future nurses. This book fills an important gap in the nursing literature."

—From the Foreword by **Claire Fagin**

This book was written to encourage nurses to become involved in the political process. The authors interviewed over 40 nurses who hold or have run for public office–from Members of Congress to local aldermen. These nurses share their experiences on everything from getting informed on the issues to getting involved in a political party, from presenting the right image to fundraising. A chapter on nurses who have made use of the public arena in the past includes figures such as Lillian Wald, Lavinia Dock, and Margaret Sanger.

Contents:
• Foreword by Claire M. Fagin
• Nurses in the Political Process
• Historical Perspective on Nurses Active in the Political Process
• Nurses in the Political Arena
• Nurses Action on Social Issues
• Negotiating the Political Process
• Creating Political Opportunities
• Appendixes

2000　200pp　0-8261-1331-1　hard

536 Broadway, New York, NY 10012 • Telephone: (212) 431-4370
Fax: (212) 941-7842 • Order Toll-Free: (877) 687-7476
Order On-line: *www.springerpub.com*

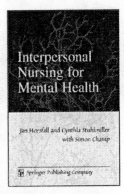

Nursing History Review

Official Journal of the American Association for the History of Nursing

Joan E. Lynaugh, PhD, FAAN, Editor

Nursing History Review is the only scholarly journal of new peer reviewed research on the history of nursing and health care in the United States and in the world. It publishes significant scholarly work in all aspects of nursing history as well as short and extended reviews of recent books along with updates on national and international activities in nursing and health care history.

Sample Contents:

- "The Steel Cocoon": Tales of the Nurses and Patients of the Iron Lung
- Blood Work: Canadian Nursing and Blood Transfusion, 1942-1990
- Care of the Maternal Breast: Techniques and Nurses' Roles, 1900-1948
- From the Private to the Public Sphere: The First Generation of Lady Nurses in England
- Florence Henderson: The Art of Open Drop Ether
- DOING THE WORK OF HISTORY—Nurses Residences: Using the Built Environment As Evidence
- Passing On More Than a Blank Disc
- BOOK REVIEWS
- FLORENCE NIGHTINGALE MUSEUM IN TURKEY

Volume 10 (2002), ISSN 1062-8061

Visit www.springerjournals.com to browse tables of contents of past issues, and to order the journal on-line!

SPRINGER PUBLISHING COMPANY • www.springerpub.com
Order Toll-Free: 877.687.7476 • Phone: 212.431.4370 • Fax: 212.941.7842

Printed in the United States
63688LVS00002B/328-342

9 780826 138828